PETERS HEALTH
SCIENCES LIBRARY
Rhode Island Hospital

PROGRESS IN CLINICAL AND BIOLOGICAL RESEARCH

Series Editors

Nathan Back Vincent P. Eijsvoogel Kurt Hirschhorn Sidney Udenfriend
George J. Brewer Robert Grover Seymour S. Kety Jonathan W. Uhr

RECENT TITLES

Vol 163: **Prevention of Physical and Mental Congenital Defects**, Maurice Marois, *Editor.* Published in 3 volumes: Part A: *The Scope of the Problem.* Part B: *Epidemiology, Early Detection and Therapy, and Environmental Factors.* Part C: *Basic and Medical Science, Education, and Future Strategies*

Vol 164: **Information and Energy Transduction in Biological Membranes**, C. Liana Bolis, Ernst J.M. Helmreich, Hermann Passow, *Editors*

Vol 165: **The Red Cell: Sixth Ann Arbor Conference**, George J. Brewer, *Editor*

Vol 166: **Human Alkaline Phosphatases**, Torgny Stigbrand, William H. Fishman, *Editors*

Vol 167: **Ethopharmacological Aggression Research**, Klaus A. Miczek, Menno R. Kruk, Berend Olivier, *Editors*

Vol 168: **Epithelial Calcium and Phosphate Transport: Molecular and Cellular Aspects**, Felix Bronner, Meinrad Peterlik, *Editors*

Vol 169: **Biological Perspectives on Aggression**, Kevin J. Flannelly, Robert J. Blanchard, D. Caroline Blanchard, *Editors*

Vol 170: **Porphyrin Localization and Treatment of Tumors**, Daniel R. Doiron, Charles J. Gomer, *Editors*

Vol 171: **Developmental Mechanisms: Normal and Abnormal**, James W. Lash, Lauri Saxén, *Editors*

Vol 172: **Molecular Basis of Cancer**, Robert Rein, *Editor.* Published in 2 volumes: Part A: *Macromolecular Structure, Carcinogens, and Oncogenes.* Part B: *Macromolecular Recognition, Chemotherapy, and Immunology*

Vol 173: **Pepsinogens in Man: Clinical and Genetic Advances**, Johanna Kreuning, I. Michael Samloff, Jerome I. Rotter, Aldur Eriksson, *Editors*

Vol 174: **Enzymology of Carbonyl Metabolism 2: Aldehyde Dehydrogenase, Aldo-Keto Reductase, and Alcohol Dehydrogenase**, T. Geoffrey Flynn, Henry Weiner, *Editors*

Vol 175: **Advances in Neuroblastoma Research**, Audrey E. Evans, Giulio J. D'Angio, Robert C. Seeger, *Editors*

Vol 176: **Contemporary Sensory Neurobiology**, Manning J. Correia, Adrian A. Perachio, *Editors*

Vol 177: **Medical Genetics: Past, Present, Future**, Kåre Berg, *Editor*

Vol 178: **Bluetongue and Related Orbiviruses**, T. Lynwood Barber, Michael M. Jochim, *Editors*

Vol 179: **Taurine: Biological Actions and Clinical Perspectives**, Simo S. Oja, Liisa Ahtee, Pirjo Kontro, Matti K. Paasonen, *Editors*

Vol 180: **Intracellular Protein Catabolism**, Edward A. Khairallah, Judith S. Bond, John W.C. Bird, *Editors*

Vol 181: **Germfree Research: Microflora Control and Its Application to the Biomedical Sciences**, Bernard S. Wostmann, *Editor*, Julian R. Pleasants, Morris Pollard, Bernard A. Teah, Morris Wagner, *Co-Editors*

Vol 182: **Infection, Immunity, and Blood Transfusion**, Roger Y. Dodd and Lewellys F. Barker, *Editors*

Vol 183: **Aldehyde Adducts in Alcoholism**, Michael A. Collins, *Editor*

Vol 184: **Hematopoietic Stem Cell Physiology**, Eugene P. Cronkite, Nicholas Dainiak, Ronald P. McCaffrey, Jiri Palek, Peter J. Quesenberry, *Editors*

Vol 185: **EORTC Genitourinary Group Monograph 2,** Fritz H. Schroeder, Brian Richards, *Editors.* Published in two volumes: Part A: *Therapeutic Principles in Metastatic Prostatic Cancer.* Part B: *Superficial Bladder Tumors*

Vol 186: **Carcinoma of the Large Bowel and Its Precursors,** John R.F. Ingall, Anthony J. Mastromarino, *Editors*

Vol 187: **Normal and Abnormal Bone Growth: Basic and Clinical Research,** Andrew D. Dixon, Bernard G. Sarnat, *Editors*

Vol 188: **Detection and Treatment of Lipid and Lipoprotein Disorders of Childhood,** Kurt Widhalm, Herbert K. Naito, *Editors*

Vol 189: **Bacterial Endotoxins: Structure, Biomedical Significance, and Detection With the Limulus Amebocyte Lysate Test,** Jan W. ten Cate, Harry R. Büller, Augueste Sturk, Jack Levin, *Editors*

Vol 190: **The Interphotoreceptor Matrix in Health and Disease,** C. David Bridges, *Editor*, Alice J. Adler, *Associate Editor*

Vol 191: **Experimental Approaches for the Study of Hemoglobin Switching,** George Stamatoyannopoulos, Arthur W. Nienhuis, *Editors*

Vol 192: **Endocoids,** Harbans Lal, Frank LaBella, John Lane, *Editors*

Vol 193: **Fetal Liver Transplantation,** Robert Peter Gale, Jean-Louis Touraine, Guido Lucarelli, *Editors*

Vol 194: **Diseases of Complex Etiology in Small Populations: Ethnic Differences and Research Approaches,** Ranajit Chakraborty, Emöke J.E. Szathmary, *Editors*

Vol 195: **Cellular and Molecular Aspects of Aging: The Red Cell as a Model,** John W. Eaton, Diane K. Konzen, James G. White, *Editors*

Vol 196: **Advances in Microscopy,** Ronald R. Cowden, Fredrick W. Harrison, *Editors*

Vol 197: **Cooperative Approaches to Research and Development of Orphan Drugs,** Melvin Van Woert, Eunyong Chung, *Editors*

Vol 198: **Biochemistry and Biology of DNA Methylation,** Giulio L. Cantoni, Aharon Razin, *Editors*

Vol 199: **Leukotrienes in Cardiovascular and Pulmonary Function,** Allan M. Lefer, Marlys H. Gee, *Editors*

Vol 200: **Endocrine Genetics and Genetics of Growth,** Costas J. Papadatos, Christos S. Bartsocas, *Editors*

Vol 201: **Primary Chemotherapy in Cancer Medicine,** D.J. Theo Wagener, Geert H. Blijham, Jan B.E. Smeets, Jacques A. Wils, *Editors*

Vol 202: **The 2-5A System: Molecular and Clinical Aspects of the Interferon-Regulated Pathway,** Bryan R.G. Williams, Robert Silverman, *Editors*

Please contact the publisher for information about previous titles in this series.

FETAL LIVER TRANSPLANTATION

FETAL LIVER TRANSPLANTATION

Proceedings of an International Symposium
Held in Pesaro, Italy
September 29–October 1, 1984

Editors

ROBERT PETER GALE
UCLA School of Medicine
Los Angeles, California

JEAN-LOUIS TOURAINE
Hôpital E. Herriot
Lyon, France

GUIDO LUCARELLI
Ospedale di Pesaro
Pesaro, Italy

ALAN R. LISS, INC. • NEW YORK

Address all Inquiries to the Publisher
Alan R. Liss, Inc., 41 East 11th Street, New York, NY 10003

Copyright © 1985 Alan R. Liss, Inc.

Printed in the United States of America

Under the conditions stated below the owner of copyright for this book hereby grants permission to users to make photocopy reproductions of any part or all of its contents for personal or internal organizational use, or for personal or internal use of specific clients. This consent is given on the condition that the copier pay the stated per-copy fee through the Copyright Clearance Center, Incorporated, 27 Congress Street, Salem, MA 01970, as listed in the most current issue of "Permissions to Photocopy" (Publisher's Fee List, distributed by CCC, Inc.), for copying beyond that permitted by sections 107 or 108 of the US Copyright Law. This consent does not extend to other kinds of copying, such as copying for general distribution, for advertising or promotional purposes, for creating new collective works, or for resale.

Library of Congress Cataloging in Publication Data
Main entry under title:

Fetal liver transplantation.

    Proceedings of the 2nd International Symposium on Fetal Liver Transplantation.
    Includes bibliographies and index.
    1. Liver—Transplantation—Congresses.
2. Hematopoiesis—Congresses. 3. Fetus—Surgery—Congresses. 4. Surgery, Experimental—Congresses.
I. Gale, Robert Peter. II. Touraine, J. L. (Jean Louis)
III. Lucarelli, Guido. IV. International Symposium on Fetal Liver Transplantation (2nd : 1984 : Pesaro, Italy) [DNLM: 1. Fetus—congresses. 2. Hematopoietic Stem Cells—congresses. 3. Liver—transplantation—congresses. W1 PR668E v.193 / WI 770 F419 1984]
RD546.F48 1985   617'.556   85-10429
ISBN 0-8451-5043-X

Contents

Contributors xi
Preface
Robert Peter Gale, Jean-Louis Touraine, and Guido Lucarelli xvii

SECTION I: EXPERIMENTAL HEMATOPOIESIS AND IMMUNE DEVELOPMENT—ANIMALS

Renewal and Differentiation of Totipotent Hematopoietic Stem Cells of the Mouse After Transplantation Into Early Fetuses
Beatrice Mintz 3

Ontogeny of the Mouse Hemopoietic System
Peter M.C. Wong, Siu Wah Chung, Connie J. Eaves, and David H.K. Chui . . . 17

Hemopoietic Stem Cell Regulators in Fetal Liver
Martine Guigon and Joanna Wdzieczak-Bakala 29

Changes in the Growth Requirements of Baboon Liver Hematopoietic Progenitors During Ontogeny
G. David Roodman 43

SECTION II: EXPERIMENTAL HEMATOPOIESIS AND IMMUNE DEVELOPMENT—MAN

Embryonic Hemopoiesis in Human Liver: Morphologic Aspects at Sequential Stages of Ontogenic Development
S. Petti, U. Testa, A.R. Migliaccio, F. Mavilio, M. Marinucci, D. Lazzaro, G. Russo, G. Mastroberardino, and C. Peschle 57

Immune Development in Human Fetal Liver
Robert Peter Gale 73

Immune Characterization of Human Fetal Tissues With Monoclonal Antibodies
M. De Biagi, M. Andreani, and F. Centis 89

Experimental Studies on Hemopoietic Stem Cells of Fetal Liver Origin and its Clinical Application
Chu-tse Wu 95

Fetal Liver: Erythropoiesis In Vivo, Sustained Granulopoiesis In Vitro
M.D. Cappellini, C.G. Potter, and W.G. Wood 113

Cryopreservation of Human Fetal Liver: Factors Influencing Granulocyte-Macrophage Colony (CFU-GM) Survival After Cryopreservation
L. Moretti, S. Stramigioli, N. Talevi, M. Bartolucci, M.T. Marchetti-Rossi, P. Polchi, A. Porcellini, and G. Lucarelli 121

Isolation of Erythroid and Myeloid Hematopoietic Progenitors From Human Fetal Liver
Stephen G. Emerson 135

HLA-Typing of Fetal Liver Cells Using Interferon Treatment In Vitro
Catherine Royo, Jean-Louis Touraine, and Hervé Bétuel 149

Regulation of In Vitro Granulopoiesis by Human Fetal Liver Stromal Cells
Y. Barak, Y. Karov, S. Levin, A. Barash, H. Ben-Hur, and M. Lancet 157

Morphological Pattern of Hematopoiesis in Human Fetal Liver
S. Sharma, M. Bhargava, and V. Kochupillai 167

SECTION III: FETAL LIVER TRANSPLANTATION—ANIMAL MODELS

Hemopoiesis and Immune Functions in Dogs Following Fetal Liver Transplantation
Otto Prümmer, Wenceslao Calvo, Christine Werner, Felix Carbonell, and Theodor M. Fliedner 175

Fetal Liver Cell Transplantation in Dogs: Results With DLA-Compatible and Incompatible Grafts
Richard Champlin, Gary Cain, Katherine A. Stitzel, and Robert Peter Gale 195

Fetal Liver Transplantation in the Mini-Pig
M. Andreani, M. De Biagi, F. Centis, M. Manna, F. Agostinelli, A. Filippetti, G. Gaudenzi, P. Muretto, C. Grianti, G. Sotti, A. Rigon, and G. Lucarelli 205

Fetal Hemopoietic-Cell Transplantation in Sheep: An Approach to the Cellular Control of Hemoglobin Switching
Christopher Bunch, W.G. Wood, and Susan J. Kelly 219

SECTION IV: FETAL LIVER TRANSPLANTATION—MAN

Fetal Liver Transplant in Aplastic Anemia and Acute Leukemia
T. Izzi, P. Polchi, M. Galimberti, C. Delfini, L. Moretti, A. Porcellini, A. Manna, G. Sparaventi, C. Giardini, E. Angelucci, P. Politi, and G. Lucarelli 237

Bone Marrow Reconstitution Following Human Fetal Liver Infusion (FLI) in Sixteen Severe Aplastic Anemia Patients
V. Kochupillai, S. Sharma, S. Francis, N.K. Mehra, A. Nanu, V. Kalra, P.S.N. Menon, and M. Bhargava 251

Fetal Liver Infusion: An Adjuvant in the Therapy of Acute Myeloid Leukemia (AML)
V. Kochupillai, S. Sharma, S. Francis, N.K. Mehra, A. Nanu, I.C. Verma, D. Takkar, S. Kumar, and U. Gokhale 267

Allogeneic Fetal Liver Transplantation in Acute Leukemia
Pei-lin Meng, Rui-gao Fei, Ding-wei Gu, Wen-zheng Yie, Ben-tie Liu, Fang Yan, You-yu Yu, Zhi-guang Mai, Bao-zhen Chen, Ling-xian Zhu, Feng Guo, and Xiao-hui Wang 281

Fetal Liver Transplantation in Hematologic Disorders
Robert Peter Gale 293

Fetal Liver Transplantation in Immunodeficiencies and Inborn Errors of Metabolism
J.L. Touraine, M.G. Roncarolo, G.L. Marseglia, G. Souillet, B. Bétend,
H. Bétuel, F. Touraine, C. Royo, N. Philippe, and R. François 299

Transplantation of T Lymphocyte Depleted Bone Marrow to Prevent Graft-Versus-Host Disease: Its Implications for Fetal Liver Transplantation
Richard E. Champlin, Ronald T. Mitsuyasu, and Robert Peter Gale 315

A Comparative Review of the Results of Transplants of Fully Allogeneic Fetal Liver and HLA-Haplotype Mismatched, T-Cell Depleted Marrow in the Treatment of Severe Combined Immunodeficiency
Richard J. O'Reilly, Dahlia Kirkpatrick, Neena Kapoor, Nancy Collins,
Joel Brochstein, Nancy Kernan, Neal Flomenberg, Marilyn Pollack,
Bo Dupont, Carlos Lopez, and Yair Reisner 327

Index 343

Contributors

F. Agostinelli, Divisione di Ematologia, Ospedale di Pesaro, Pesaro 61100, Italy **[89, 205]**

Marco Andreani, Divisione di Ematologia, Ospedale di Pesaro, Pesaro 61100, Italy **[89, 205]**

Emanuale Angelucci, Divisione di Ematologia, Ospedale di Pesaro, Pesaro 61100, Italy **[237]**

Y. Barak, Pediatric Research Institute, Kaplan Hospital, Rehovot 76100, Israel **[157]**

A. Barash, Department of Obstetrics and Gynecology, Kaplan Hospital, Rehovot 76100, Israel **[157]**

M. Bartolucci, Divisione di Ematologia, Ospedale di Pesaro, Pesaro 61100, Italy **[121]**

H. Ben-Hur, Kaplan Hospital, Rehovot 76100, Israel **[157]**

B. Bétend, Transplantation and Immunobiology Unit, INSERM U80, Hôpital Edouard Herriot, 69374 Lyon Cedex 8, France **[299]**

Hervé Bétuel, Centre de Transfusion Sanguine de Gerland, 69342 Lyon Cedex 7, France **[149, 299]**

M. Bhargava, Department of Medical Oncology, All-India Institute of Medical Sciences, New Delhi 110 029, India **[167, 251]**

Joel Brochstein, Memorial Sloan-Kettering Cancer Center, New York, NY 10021 **[327]**

Christopher Bunch, Nuffield Department of Clinical Medicine, University of Oxford, John Radcliffe Hospital, Headington, Oxford OX3 9DU, England **[219]**

Gary Cain, Laboratory for Energy Related Health Research, University of California–Davis, Davis, CA 95616 **[195]**

Wenceslao Calvo, Department of Clinical Physiology and Occupational Medicine, University of Ulm, D-7900 Ulm, Federal Repulic of Germany **[175]**

M.D. Cappellini, Instituto di Clinica Medica III, University of Milan, Milan 20122, Italy **[113]**

Felix Carbonell, Department of Clinical Physiology and Occupational Medicine, University of Ulm, D-7900 Ulm, Federal Republic of Germany **[175]**

Filippo Centis, Divisione di Ematologia, Ospedale di Pesaro, Pesaro 61100, Italy **[89, 205]**

Richard E. Champlin, Department of Medicine, Division of Hematology/ Oncology, UCLA Center for the Health Sciences, Los Angeles, CA 90024 **[195, 315]**

Bao-zhen Chen, Department of Hematology, Changhai Hospital, Shanghai 201903, China **[281]**

David H.K. Chui, Department of Pathology, McMaster University, Hamilton, Ontario L8N 3Z5, Canada **[17]**

The number in brackets is the opening page number of the contributor's article.

Siu-Wah Chung, Department of Pathology, McMaster University, Hamilton, Ontario L8N 3Z5, Canada and Terry Fox Laboratory, British Columbia Cancer Research Centre, Vancouver, British Columbia V5Z 1L3, Canada [17]

Nancy Collins, Memorial Sloan-Kettering Cancer Center, New York, NY 10021 [327]

Massimo De Biagi, Division of Hematology, Pesaro Hospital, Pesaro 61100, Italy [89, 205]

Costante Delfini, Divisione di Ematologia, Ospedale di Pesaro, Pesaro 61100, Italy [237]

Bo Dupont, Memorial Sloan-Kettering Cancer Center, New York, NY 10021 [327]

Connie J. Eaves, Terry Fox Laboratory, British Columbia Cancer Research Centre, Vancouver, British Columbia V5Z 1L3, Canada [17]

Stephen G. Emerson, Division of Hematology, Brigham and Women's Hospital; Hematology/Oncology, Dana-Farber Cancer Institute and Children's Hospital; and Departments of Medicine and Pediatrics, Harvard Medical School, Boston, MA 02115 [135]

Rui-gao Fei, Department of Hematology, Changhai Hospital, Shanghai 201903, China [281]

A. Filippetti, Divisione di Ematologia, Ospedale di Pesaro, Pesaro 61100, Italy [205]

Theodor M. Fliedner, Department of Clinical Physiology and Occupational Medicine, University of Ulm, D-7900 Ulm, Federal Republic of Germany [175]

Neal Flomenberg, Memorial Sloan-Kettering Cancer Center, New York, NY 10021 [327]

Santhosh Francis, Department of Medical Oncology, All-India Institute of Medical Sciences, New Delhi 110 029, India [251, 267]

R. François, Transplantation and Immunobiology Unit, INSERM U80, Hôpital Edouard Herriot, 69374 Lyon Cedex 8, France [299]

Robert Peter Gale, Department of Medicine, Division of Hematology and Oncology, UCLA School of Medicine, Center for the Health Sciences, Los Angeles, CA 90024 [xvii, 73, 195, 293, 315]

Mariella Galimberti, Divisione di Ematologia, Ospedale di Pesaro, Pesaro 61100, Italy [237]

G. Gaudenzi, Veterinary Surgeon, Pesaro, Italy [205]

Claudio Giardini, Divisione di Ematologia, Ospedale di Pesaro, Pesaro 61100, Italy [237]

U. Gokhale, Department of Medicine, All-India Institute of Medical Sciences, New Delhi 110 029, India [267]

C. Grianti, Servizio di Anatomia Patologica, Pesaro, Italy [205]

Ding-wei Gu, Department of Hematology, Changhai Hospital, Shanghai 201903, China [281]

Martine Guigon, Unité de Recherches sur la Cinétique Cellulaire INSERM U250, Institut Gustave-Roussy, Villejuif 94805, France [29]

Feng Guo, Department of Hematology, Changhai Hospital, Shanghai 201903, China [281]

Contributors / xiii

Teodosio Izzi, Divisione di Ematologia, Ospedale di Pesaro, Pesaro 61100, Italy **[237]**

V. Kalra, Department of Pediatrics, All-India Institute of Medical Sciences, New Delhi 110 029, India **[251]**

Neena Kapoor, Memorial Sloan-Kettering Cancer Center, New York, NY 10021 **[327]**

Y. Karov, Pediatric Research Institute, Kaplan Hospital, Rehovot 76100, Israel **[157]**

Susan J. Kelly, MRC Molecular Haematology Unit, Nuffield Department of Clinical Medicine, University of Oxford, John Radcliffe Hospital, Headington, Oxford OX3 9DU, England **[219]**

Nancy Kernan, Memorial Sloan-Kettering Cancer Center, New York, NY 10021 **[327]**

Dahlia Kirkpatrick, Memorial Sloan-Kettering Cancer Center, New York, NY 10021 **[121,327]**

Vinod Kochupillai, Department of Medical Oncology, All-India Institute of Medical Sciences, New Delhi 110 029, India **[167, 251, 267]**

S. Kumar, Department of Blood Transfusions, All-India Institute of Medical Sciences, New Delhi 110 029, India **[267]**

M. Lancet, Kaplan Hospital, Rehovot 76100, Israel **[157]**

D. Lazzaro, Instituto Patologia Generale, University of Rome "La Sapienza", Rome, Italy **[57]**

S. Levin, Kaplan Hospital, Rehovot 76100, Israel **[157]**

Ben-tie Liu, Department of Hematology, Changhai Hospital, Shanghai 201903, China **[281]**

Carlos Lopez, Memorial Sloan-Kettering Cancer Center, New York, NY 10021 **[327]**

Guido Lucarelli, Divisione di Ematologia, Ospedale di Pesaro, Pesaro 61100, Italy **[xvii, 121, 205, 237]**

Zhi-guang Mai, Department of Hematology, Changhai Hospital, Shanghai 201903, China **[281]**

Annunziata Manna, Divisione di Hematologia, Ospedale di Pesaro, Pesaro 61100, Italy **[237]**

M. Manna, Divisione di Ematologia, Ospedale di Pesaro, Pesaro 61100, Italy **[205]**

M.T. Marchetti-Rossi, Divisione di Ematologia, Ospedale di Pesaro, Pesaro 61100, Itlay **[121]**

M. Marinucci, Department of Hematology, Istituto Superiore di Sanità, Rome 00161, Italy **[57]**

G.L. Marseglia, Transplantation and Immunobiology Unit, INSERM U80, Hôpital Edouard Herriot, 69374 Lyon Cedex 8, France **[299]**

G. Mastroberardino, Division of Obstetrics and Gynecology, Ospedale Generale, Avellino, Italy **[57]**

F. Mavilio, Department of Hematology, Istituto Superiore di Sanità, Rome 00161, Italy **[57]**

N.K. Mehra, Department of Anatomy, All-India Institute of Medical Sciences, New Delhi 110 029, India **[251, 267]**

Pei-lin Meng, Department of Hematology, Changhai Hospital, Shanghai 201903, China **[281]**

P.S.N. Menon, Department of Pediatrics, All-India Institute of Medical Sciences, New Delhi 110 029, India **[251]**

A.R. Migliaccio, Department of Hematology, Istituto Superiore di Sanità, Rome 00161, Italy **[57]**

Beatrice Mintz, Institute for Cancer Research, Fox Chase Cancer Center, Philadelphia, PA 19111 **[3]**

Ronald T. Mitsuyasu, UCLA Transplantation Biology Program, Division of Hematology/Oncology, UCLA Center for the Health Sciences, Los Angeles, CA 90024 **[315]**

Luciano Moretti, Divisione di Ematologia, Ospedale di Pesaro, Pesaro 61100, Italy **[121, 237]**

P. Muretto, Servizio di Anatomia Patologica, Pesaro, Italy **[205]**

A. Nanu, Department of Blood Transfusions, All-India Institute of Medical Sciences, New Delhi 110 029, India **[251, 267]**

Richard J. O'Reilly, Memorial Sloan-Kettering Cancer Center, New York, NY 10021 **[327]**

Cesare Peschle, Department of Hematology, Istituto Superiore di Sanità, Rome 00161, Italy **[57]**

Stefano Petti, Department of Hematology, Istituto Superiore di Sanità, Rome 00161, Italy **[57]**

N. Philippe, Transplantation and Immunobiology Unit, INSERM U80, Hôpital Edouard Herriot, 69374 Lyon Cedex 8, France **[299]**

Paola Polchi, Divisione di Ematologia, Ospedale di Pesaro, Pesaro 61100, Italy **[121, 237]**

Patrizia Politi, Divisione di Ematologia, Ospedale di Pesaro, Pesaro 61100, Italy **[237]**

Marilyn Pollack, Memorial Sloan-Kettering Cancer Center, New York, NY 10021 **[327]**

Adolfo Porcellini, Divisione di Ematologia, Ospedale di Pesaro, Pesaro 61100, Italy **[121, 237]**

C.G. Potter, Nuffield Department of Clinical Medicine, University of Oxford, John Radcliffe Hospital, Headington, Oxford OX3 9DU, England **[113]**

Otto Prümmer, Department of Clinical Physiology and Occupational Medicine, University of Ulm, D-7900 Ulm, Federal Republic of Germany **[175]**

Yair Reisner, Memorial Sloan-Kettering Cancer Center, New York, NY 10021 **[327]**

A. Rigon, Servizio di Radiologia, Padova, Italy **[205]**

M.G. Roncarolo, Transplantation and Immunobiology Unit, INSERM U80, Hôpital Edouard Herriot, 69374 Lyon Cedex 8, France **[299]**

G. David Roodman, Research Service, Audie Murphy Memorial Veterans Administration Hospital, San Antonio, TX 78284 **[43]**

Catherine Royo, Transplantation and Immunobiology Unit, INSERM U80, Hôpital Edouard Herriot, 69374 Lyon Cedex 8, France **[149, 299]**

G. Russo, Istituto di Patologia Medica VI, University of Rome "La Sapienza", Rome, Italy **[57]**

Subhadra Sharma, Department of Medical Oncology, All-India Institute of Medical Sciences, New Delhi 110 029, India **[167, 251, 267]**

G. Sotti, Servizio di Radiologia, Padova, Italy **[205]**

G. Souillet, Transplantation and Immunobiology Unit, INSERM U80, Hôpital Edouard Herriot, 69374 Lyon Cedex 8, France **[299]**

Giovanni Sparaventi, Divisione di Ematologia, Ospedale di Pesaro, Pesaro 61100, Itlay [237]

Katherine A. Stitzel, Laboratory for Energy Related Health Research, University of California–Davis, Davis, CA 95616 [195]

Stefania Stramigioli, Divisione di Ematologia, Ospedale di Pesaro, Pesaro 61100, Italy [121]

D. Takkar, Department of Obstetrics–Gynecology, All-India Institute of Medical Sciences, New Delhi 110 029, India [267]

N. Talevi, Divisione di Ematologia, Ospedale di Pesaro, Pesaro 61100, Italy [121]

Ugo Testa, Department of Hematology, Istituto Superiore di Sanità, Rome 00161, Italy [57]

F. Touraine, Transplantation and Immunobiology Unit, INSERM U80, Hôpital Edouard Herriot, 69374 Lyon Cedex 8, France [299]

Jean-Louis Touraine, Transplantation and Immunobiology Unit, INSERM U80, Hôpital Edouard Herriot, 69374 Lyon Cedex 8, France [xvii,149,299]

I.C. Verma, Department of Pediatrics, All-India Institute of Medical Sciences, New Delhi 110 029, India [267]

Xiao-hui Wang, Department of Hematology, Changhai Hospital, Shanghai 201903, China [281]

Joanna Wdzieczak-Bakala, Unité de Recherches sur la Cinétique Cellulaire INSERM U250, Institut Gustave-Roussy, Villejuif 94805, France [29]

Christine Werner, Department of Clinical Physiology and Occupational Medicine, University of Ulm, D-7900 Ulm, Federal Republic of Germany [175]

Peter M.C. Wong, Department of Pathology, McMaster University, Hamilton, Ontario L8N 3Z5, Canada and Terry Fox Laboratory, British Columbia Cancer Research Centre, Vancouver, British Columbia V5Z 1L3, Canada; present address: National Institutes of Health, Bethesda, MD 20205 [17]

W.G. Wood, MRC Molecular Haematology Unit, Nuffield Department of Clinical Medicine, University of Oxford, John Radcliffe Hospital, Headington, Oxford OX3 9DU, England [113,219]

Chu-tse Wu, Department of Experimental Hematology, Institute of Radiation Medicine, Beijing, China [95]

Fang Yan, Department of Hematology, Changhai Hospital, Shanghai 201903, China [281]

Wen-zheng Yie, Department of Hematology, Changhai Hospital, Shanghai 201903, China [281]

You-yu Yu, Department of Hematology, Changhai Hospital, Shanghai 201903, China [281]

Ling-xian Zhu, Department of Hematology, Changhai Hospital, Shanghai 201903, China [281]

Preface

The First International Symposium on Fetal Liver Transplantation was held in Pesaro, Italy in 1979. The meeting and its publication summarized the current state of research on the hematopoietic, immune, and clinical aspects of fetal liver development and transplantation and defined areas for future investigators.

Since 1979, there have been considerable advances in several fields closely related to fetal liver transplantation. These include new understanding of hematopoietic and lymphoid stem cells and growth regulatory factors, the development of monoclonal antibodies to T and B lymphocytes, and a clearer definition of the results and problems in bone marrow transplantation in man. Much of these data and techniques have recently been applied to fetal liver transplantation with interesting and important results. Animal models of fetal liver transplantation have also advanced considerably. Increasing numbers of fetal liver transplants have been performed in patients with immune deficiency disease, aplastic anemia, and leukemia.

Because of these important recent advances we felt it timely to convene a Second International Symposium on Fetal Liver Transplantation. This was held in Pesaro, Italy from September 29 to October 1, 1984.

This publication represents a comprehensive review of the field. It includes studies presented at the meeting as well as research from scientists working in closely related fields. We hope it will serve as a useful reference for scientists and clinicians interested in fetal liver transplantation and its related disciplines.

Fetal liver is a unique organ with much to teach us regarding the development and regulatory aspects of hematopoiesis and the immune system. We hope the studies summarized in this book will encourage others to enter into this exciting and expanding area of research.

> **Robert Peter Gale, M.D., Ph.D.**
> Los Angeles, California
>
> **Jean-Louis Touraine, M.D.**
> Lyon, France
>
> **Guido Lucarelli, M.D.**
> Pesaro, Italy

SECTION I
EXPERIMENTAL HEMATOPOIESIS AND IMMUNE DEVELOPMENT–ANIMALS

RENEWAL AND DIFFERENTIATION OF TOTIPOTENT HEMATOPOIETIC
STEM CELLS OF THE MOUSE AFTER TRANSPLANTATION INTO EARLY
FETUSES

Beatrice Mintz, Ph.D.

Institute for Cancer Research
Fox Chase Cancer Center
Philadelphia, PA   19111

INTRODUCTION

Hematopoiesis in mammals occurs first in the yolk sac of the embryo, then in the fetal liver and, starting around the time of birth, chiefly in the bone marrow and to some extent in the spleen. It remains uncertain whether the hematopoietic stem cells in the yolk sac give rise to those in the fetal liver. What is clear is that stem cells from the fetal liver progress to the bone marrow and are the direct antecedents of the definitive blood cells produced in the marrow. There are many basic questions, concerning the stem cells and the control of their development, to which answers must be obtained chiefly from experiments in the developing organism itself. Some of these will be addressed here.

Laboratory mice have continued to be the species of choice for *in vivo* experiments, including those involving transplantation, because of the availability of different genetically uniform strains and of many known genetic markers affecting blood cell differentiation and immunological parameters. Although some other species of mammals may present closer clinical parallels to human hematopoiesis, and ultimately to transplantation regimens, it seems likely that the underlying "rules of the game," dictated by genetic considerations, will be most readily discovered where the genetic composition of the subjects can be controlled.

For many years, the *in vivo* developmental potential

of blood-forming cells of the mouse has been assayed by introducing cells from bone marrow or fetal liver into adults, usually after irradiation of the host, and examining the colonies (clones) formed in the spleen (Till, McCulloch 1961). This approach has yielded much useful information and has testified to the pluripotency of the colony-forming stem cells, designated CFU-S, at least in myeloid differentiation. Nevertheless, the irradiated adult spleen is not the usual tissue environment for stem cell differentiation -- a fact which may account for the paucity of lymphoid development and the relatively limited self-renewal capacity of CFU-S (Paige et al. 1979; Siminovitch et al. 1963).

I was therefore interested in devising an experimental arrangement whereby genetically marked hematopoietic stem cells could encounter the characteristic sequence and ages of tissue environments throughout life, in unirradiated hosts, starting prenatally in the early hepatic phase of blood formation and continuing in the bone marrow. The method that proved to be successful was microinjection *in utero* into a small efferent blood vessel of the fetal placenta (Fleischman, Mintz 1979). The injected cells circulate quickly into the fetus and lodge in the fetal liver. The use of recipients with W-series mutations, known to cause a hematopoietic stem cell defect as well as macrocytic anemia, confers a competitive advantage upon normal donor stem cells, even when very few of the normal cells are present in the inoculum and reach the recipient's liver. Blood lineages originating from donor cells can then be monitored by tissue-specific markers distinguishing donor and host strains, *e.g.*, hemoglobin electrophoretic differences in erythrocytes, large lysosomal granules (of the *beige* genotype) in donor or host granulocytes, allotype differences in immunoglobulins produced by B-lymphocytes, etc.

We have used the transplacental route to introduce fetal liver cells into fetuses and to compare their *in vivo* developmental capacity with that of adult bone marrow cells similarly introduced into a fetal environment.

DEVELOPMENTAL POTENTIAL OF FETAL LIVER HEMATOPOIETIC STEM CELLS

Inoculation, via the placenta, of a suspension of mouse fetal liver cells into completely allogeneic fetuses often results in permanent establishment of donor-derived blood cell lineages (Fleischman, Mintz 1979). There are no adverse immunological consequences, a fact that is not surprising, in view of the immunological immaturity of both donor and host.

The developmental potential of individual hematopoietic stem cells cannot be tested by seeding hosts with single stem cells. The standard inoculum of $1-2 \times 10^5$ unfractionated fetal liver cells used in all our injections probably contains less than 40 stem cells (Metcalf, Moore 1971). These are not recognizable, have not been isolated, and would undoubtedly fare badly in very dilute suspensions if one were to attempt a conventional limiting-dilution experiment. We have therefore utilized instead a series of different W-mutant recipients with decreasing severity of their endogenous stem-cell defect (Fleischman et al. 1982). In this series, the most severely afflicted members (W/W, ordinarily lethal within a few days after birth) are most frequently seeded and provide a measure of our best technical success: Approximately 50-60% of the W/W animals born from heterozygous parents are seeded with donor-strain cells; many of these individuals then have a normal lifespan free of anemia. Viable but anemic genotypes (e.g., W^v/W^v) are less frequently seeded. Mutants with a very mild defect (e.g., W^f/W^f or $W^v/+$) are infrequently seeded (approximately 5-10% of cases). (Presence of donor-strain cells rarely occurs, and is likely to be temporary, in $+/+$ recipients.) Thus, the graded host series, rather than changes in concentration of injected stem cells, furnishes the equivalent of a limiting-dilution experiment, with recipients such as W^f/W^f only marginally likely to be seeded, probably by single stem cells or very few. These near-normal mutants provide very little advantage to, and little available hepatic space for, normal donor stem cells. The fact that replacement of host- by donor-derived blood cells occurs more rapidly in W/W than in W^f/W^f or $W^v/+$ lends further support to this view. Evidence that even in the most favorable W/W hosts only small numbers of donor stem cells become established is seen in direct examination of fetal livers a week after transplacental injection: against the very pale tissue background characteristic of *W/W*, dark-red foci representing colonies from normal donor stem cells are readily apparent, and are very few in number.

Monitoring of replacement in the erythroid lineage, by means of hemoglobin electrophoretic variants distinguishing donor and host inbred strains, has proved to be a reliable and sensitive indicator of replacement at the stem cell level. In view of the known mouse erythrocyte lifespan of 6-7 weeks (Russell, Bernstein 1966), persistence of donor-type erythrocytes for 8 weeks or longer indicates formation from an ongoing source capable of self-renewal as well as differentiation into erythroid cells (Fleischman *et al.* 1982). Moreover, these cases are accompanied by donor-type cells in other blood lineages. Those tested include other myeloid cells (polymorphonuclear neutrophils were detected by the giant lysosomal granules typical of the *beige* genotype) and lymphoid cells (T- and B-lymphocytes). Based on long-term monitoring of erythrocyte genotypes, some experimental animals were found to undergo what was classified as *complete* replacement, with close to 100% of their erythrocytes of the donor strain; others had replacement described as *limited*, either in amount or duration (but enduring for more than 8 weeks); others were only *transiently* replaced. The *complete* and *limited* replacement classes are interpreted as attributable to successful donor stem cell engraftment, with self-renewal, to maintain the stem cell pool, and differentiation. Quantitative measurements of non-erythroid donor-type lineages, especially with immunoglobulin allotype markers, demonstrated that *complete* and *limited* replacement by donor-strain erythroid cells was invariably accompanied by a progressive and coordinate shift to donor-strain cells in the other blood lineages. Replacement is, nevertheless, generally relatively more extensive in the erythroid lineage, as would be expected in view of the selection favoring normal erythroid cells, in addition to normal stem cells (but not other lineages), in these *W*-anemic hosts.

From the evidence summarized above, the conclusion is reached that the stem cells found in fetal liver and successfully transplanted in these experiments are *totipotent hematopoietic stem cells* (THSC), *i.e.*, cells ancestral to the definitive myeloid and lymphoid lineages and capable of sustained self-renewal and regulated

differentiation for more than two years (Fleischman et al.
1982). Some other evidence for totipotent stem cells has
been presented but has heretofore depended on the use of
radiation-induced chromosomal markers (Wu et al. 1968).
Despite suggestions that separate myeloid and lymphoid stem
cells exist (Abramson et al. 1977), our data from prenatal
grafting, with normal unirradiated cells in unirradiated
hosts, provides no evidence in support of separate myeloid
and lymphoid stem cells (Fleischman et al. 1982).

MONOCLONAL DERIVATION OF MYELOID AND LYMPHOID LINEAGES FROM TOTIPOTENT HEMATOPOIETIC STEM CELLS

More direct verification of the presence of totipotent
hematopoietic stem cells, within the framework of the
developing organism, was sought by offering to fetal recipients a "choice" from a mixture of 2 normal strains of
fetal liver cells (Mintz et al. 1984). The assumption
being tested here is that if many donor cells were engrafted in each recipient, it is unlikely that any mouse would
escape seeding by both donors, whereas single-cell seeding
-- especially in a marginally defective host such as W^f/W^f
-- would tend to lead to retention of one or the other
donor strain more frequently than both. From 236 W^f/W^f
injected fetuses, 11 mice were found to have donor stem-
cell engraftment (monitored for at least 8 weeks in the
erythroid population and verified in some other blood lineages). This frequency (5%) is similar to the frequency of
engraftment (6%) previously found (Fleischman et al. 1982)
when only one strain of fetal liver cells was administered
to W^f/W^f fetuses in the same size inoculum. Eight of the
11 engrafted animals had donor-strain cells of only one or
the other strain and 3 mice had both strains. Computerized
statistical models, taking into account the possibility
that an animal with only one donor genotype might nevertheless have received two (or more) donor cells of the same
strain, showed that some animals must have been seeded by
only a single donor cell ($p = 0.1$); and that the frequency
of this event was at least 20% (90% confidence) and most
likely 50% of the cases (Mintz et al. 1984). In a smaller
group of W/W recipients in the same study, some hosts were
found to be seeded by at most 2 cells ($p = 0.1$) and
single-cell seeding could not be ruled out.

These results strongly reinforce the conclusion (Fleischman, Mintz 1979; Fleischman et al. 1982) that the developmentally primitive stem cells from which myeloid and lymphoid cell types originate are THSC. In support of this conclusion are the observations that hematopoiesis in adult irradiated or postnatal W-hosts can be restored from a small number of bone marrow cells (Micklem et al. 1975; Abramson et al. 1977; Boggs et al. 1982).

CLONAL SUCCESSION LEADING TO A HIERARCHY OF TOTIPOTENT HEMATOPOIETIC STEM CELLS

The occurrence prenatally of seeding by individual stem cells, in the experiment referred to above (Mintz et al. 1984), uniquely enables stem cell pedigrees to be examined in the normal developmental progression within individuals. This becomes especially revealing in those animals with two or three blood-cell genotypes of donor/ host origin. Of 7 mice with multiple genotypes (again

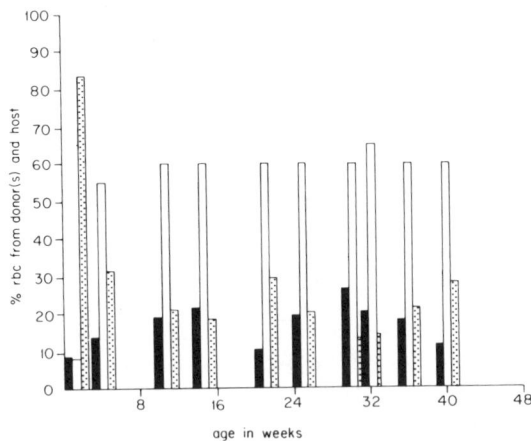

Fig. 1. In this W^f/W^f-C3H host, two donor strains of normal fetal liver hematopoietic stem cells were seeded prenatally. Erythrocyte genotypes at postnatal ages are shown. The C57BL/6 donor strain (solid bars) and the host strain (stippled bars) show a complementary rise and fall for two cycles of approximately 20 weeks each. The BALB/c donor strain contribution (open bars) remains stable. (From Mintz et al. 1984).

monitored in the erythroid lineage) over a long period of time, a complementary rise and fall was observed in the subpopulations of genetically different cells. These cycles had a periodicity of approximately 20-30 weeks. In one example (Fig. 1), one of the donor types (C57BL/6) underwent two cycles of increase and decrease, with the host type inversely decreasing and increasing; the other donor type (BALB/c) remained constant. The complementary nature of the changes indicates physiologically regulated responsiveness.

This decline and resurgence, as well as the temporary disappearance and reappearance (in the circulation) of a donor strain in some hosts, suggest that the stem cell population is hierarchical. The hierarchy appears to consist of an actively proliferating but ephemeral compartment, whose differentiated products are more immediately visible, and a "hidden" reserve compartment. A waxing-and-waning wave of red blood cells would then

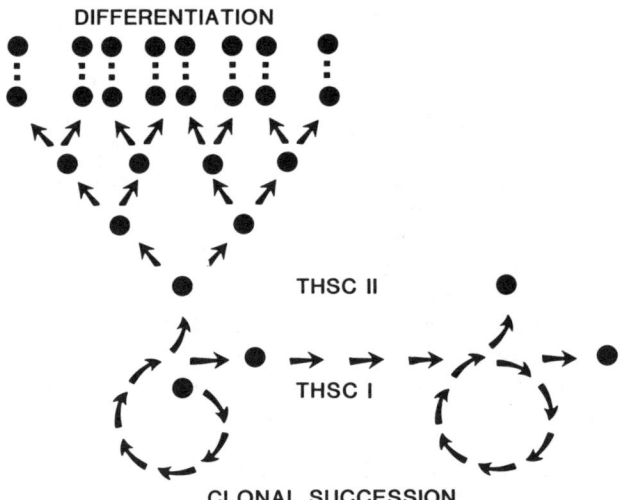

Fig. 2. A diagrammatic representation of two postulated THSC compartments. Cells in the THSC I class are slowly cycling and have long-term renewal potential; those in the THSC II class arise successively as clones that expand rapidly, have decreasing renewal potential, and give rise to differentiated progenitor cells. (The diagram does not literally represent details of kinetics.)

represent the differentiated products of a clone in the active compartment with a maximum lifespan of some 20-30 weeks. It must then be replaced from a smaller reserve of more quiescent, slowly dividing, and more long-lived cells that are the hematopoietic founder cells or their direct lineal descendants. I have here for convenience termed the reserve compartment "THSC I" and the active compartment "THSC II" (Fig. 2). However, it should be emphasized that this distinction is to some extent arbitrary, inasmuch as the THSC II compartment is likely to consist of a heterogeneous series of cells with gradual changes in their renewal potential and other stem-cell properties.

The hypothesis of clonal succession, first proposed by Kay (1965), describes a model which our data seem to substantiate: small numbers of primitive stem cells that are relatively quiescent are sequentially triggered to produce large amplifying clones. The stem cell population is thus heterogeneous, with an "age structure" of gradually decreasing self-renewal capacity and increasing proliferative activity, progressing toward differentiation, as postulated (Hellman et al. 1978).

TOTIPOTENT HEMATOPOIETIC STEM CELLS IN ADULT BONE MARROW

The results of transplacental inoculation of genetically marked cells from adult bone marrow into early W-mutant fetuses showed that THSC capable of seeding the fetal liver, progressing to the bone marrow, and undergoing sustained self-renewal and differentiation are still present; coordinate donor derivation of the various myeloid and lymphoid lineages was also confirmed by tissue-specific and strain-specific markers (Fleischman, Mintz 1984).

However, if host and donor have histocompatibility differences, specifically at the $H-2$ locus, the graft apparently may successfully seed the fetal liver but usually then fails to become well established in the bone marrow. This is in contrast to the fact that THSC from allogeneic fetal liver not only fare as well as syngeneic THSC in the livers of fetal recipients but also subsequently prosper in the bone marrow (Fleischman et al. 1982). Although syngeneic THSC from adult marrow (with only such markers as hemoglobin-type differing in donor and host) are able to seed and populate the recipients, fully allogeneic marrow cells (*e.g.*, C3H ($H-2^k$) donors → W/W^v-C57BL/6 ($H-2^b$) hosts) only rarely continue to proliferate and develop for long periods (Fleischman, Mintz 1984). The crucial role of the major histocompatibility genetic region was demonstrated by the following experiments: $H-2$ compatibility even when other histocompatibility loci were incompatible, resulted in successful long-term renewal and differentiation, *e.g.*, in (C3H x C57BL/6)F_1 → W/W^v-C57BL/6, also in C3H.SW ($H-2^b$) → W/W^v-C57BL/6 ($H-2^b$), and in $H-2^k$-C57BL/6 → W/W^f-(C3H ($H-2^k$) x C57BL/6)F_1. On the other hand, congenic donor-host associations with only $H-2$ incompatibility were not sustained, *e.g.*, $H-2^k$-C57BL/6 → W/W^v-C57BL/6.

It is especially noteworthy that the unsuccessful cases with $H-2$ donor-host differences did not display any signs of graft-*versus*-host disease and did not appear to be undergoing actual rejection of the graft. Rather, there was a marked reduction in the establishment of THSC in the marrow and in their proliferation and differentiation there.

PROGRESSIVE DEVELOPMENTAL HETEROGENEITY OF TOTIPOTENT HEMATOPOIETIC STEM CELLS

We have found several lines of evidence that THSC are a heterogeneous rather than a uniform class, and that they become more heterogeneous as hematopoietic development progresses from liver to bone marrow. One phenotype that changes is the capacity for self-renewal, which diminishes progressively. This can be concluded from the fact that THSC from adult bone marrow generally sustained their renewal for a shorter time than THSC from fetal liver, after transplantation into fetuses, even when syngeneic donor marrow was used (Fleischman, Mintz 1984; Fleischman *et al.* 1982). These results reflect the careers of individual THSC or are, at most, assays of very small numbers seeded in individual fetal hosts. Our conclusion, that stem cells in fetal liver have a higher intrinsic capacity for self-renewal than those in bone marrow, is in agreement with many previous reports based on the use of irradiated adult hosts (*e.g.*, Micklem *et al.* 1972), although contrary claims have been made (Harrison *et al.* 1984).

Marrow THSC have also undergone partial histocompatibility restriction (as summarized above) in relation to their environment, while fetal liver THSC have not.

Another phenotypic change is that marrow THSC, even when experimentally placed in a fetal environment, have lost the capacity to generate erythroid cells on which the erythrocyte-specific and fetal-specific antigen, Ft, is expressed (Blanchet et al. 1982).

These observations lend further support to the interpretation deduced from the complementary rise and fall of co-existing genotypes (Mintz et al. 1984) and diagrammatically represented in Fig. 2. According to this view, differentiation does not proceed in a single step from THSC to special progenitor cells. Rather, the THSC II class subsumes progressive maturational changes in gene expression which are, nevertheless, consistent with some appreciable degree of self-renewal and with totipotency for myeloid and lymphoid differentiation. It seems reasonable to expect that the THSC II class would continue to become more numerous (relative to THSC I) as the hematopoietic system expands during development; and that THSC obtained from adult bone marrow would be likely to include more THSC II with reduced renewal potential than a comparable sample from fetal liver. Moreover, even if prolonged *in vitro* culture of hematopoietic stem cells becomes feasible, it may not achieve the desired result of providing a rich source of THSC capable of extensive self-renewal, if cells of the THSC II class soon predominate.

AUTONOMOUS *versus* ENVIRONMENTAL CONTROL OF STEM CELL DEVELOPMENT

The concept of a hematopoietic microenvironment crucial for stem cell development has been well substantiated, *e.g.*, in the case of the series of *steel* mouse mutations. These are due to a defect in the tissue environment rather than a defect in the stem cells themselves, as is the case in the *W*-mutations (McCulloch et al. 1965; Altus et al. 1971; Fried et al. 1973). We have investigated the status and possible transplantability of the early hematopoietic microenvironment by transplacental inoculation of normal fetal liver cells into *steel* mutant early fetuses (Okamoto et al. in press). Donor THSC were able to lodge in the livers and to progress to the bone marrow. However, self-renewal and differentiation remained very limited. The microenvironmental defect in *steel* is thus present from the very inception of hepatic hematopoiesis. Although some studies (*e.g.*, Friedenstein *et al.* 1978; Keating *et al.* 1982) have implied possible transplantability of non-stem cells of marrow origin, our experiments with *steel*, and postnatal graft tests by others, indicate that the relevant "stromal" cells in this case are not transplantable.

On the other hand, the capacity of THSC to generate erythrocytes with the cell-specific and fetal-specific Ft antigen is autonomously controlled in the stem cells, rather than in the tissue environment, as already stated: Transplantation of adult mouse marrow THSC to fetuses yields donor-derived, apparently normal, erythrocytes, but they lack the Ft antigen during the period when it is ordinarily present (Blanchet *et al.* 1982). Grafting of adult sheep bone marrow cells to sheep fetuses has also yielded erythrocytes with an adult phenotype: They continue to produce adult globins (Zanjani *et al.* 1982).

A further example of cell-automous, rather than environmental control of hematopoietic development concerns the normal developmental decrease in production of the "minor" hemoglobin relative to the "major" one, found in mice of the *diffuse*-hemoglobin genotype. The relatively high early level of the minor type has been interpreted as "fetal-specific", and yet inducible in adults (Alter *et al.* 1981). However, our results, based on transplanting *diffuse*-strain marrow into non-*diffuse* fetuses, demonstrate that the hemoglobin ratio favoring the minor type is not determined by the environment, is not fetal-specific, and is likely simply to reflect accelerated cell proliferation (Blanchet *et al.* 1982).

MHC CONTROL OF STEM CELL PROLIFERATION AND DEVELOPMENT IN BONE MARROW

The adverse effect of certain histocompatibility differences (termed allogeneic and hybrid resistance) on bone marrow grafts in irradiated recipients has been extensively considered by Cudkowicz and colleagues and ascribed to special H-2D-linked recessive hematopoietic histocompatibility genes that are tissue-specific (reviewed by Cudkowicz, Nakamura 1983). Recent experiments by Drizlikh et al. (1984) suggest that both class I (K and D) and class II (I-A and I-E) major histocompatibility complex genes, rather than hypothetical hematopoietic histocompatibility genes, are responsible.

The usual occurrence of graft failures of allogeneic bone marrow cells, but not of fetal liver cells, after introduction into fetuses (Fleischman et al. 1982; Fleischman, Mintz 1984) may ultimately prove to have a similar explanation. Some differences in our results, compared to those of others, suggest that introduction of cells via fetal rather than postnatal recipients may help to unravel the resistance mechanisms. For example, some combinations that are resisted in the postnatal grafts appear to be acceptable after marrow introduction into fetuses. Further experiments with intraplacental grafts may clarify these and other questions basic to hematopoiesis.

ACKNOWLEDGEMENT

This work was supported by grants HD-10646, CA-06927, and RR-05539 from the U.S. Public Health Service, and by an appropriation from the Commonwealth of Pennsylvania.

REFERENCES

Abramson S, Miller RG, Phillips RA (1977). The identification in adult bone marrow of pluripotent and restricted stem cells of the myeloid and lymphoid systems. J Exp Med 145:1567.
Alter BP, Campbell AS, Friend C (1981). Increased mouse minor hemoglobin *in vivo* and *in vitro*: a model for hemoglobin regulation. Blood 58:66a.
Altus MS, Bernstein SE, Russell ES, Carsten AL, Upton AC (1971). Defect extrinsic to stem cells in spleens of steel anemic mice (36032). Proc Soc Exp Biol Med 138;985.
Blanchet JP, Fleischman RA, Mintz B (1982). Murine adult hematopoietic cells produce adult erythrocytes in fetal recipients. Dev Genet 3:197.

Boggs DR, Boggs SS, Saxe DF, Gress LA, Canfield DR (1982). Hematopoietic stem cells with high proliferative potential. Assay of their concentration in marrow by the frequency and duration of cure of W/W^v mice. J Clin Invest 70:242.

Cudkowicz G, Nakamura I (1983). Genetics of the murine hemopoietic-histocompatibility system: An overview. Transplant Proc 15:2058.

Drizlikh G, Schmidt-Sole J, Yankelevich B (1984). Involvement of the K and I regions of the H-2 complex in resistance to hemopoietic allografts. J Exp Med 159:1070.

Fleischman RA, Custer RP, Mintz B (1982). Totipotent hematopoietic stem cells: Normal self-renewal and differentiation after transplantation between mouse fetuses. Cell 30:351.

Fleischman RA, Mintz B (1979). Prevention of genetic anemias in mice by microinjection of normal hematopoietic stem cells into the fetal placenta. Proc Natl Acad Sci USA 76:5736.

Fleischman RA, Mintz B (1984). Development of adult bone marrow stem cells in H-2-compatible and -incompatible mouse fetuses. J Exp Med 159:731.

Fried W, Chamberlin W, Knospe WH, Husseini S, Trobaugh FE Jr (1973). Studies on the defective haematopoietic microenvironment of Sl/Sl^d mice. Brit J Haematol 24:643.

Friedenstein AJ, Ivanov-Smolenski AA, Chajlakjan RK, Gorskaya UF, Kuralesova AI, Latzinik NW, Gerasimow UW (1978). Origin of bone marrow stromal mechanocytes in radiochimeras and heterotopic transplants. Exp Hematol 6:440.

Harrison DE, Astle CM, Lerner C (1984). Ultimate erythropoietic repopulating abilities of fetal, young adult, and old adult cells compared using repeated irradiation. J Exp Med 160:759.

Hellman S, Botnick LE, Hannon EC, Vigneulle RM (1978). Proliferative capacity of murine hematopoietic stem cells. Proc Natl Acad Sci USA 75:490.

Kay HEM (1965). How many cell-generations? Lancet 2:418.

Keating A, Singer JW, Killen PD, Striker GE, Salo AC, Sanders J, Thomas ED, Thorning D, Fialkow PJ (1982). Donor origin of the *in vitro* haematopoietic microenvironment after marrow transplantation in man. Nature 298:280.

McCulloch EA, Siminovitch L, Till JE, Russell ES, Bernstein SE (1965). The cellular basis of the genetically determined hemopoietic defect in anemic mice of genotype Sl/Sl^d. Blood 26:399.

Metcalf D, Moore MAS (1971). "Haemopoietic Cells," Amsterdam: Elsevier/North Holland, 550 pp.

Micklem HS, Ford CE, Evans EP, Ogden DA (1975). Compartments and cell flows within the mouse haemopoietic system. I. Restricted interchange between haemopoietic sites. Cell Tissue Kinet 8:219.

Micklem HS, Ford CE, Evans EP, Ogden DA, Papworth DS (1972). Competitive *in vivo* proliferation of foetal and adult haematopoietic cells in lethally irradiated mice. J Cell Physiol 79:293.

Mintz B, Anthony K, Litwin S (1984). Monoclonal derivation of mouse myeloid and lymphoid lineages from totipotent hematopoietic stem cells experimentally engrafted in fetal hosts. Proc Natl Acad Sci USA In press.

Okamoto T, Anthony K, Mintz B Abnormal development of genetically normal fetal hematopoietic stem cells in *steel* mutant mouse fetuses. Dev Biol In press.

Paige CJ, Kincade PW, Moore MAS, Lee G (1979). The fate of fetal and adult B-cell progenitors grafted into immunodeficient CBA/N mice. J Exp Med 150:548.

Russell ES, Bernstein SE (1966). Blood and blood formation. In Green EL (ed): "Biology of the Laboratory Mouse," New York: McGraw-Hill, pp. 351-372.

Siminovitch L, McCulloch EA, Till JE (1963). The distribution of colony-forming cells among spleen colonies. J Cell Comp Physiol 62:327.

Till JE, McCulloch EA (1961). A direct measure of the radiation sensitivity of normal mouse marrow cells. Radiat Res 14:213.

Wu AM, Siminovitch L, Till JE, McCulloch EA (1968). Cytological evidence for a relationship between normal hematopoietic colony-forming cells and cells of the lymphoid system. J Exp Med 127:455.

Zanjani ED, Lim G, McGlave PB, Clapp JF, Mann LI, Norwood TH, Stamatoyannopoulos G (1982). Adult haematopoietic cells transplanted to sheep fetuses continue to produce adult globins. Nature 295:244.

ONTOGENY OF THE MOUSE HEMOPOIETIC SYSTEM

Peter MC Wong*†∇, Siu Wah Chung*†,
Connie J Eaves†, David HK Chui*
*Department of Pathology, McMaster University,
Hamilton, Ontario; †Terry Fox Laboratory, B.C.
Cancer Research Centre, Vancouver, B.C.

The hemopoietic system has been widely used as a model for studies of lineage restriction and cellular differentiation. Within the erythroid pathway, analysis of globin gene expression has revealed a well defined developmentally regulated pattern. Characterization of hemopoietic progenitor populations during embryogenesis by assessment of their differentiation potential in vitro offers an approach to the investigation of mechanisms that result in the normal erythropoietic developmental pattern. In the mouse hemopoiesis begins in the extra-embryonic yolk sac, followed by the fetal liver, spleen and bone marrow (Metcalf, Moore 1971; Russell 1979).

In the developing mouse embryo, blood islands first appear in the yolk sac on the seventh day of gestation (Russell 1979). These consist initially of aggregates of undifferentiated blast cells, but shortly thereafter cohorts of large, differentiating erythroblasts become apparent. These "primitive" erythroblasts are rapidly released into the circulation, which is completely established by the ninth day of gestation (Haar, Ackerman 1971; Russell 1979). There they continue to proliferate and mature in a relatively synchronous manner but remain nucleated until the 14-15th day of gestation, after which they are no longer detected (Metcalf, Moore 1971). Initially these primitive erythroblasts synthesize

---

∇Present Address: Bldg. 10, Room 7C103, National Institutes of Health, Bethesda, Maryland 20205

primarily embryonic hemoglobins, i.e. HbEI (x_2y_2), HbEII (α_2y_2) and HbEIII (α_2z_2), but as development proceeds, an increasing amount of adult hemoglobin, HbA, also becomes detectable in them (Brotherton et al 1979).

Shortly after the tenth day of gestation, formation of the fetal liver begins. At this time, immature "definitive" erythroblasts are found within the fetal hepatic parenchyma (Rifkind et al 1969) and by the twelfth day of gestation, enucleated erythrocytes, are released into the circulation. These cells contain HbA only (Barker 1968).

These changes in the phenotype of erythrocytes produced at different stages of embryogenesis and the associated shift of erythrocyte production from the yolk sac to the fetal liver raise a number of fundamental questions about the relationship of these two events. First, at what level of progenitor cell differentiation is the capacity for primitive versus definitive erythrocyte production fixed? Second, does all hemopoiesis derive from a single stem cell population of yolk sac origin, or are there separately produced intra-embryonic hemopoietic stem cells that colonize the fetal liver? To approach these questions we have undertaken a series of studies in which conditions that support the growth of colonies of primitive and definitive erythroblasts in vitro have been defined and then used to analyze the potentialities of clonogenic pluripotent and erythropoietic progenitors present in the yolk sac, early fetal circulation and fetal liver between 7 and 13 days of gestation.

FETAL HEPATIC ERYTHROPOIESIS (DAYS 11-13 OF GESTATION)

Progenitor cells present in the fetal liver of 11 to 13-day old embryos were first tested for their ability to produce primitive as well as definitive erythroblasts by assessment of the type of hemoglobin present in the colonies to which they give rise in methylcellulose cultures containing 1-2 units/ml of erythropoietin (Ep) and pokeweed mitogen stimulated spleen cell conditioned medium (SCCM) at a final concentration of 20%. These conditions support the formation within 6-8 days of high numbers of large erythroid colonies and a significant proportion of these contain cells of other lineages (Johnson, Metcalf 1977; Wong et al 1983). For both colony types plating efficiency was shown to be dependent of the number of cells plated. Such 6 to 8-day old cultures were harvested in bulk and hemolysates prepared from the cells that had been produced. The hemolysates were then evaluated by a sensitive native polyacrylamide gel isoelectric focusing procedure that was capable of detecting as little as 300 ng of hemoglobin per band. No evidence of HbE was detected even when a six fold excess of hemolysate was added to each lane (Wong et al 1983).

Because of studies indicating that the tumor promoter, 12-0-tetradecanoylphorbol 13-acetate (TPA) can induce the differentiation of some early hemopoietic progenitor cells in vitro (Fibach et al 1980), we investigated whether TPA might also stimulate early erythroid and multipotent progenitor cells from fetal liver to produce primitive, HbE-synthesizing erythroblasts. Inclusion of TPA at a final concentration of $10^{-7}M$ in the methylcellulose culture medium resulted in a two fold increase in the number of large (pure and mixed) erythroid colonies obtained and a five fold increase in the amount of hemoglobin produced in 13-day old fetal liver cell cultures. Nevertheless, an analysis of all hemolysates from these cultures again showed only hemoglobin bands with the same migration pattern as that of the HbA (Wong et al 1983).

These experiments suggest that even the earliest pluripotent and erythropoietic progenitors detectable in the fetal liver appear to be committed to the production of definitive (exclusively HbA synthesizing) erythroblasts. However, the possibility that a small amount of embryonic hemoglobin might be produced by some fetal erythroblasts could not be ruled out. To address this latter possibility, specific rabbit anti-mouse HbA and HbE antisera were prepared and conjugated with fluorescein and rhodamine, respectively. Double immunofluorescence staining of fetal hepatic erythroblasts obtained from 12-day old embryos indicated the presence of HbA but not HbE (Wong et al 1983). Taken together, these data suggest that HbE synthesis is normally restricted to the primitive erythroblast and that progenitors capable of producing primitive erythroblasts are not present in the fetal liver.

HEMOPOIETIC PROGENITORS PRESENT IN THE CIRCULATION AND IN THE YOLK SAC PRIOR TO THE ESTABLISHMENT OF THE FETAL LIVER

A similar series of experiments were undertaken to determine the types of progenitors that might be found in the embryonic circulation at a time when the fetal hepatic organ is not yet formed. Accordingly, embryonic peripheral blood cells were obtained from 9- and 10-day old embryos and placed in both plasma clot and methylcellulose cultures under the same conditions described above for the assessment of fetal liver progenitors. After 6-8 days large erythroid and erythroid-mixed colonies were observed indicating the presence of early erythroid and pluripotent progenitors in the circulation of these very young embryos (Chui et al 1981a; Chui et al 1981b). To examine the types of hemoglobins present in the erythroid cells that had been produced in these colonies, ^{3}H-leucine or ^{59}Fe-transferrin was added to the cultures on day 6 or 7 and 1-2 days later hemolysates were prepared from the harvested cells. These were then analyzed using ion exchange chromatography or native gel electrophoresis plus autoradiography, respectively. Only HbA was detected even when excess hemolysate was added and the sensitivity of the autoradiographic detection limit increased by lengthening the exposure time (Wong et al 1982). Analysis of hemolysates prepared from 4-day old cultures also failed to reveal any evidence that HbE might be produced at earlier times. Similar results were reported by Cudennec et al (1981).

These experiments suggest that pluripotent and restricted erythropoietic progenitors committed to definitive erythroblast production are released into the circulation even before the fetal liver begins to develop. To examine the possibility that this conclusion might be biased by the use of conditions optimized for the support of definitive erythropoiesis, i.e. the addition of Ep and adult spleen cell derived SCCM, additional cultures were set up in which an attempt was made to reproduce more closely conditions prevailing in the embryo. To achieve this, embryonic fluid (EF) from the excoelomic cavity of 10-day old conceptuses was added in place of SCCM. These experiments showed that EF appears to contain an activity similar to that in adult SCCM, that is able to stimulate or enhance the formation of erythroid colonies from 9-day old circulating progenitors. Analysis of hemolysates from the erythroid cells produced in these EF containing cultures again revealed the presence of HbA only (Wong et al 1982; Chui et al 1981b). It was recently reported that mouse yolk sacs can produce factors capable of inducing erythroid burst forming growth in vitro (Labastie et al 1984).

A high frequency of clonogenic progenitors of definitive erythroblasts was also demonstrated in the 9- to 10-day old yolk sac (Wong et al 1982; unpublished data). Release of some of these into the circulation would appear the likely explanation for their simultaneous presence in the embryonic blood stream.

ERYTHROPOIESIS IN THE YOLK SAC OF 7- AND 8-DAY OLD CONCEPTUSES

Initial attempts to detect clonogenic precursors of primitive erythroblasts in culture showed that physical or enzymatic disaggregation of tissues from very young (early day 8) conceptuses yielded no or very few colonies. However, when small tissue fragments were cultured in the presence of 2 units/ml of Ep, numerous clusters of erythroblasts were observed 6 days later. Analysis of hemolysates from these clusters showed only HbE to be present (Fig. 1, lane 2) suggesting that primitive erythroblast production in vitro had been achieved. In cultures containing SCCM but no Ep, this erythropoietic growth appeared to be markedly reduced and the amount of hemoglobin present was insufficient to obtain detectable bands on isoelectric focussing gels (Fig. 1, lane 3). On the other hand addition of both SCCM and Ep to the culture medium appeared to greatly increase the number of erythroid clusters produced and subsequent analysis of their hemolysates showed that HbA as well as HbE had been produced under these conditions (Fig. 1, lane 4). Moreover, when tissue fragments from slightly older (day 8 1/2) conceptuses were cultured, addition of Ep alone appeared sufficient to support a small amount of HbA production as well as HbE. However, Ep plus SCCM again resulted in a marked and selective enhancement of the amount of HbA detected in culture hemolysates (Wong, Chui 1982).

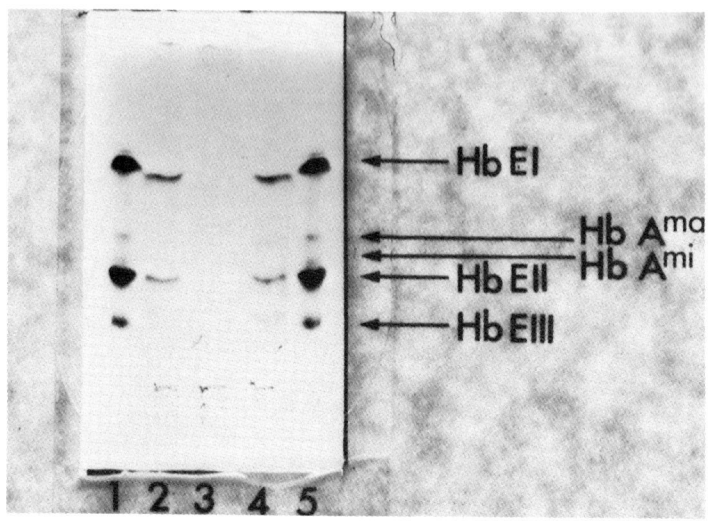

FIGURE 1

Isoelectric focusing of hemolysates of cells from 6-day old cultures of embryonic tissues from 8-day old conceptuses with an average ECL of 0.89 mm. Controls (lanes 1 and 5) show hemolysates of day 13 peripheral blood; lane 2, a hemolysate from cultures containing 2 units of Ep per ml only; lane 3, a hemolysate from cultures containing 20% SCCM only; lane 4, a hemolysate from cultures with both 2 units/ml of Ep and 20% SCCM.

These findings suggest the formation of two types of erythroid precursors, appearing at different times during development, responsive to different factors, and distinguished by the presence or absence of HbE in their erythroblast progeny. Additional support for program selection at the level of a precursor cell was obtained by immunofluorescent studies of the erythroblasts produced in the presence or absence of SCCM. In the absence of SCCM, most of the erythroid cells produced showed positive staining with anti-HbA as well as with anti-HbE (Wong, Chui

1982). When cultures contained both Ep and SCCM, a large additional population of erythroid cells that stained exclusively with anti-HbA was detected.

Subsequent studies (Wong et al 1984) showed that a variety of viable clonogenic hemopoietic precursors could be isolated from 7- to 8-day old conceptuses when these were incubated in a 0.1% collagenase solution if 20% fetal calf serum was also present (Table 1). On the other hand, assays of cells from older (9-10 day old) embryos dissociated by collagenase showed no qualitative or quantitative difference when the fetal calf serum was omitted from the collagenase solution. Time course studies of the colonies obtained in assays of cells from day 7 or day 8 conceptuses also showed differences from the kinetic pattern typical of cultures established from older (more than 10-day old) embryos. In particular, a small erythroid colony similar to those derived from adult or fetal liver CFU-E was the predominant type of colony obtained when Ep only was present (Wong et al 1984). However, in contrast to colonies derived from adult or fetal liver CFU-E which reach peak numbers on the 2nd day of incubation (Gregory et al 1976; Chui et al 1978) these small clusters arising in the assays of day 7 and 8 conceptuses increased in number until the 4th day of incubation and then declined. Progenitors of such colonies were not detectable when cells from 10-day old (or more) conceptuses were cultured. Inclusion of SCCM in the culture medium used to assay clonogenic cells from 8-day old conceptuses stimulated the formation of additional, larger erythroid colonies as well as some colonies of mixed cellularity. If, however, only SCCM was added and no Ep, then some, albeit very few erythroid colonies were obtained and hemoglobinization was very poor.

Immunofluorescent analysis of the erythroblasts present in individual colonies obtained in these assays of 7- to 8-day conceptuses showed that most colonies contained cells that were positive for both HbE and HbA. A few of the precursors present in day 8 conceptuses, and almost all of the erythroid precursors present in day 9 embryos yielded colonies that were positive for HbA only (Wong et al 1984).

Table 1. Progenitors detectable in methylcellulose culture from yolk sac cells of 8-day old conceptuses disaggregated by collagenase in the presence or absence of fetal calf serum (FCS)

FCS	Colonies per 9×10^3 [a]				
	CFU-E	BFU-E (small bursts)	BFU-E (large bursts)	E-mix	non-E
+[b]	35,27,24	10,13,8	6,6,7	1,4,4	4,12,3
−[c]	6,3,0	5,1,1	3,3,4	4,3,1	1,5,3

Treatment of collagenase in the presence of FCS was done by placing 4 yolk sacs of 8-day old conceptuses in 8 ml of a 0.1% collagenase solution in α-medium containing 20% FCS and incubating for 3 hours with occasional shaking. Treatment of collagenase in the absence of FCS was done by placing 4 yolk sacs in 8 ml of the same collagenase solution but without FCS and incubating in this case for 20 min. Values shown are counts in replicate assay dishes from a single representative experiment.

[a] Assays were scored on Day 6 at which time a unique type of CFU-E-like cluster could still be readily scored (see text, for further details).

[b] The average egg cylindrical length (ECL) of the conceptuses used in this condition was 1.5 mm (1.4-1.6 mm). 9×10^3 cells plated per dish.

[c] The average ECL of the conceptuses used in this situation was 1.3 mm (1.2-1.4 mm). The actual plating cell concentration was 7×10^3 cells per dish.

The apparent association between the age of the conceptus, colony maturation kinetics, SCCM dependence and the production of either primitive or definitive erythroblasts suggests that two separate developmental lines may diverge very early within the yolk sac - one line consisting of low proliferative potential progenitors of primitive erythroblasts, and the other consisting of pluripotent progenitors whose erythroid progeny will be exclusively of the definitive type. The fact that the latter type of progenitor is present at high concentration in 8-day old conceptuses at a stage when the circulation is not quite complete, provides strong evidence for their origin in the yolk sac. On the other hand, there is data from avian studies (Dieterlenn-Lievre, Martin 1981; Lassila et al 1982) to indicate that definitive hemopoietic stem cells may arise de novo in the embryo itself and not by colonization from yolk sac elements. If this were so in the developing mouse also, then it should be possible to demonstrate the presence of definitive precursors in the embryo at a time preceding the completion of the circulation. Experiments were therefore undertaken to assay separately cells from the extra-embryonic yolk sac and cells from the embryo proper of day 8 conceptuses. These showed that virtually all of the erythroid colonies obtained were generated in assays of the yolk sac samples (Wong et al 1984).

SUMMARY AND CONCLUSIONS

In summary, we have shown that clonogenic precursors of both primitive and definitive erythroblasts can be isolated from early stage mouse conceptuses and stimulated to form colonies in standard methylcellulose cultures containing Ep and SCCM. These two types of precursors appear to differ not only in their ability to produce HbE-synthesizing progeny, but also in their innate sensitivity to physical or enzymatic treatment, and in their maturation kinetics and differential responsiveness to SCCM. On the basis of sequential studies of the distribution of these precursors in the yolk sac, early circulation and fetal liver it appears most likely that in the mouse, both primitive and definitive hemopoietic cells originate extra-embryonically in the yolk sac blood islands. We suggest that commitment to primitive erythropoiesis is an early transient event that leads to the rapid and exclusive production of primitive erythroblasts. All other cells become committed to definitive erythropoiesis and this decision may precede actual restriction of differentiation potential to the erythroid lineage. As a result only definitive pluripotent stem cells enter the circulation and hence seed the other hemopoietic tissues.

ACKNOWLEDGEMENT

This work was supported by research grants from the Medical Research Council of Canada to DHK Chui and CJ Eaves, and from the National Cancer Institute of Canada to CJ Eaves with core support from the British Columbia Cancer Foundation and the Cancer Control Agency of British Columbia. CJ Eaves is a Research Associate of the NCI of Canada, SW Chung was an MRC Postdoctoral Fellow and PMC Wong is a Postdoctoral Fellow of the NCI of Canada. The secretarial assistance of M Coulombe is gratefully acknowledged.

REFERENCES

Barker JE (1968). Development of the mouse hemopoietic system. I. Types of hemoglobin produced in embryonic yolk sac and liver. Dev Biol 18:14.
Brotherton TW, Chui DHK, Gauldie J, Patterson M (1979). Hemoglobin ontogeny during normal mouse fetal development. Proc Natl Acad Sci USA 76:2853.
Chui DHK, Liao SK, Walker K (1978). Fetal erythropoiesis in Steel mutant mice. III. Defect in differentiation from BFU-E to CFU-E during early development. Blood 51:539.
Chui DHK, Wong PMC, Clarke BJ (1981a). Developmental hemoglobins in the mouse Adv Physiol Sci 6:133.
Chui DHK, Wong PMC, Clarke BJ, Carr DH (1981b). Murine embryonic erythropoiesis: Adult hemoglobin is synthesized in BFU-E derived erythroid colonies in vitro. In: Stamatoyannopoulos G & Nienhuis AW (eds): "Hemoglobin in Development and Differentiation", New York: Alan R. Liss, p 171.
Cudennec CA, Thiery JP, LeDouarin NM (1981). In vitro induction of adult erythropoiesis in early mouse yolk sac. Proc Natl Acad Sci 78:2412.

Dieterlenn-Lievre F, Martin C (1981). Diffuse intraembryonic hemopoiesis in normal and chimeric avian development. Dev Biol 88:180.

Fibach E, Marks PA, Rifkind RA (1980). Tumor promoters enhance myeloid and erythroid colony formation by normal mouse hemopoietic cells. Proc Natl Acad Sci USA 77:4152.

Gregory CJ (1976). Erythropoietin sensitivity as a differentiation marker in the hemopoietic system: Studies of three erythropoietic colony responses in culture. J Cell Physiol 89:289.

Haar JL, Ackerman (1971). A phase and electron microscopic study of vasculogenesis and erythropoiesis in the yolk sac of the mouse. Anat Rec 170:199.

Johnson GR, Metcalf D (1977). Pure and mixed erythroid colony formation in vitro stimulated by spleen conditioned medium with no detectable erythropoirtin. Proc Natl Acad Sci USA 74:3879.

Labastie M-C, Thiery J-P, Le Douarin NM (1984). Mouse yolk sac and intraembryonic tissues produce factors able to elicit differentiation of erythroid burst-forming units and colony-forming units, respectively. Proc Natl Acad Sci USA 81:1453.

Lassila O, Martin C, Toivanen P, Dieterlen-Lievre (1982). Erythropoiesis and lymphopoiesis in the chick yolk-sac embryo chimeras: contribution of yolk sac and intraembryonic stem cells. Blood 59:377.

Metcalf D, Moore MAS (1971). "Hemopoietic Cells." North-Holland Publishing Co, p 172.

Rifkind RA, Chui DHK, Epler H (1969). An ultrastructural study of early morphogenetic events during the establishment of fetal hepatic erythropoiesis. J Cell Biol 40:343.

Russell ES (1979). Hereditary anemias of the mouse: a review for geneticists. Adv in Genet 20:357.

Wong PMC, Chui DHK (1982). Hemoglobin switching during murine early embryonic development. Blood 60:59a.

Wong PMC, Chung SW, Chui DHK, Eaves CJ (1984). Yolk-sac derivation of progenitors of both primitive and definitive hemopoietic cells. Blood 64:120a.

Wong PMC, Chung SW, White JS, Reicheld SM, Patterson M, Clarke BJ, Chui DHK (1983). Adult hemoglobins are synthesized in murine fetal hepatic erythropoietic cells. Blood 62:1280.

Wong PMC, Clarke BJ, Carr DH, Chui DHK (1982). Adult hemoglobins are synthesized in erythroid colonies in vitro derived from murine circulating hemopoietic progenitor cells during embryonic development. Proc Natl Acad Sci USA 79:2952.

HEMOPOIETIC STEM CELL REGULATORS IN FETAL LIVER

Martine Guigon and Joanna Wdzieczak-Bakala.

Unité de Recherches sur la Cinétique Cellulaire
INSERM U250, Institut Gustave-Roussy
Villejuif, France

FETAL LIVER HEMOPOIESIS

Fetal liver is a heterogeneous population of cells consisting of parenchymal cells, epithelial cells, tissue macrophages or Kupfer cells and various blood cells. It is generally considered as an erythropoietic organ and indeed, it contains a high percentage of nucleated erythroid cells, which is about 50-55 % in 14 day mouse fetal liver as compared to 20-25 % in adult bone marrow (Rich, Kubanek 1976). It also contains the progenitors of the erythroid series (Rich, Kubanek, 1976, 1979 ; Zucali, Ulatowski, Mirand 1980) and is the main source of erythropoietin (Gallien-Lartigue 1966 ; Cole, Paul 1966 ; Zanjani, Mann, Burlington, Gordon, Wassermann 1974). The kinetics of the erythroid system in fetal liver has been extensively studied by Tarbutt and Cole (1970) who have reported two distinct phases in fetal erythropoiesis, corresponding to periods of sensitivity and non-sensitivity to erythropoietin respectively.

Fetal liver contains pluripotent stem cells and the progenitors of the granulomacrophagic series (GM-CFC) (Metcalf, Moore 1971). In mice, pluripotent stem cells, called CFU-S (colony forming unit in the spleen) because of their capacity to form colonies in the spleen of irradiated mice, appear first in the liver on the 10th day of gestation. Their number increases rapidly to reach a maximum on the 18th day. GM-CFC, progenitors of the granulomacrophagic lineage, also appear on the 10th day of gestation and the population increases rapidly to reach a

peak on the 13th day. By day 14, the number of GM-CFC drops abruptly and remains low until day 17, with some oscillatory changes until birth. Therefore, according to Metcalf and Moore (1971), liver hemopoiesis can be divided into 3 phases :
- an initial phase of maximum growth rate between 10-13 day's gestation when GM-CFC outnumber CFU-S by 12-17 : 1,
- an intermediate plateau phase between 13 days and birth with a more constant ratio of GM-CFC's to CFU-S (4-6 :1),
- and a terminal postnatal decline phase where loss of CFU-S initially occurs more rapidly than GM-CFC.

Moreover Jonhnson and Metcalf reported in 1977 that mouse fetal liver contained cells giving rise to pure and mixed erythroid colonies when stimulated by pokeweed mitogen spleen conditioned medium. The number of these colonies declined in frequency with advancing fetal age. More recently, hemopoietic progenitors have been purified by cell sorting and the majority of pluripotent stem cells were clearly separated from the progenitors (Nicola, Metcalf, von Melchner, Burgess 1982).

However the situation observed in mice can be different in other species. Moore and Williams (1973) have reported differences in fetal GM-CFC proliferation in species of short gestation (mouse, rat, rabbit) as compared to species of long gestation (human, monkey, calf, lamb, guinea-pig).

The existence of megakaryocyte progenitors (CFU-M) in fetal liver was first demonstrated by Vainchencker, Guichard and Breton-Gorius (1979). Fetal colonies differed from adult colonies in being more numerous and also in having a higher proportion of mixed colonies, observed in cultures carried out on 20 week - old human fetuses. In fetal cells, megakaryocytes often reached a more complete maturation than in adult marrow, proceeding as far as platelet shedding.
To our knowledge, no data are available concerning the progenitors of the lymphoid lineage in fetal liver.

It should be emphasized that in fetal liver, the number and rate of proliferation of the pluripotent and unipotent stem cells are generally similar or even higher than in adult marrow. Some differences have been reported, however, between fetal and adult hematopoietic stem cells, such as differences in sensitivity to erythropoietin (Tarbutt, Cole 1970 ; Rich, Kubanek 1976) and differences in megakaryocyte differentiation (Vainchencker, Guichard, Breton-Gorius 1979).

Murine stem cell proliferation has been shown in adult animals to be regulated by a balance between stimulators and inhibitors, which have been reported to be long range (Frindel, Croizat, Vassort 1976 ; Sainteny, Frindel 1981 ; Frindel, Guigon 1977) or short range (Lord, Mori, Wright, Lajtha 1976; Lord, Mori, Wright 1977). It was of interest to know whether such modulators were present in the fetal liver as in bone marrow and whether adult stem cells could respond to these factors.

PLURIPOTENT STEM CELL REGULATORS

Inhibitors

We have previously demonstrated that fetal calf bone marrow contains a substance capable of preventing entry of adult marrow CFU-S into DNA synthesis after irradiation or chemotherapy (Frindel, Guigon 1977 ; Guigon, Frindel 1978). When administered during a sequential treatment of a phase-specific drug, cytosine arabinoside (Ara-C), it can increase significantly the number of surviving CFU-S (Guigon, Enouf, Frindel 1980). Moreover, it increases the survival of mice having received lethal doses of the same drug (Guigon, Mary, Enouf, Frindel 1982). These results indicate that CFU-S inhibitors are able to protect bone marrow against the effect of a myelotoxic drug, which is of major importance in cancer therapy.

This factor is a dialysable molecule (MW below 2000D). The first steps of purification, using Biogel P2 chromatography and high pressure liquid chromatography lead to a inhibitory fraction active at a dose of 150 ng/mouse. It is a cationic molecule containing sulfhydryl groups (Wdzieczak-Bakala, Lenfant, Guigon 1984). Further purification is now being carried out.

Since the content of this inhibitor in fetal calf marrow is very low (1 mg of inhibitory fraction extracted from 4 g of fetal marrow) and since fetal calf marrow is not easily available in large amounts, we have looked for the presence of CFU-S inhibitor in fetal calf liver (Guigon, Wdzieczak-Bakala, Mary, Lenfant, 1984).

Fetal calf livers were collected from 6-7 month-old fetuses and kept frozen at -20°C. A delipidated powder was prepared by three extractions of the tissue with cold acetone (10 ml/g tissue) and one extraction with cold butanol (2 ml/g tissue). After air-drying, the powder kept its activity for several months when stored at -20°C. The delipidated powder was extracted with 10 ml/g of 10^{-2}M acetic acid containing 10^{-2}M mercaptoethanol. After centrifugation at 10,000 g for 30 minutes, the supernatant was ultrafiltered on Amicon PM10 membranes ; the ultrafiltrate was lyophilised. The yield was about 2 mg/g liver.

The low molecular weight fractions were chromatographed on a Biogel P-2 (Biorad 200-400 mesh) column (2.5 x 100 cm) using 10^{-2}M acetic acid as eluent, at a flow rate of 1 ml/min. The eluted fractions were collected according to the elution profile. The void volume (Vo = 180 ml) was determined by Dextran Blue (Pharmacia). Optical density measurements gave yields of 80-90 %. Figure 1 summarizes the different steps of preparation of the fetal liver CFU-S inhibitor, which is slightly different from the technique used to prepare the marrow extracted inhibitor (Wdzieczak-Bakala, Guigon, Lenfant, Frindel 1983). The elution profile (Figure 2) indicates that the inhibitory fraction was eluted at the elution volume Ve/Vo 1.2-1.8.

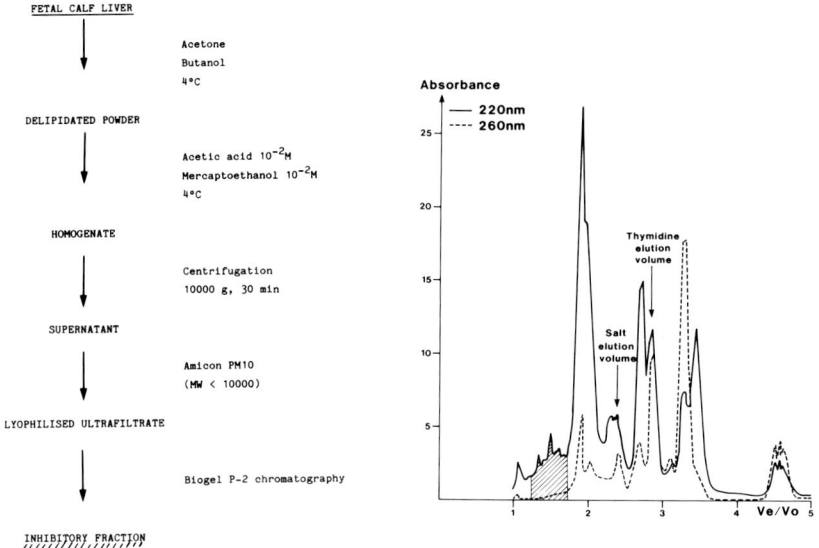

Figure 1

Figure 2

Figure 1.-Preparation of the inhibitory fraction from fetal calf liver.
Figure 2.- Biogel P-2 chromatography of fetal calf liver. The chromatography was performed on a 2.5 x 100 cm column in 10^{-2}M acetic acid. The elution rate was 1 ml/min. (Vo=180 ml). The absorbance was evaluated at 220 nm (corresponding to peptide-bound wavelength absorbance and at 260 nm (corresponding to nucleoside absorbance).

At each step of the purification, fractions were assayed in vivo in mice by determining the inhibition of the entry of CFU-S into DNA synthesis using the method of ^{3}HTdR suicide (Becker, Mc Culloch, Siminovitch, Till, 1965). Experiments were carried out on two strains of mice, C3H and Balb/c. Male and female specific pathogen free (SPF) mice Ola mice aged 2 to 3 months were used.

Adult SPF mice normally have quiescent CFU-S, so it was necessary to trigger them into the cell cycle, before measuring the effect of the inhibitor. This was achieved by giving mice one injection (i.p.) of Cytosine arabinoside (Ara-C) at a dose of 500 mg/kg. 8 hours later, about 30 % CFU-S are in S phase. The inhibitor dissolved in saline was administered (i.p.), 6 hours after the Ara-C injection, just before the CFU-S start synthesizing DNA. The control group received the same volume of saline. 8 hours after the drug injection, mice were killed and their bone marrow harvested. CFU-S were measured according to the technique of Till and Mc Culloch (1961) and their percentage in DNA synthesis was determined by the thymidine suicide method of Becker, McCulloch, Siminovitch, Till (1965). For each experimental point, we used 3 donor mice and 16 lethally irradiated recipient mice (9 and 7.5 Gy ^{60}Co for C3H and Balb/c respectively). Bone marrow was flushed out of femurs and tibias in 199 medium using a syringe and needle. The medullary suspension was divided into two aliquots, to one of which was added 200 µCi of tritiated thymidine (specific activity 25 Ci/mM) in 2 ml of 199 medium(A). Both aliquots (A and B) were incubated at 37°C for 20 minutes. Then 8 ml of cold 199 medium were added to each vial to stop further incorporation of tritiated thymidine and to dilute the concentration of cells to about 4.0×10^5 ml. 0.2 ml of each vial was injected into the retroorbital sinus of lethally irradiated recipient mice under aether anesthesia. Nine days later, the mice were killed, their spleens removed and fixed in Bouin' solution. Splenic nodules were counted 24 hours later. The percentage of CFU-S in DNA synthesis was calculated according to the following formula :

$$\% \text{ in } S = \frac{\text{Number of nodules (B)} - \text{Number of nodules (A)}}{\text{Number of nodules (B)}} \times 100$$

As shown in Table 1, a dose as low as 0.1 µg/mouse inhibits the entry of CFU-S into S phase. Moreover the fetal liver extract is not toxic since there is no difference in the number of splenic colonies in the treated and in the control group.

Dose of inhibitor (μg)	n	% of CFU-S in S phase		Statistical Significance
		Ara-C	Ara-C + inhibitor	
0.1	1	56 ± 6	31 ± 13	$p < 0.05$
1	4	45 ± 4	30 ± 6	$p < 0.025$
5	2	37 ± 9	2 ± 12	$p < 0.01$
10	5	41 ± 4	16 ± 6	$p < 0.001$
37	2	36 ± 6	3 ± 10	$p < 0.005$

Table 1.- Mean number and standard error of the percentage of CFU-S in S phase with and without different doses of fetal liver inhibitor. Statistical significance corresponds to the unilateral comparison of the inhibitory effect to zero ; n = number of experiments.

To test the specificity of this CFU-S inhibitor, it was assayed on GM-CFC, progenitors of the granulomacrophagic series. GM-CFC were studied according to the technique of Worton, McCulloch, Till (1969) using methylcelulose, horse serum and a source of stimulating factor, either post endotoxin serum or abdominal wall CSF (Horiuchi, Ichikawa 1977). The percentage in DNA synthesis was determined by the suicide with hydroxyurea (Sinclair 1967). The CFU-S inhibitor had no effect on the number or the percentage in S phase of medullar GM-CFC (Table 2).

	n	Mean No. of GM-CFC/10^5 ¢		% of GM-CFC in S phase
		Without HU	WIth HU	
Control	3	101 ± 3	72 ± 3	29 ± 4
Fetal liver inhibitor	3	104 ± 3	80 ± 3	23 ± 4

Table 2. Mean and standard error of the number of GM-CFC (with and without hydroxyurea HU) and of the percentage of these cells in S phase with or without the liver inhibitor, calculated from 3 experiments.

Therefore, the CFU-S inhibitor present in fetal liver is very similar to the inhibitor extracted from fetal calf bone marrow. Both are small molecules, contrary to the CFU-S inhibitor found in adult mouse and rat marrow (Lord, Mori, Wright, Lajtha 1976 ; Cork, Anderson, Thomas, Brynmor, Riches 1981) and in human marrow (Wright, Sheridan, Moore 1980). They are not species specific at least from high species to low species and they seem to be specific for CFU-S. Further studies are now necessary to determine the chemical nature of the active molecule.

Although fetal liver is a rapidly proliferating hematopoietic tissue, the presence of an inhibitor is not surprising, since it has been shown in adult marrow that, irrespective of the proliferative activity of the CFU-S, haemopoietic tissues contain both inhibitor and stimulator-producing cells (Wright, Garland, Lord 1979) and that it is the relative level of each factor that influences CFU-S kinetics.

Stimulators

We have not looked for a stimulator in the fetal calf liver but it has been reported (Cork, Wright, Riches 1982) that supernatants of human fetal liver of 11 to 18 weeks of gestation contains a stimulator of murine CFU-S. This stimulator has a molecular weight of 30,000-50,000 D and is produced by adherent cells. It therefore appears to be similar to the CFU-S stimulator detected in adult mouse marrow (Lord, Mori, Wright 1977).

UNIPOTENT STEM CELL REGULATORS OF THE MYELOID LINEAGE

GM-CFC Inhibitors

An inhibitor of GM-CFC proliferation has been found to be present in the supernatant of early human fetal liver, between 11 and 13 weeks of gestation, but not at later times (Cork, Wright, Riches 1982). This inhibitor, produced by non-adherent fetal liver cells, reduced the proportion of GM-CFC synthetizing DNA, but did not decrease the number of colonies formed.

It is a high molecular weight substance (MW 100,000 D), different from the myelopoiesis inhibiting peptide present in human granulocytes, which was recently identified and synthetized (Paukovits, Paukovits, Laerum, Hinterberger 1980 ; Paukovits, Laerum 1982 ; Laerum, Paukovits 1984).

The GM-CFC inhibitor present in fetal liver is different from prostaglandin E (Kurland, Moore 1977 ; Kurland, Broxmeyer, Pelus, Bockman, Moore 1978), but is very similar to the leukemia-associated inhibitor (LAI) described by Olofsson and Olsson (1980 a-b), which has been shown to be acid isoferritin (Broxmeyer, Bognacki, Dorner, Sousa 1981).

GM-CFC Stimulators

Cork, Wright, Riches (1982) have also reported that the supernatant from late human fetal liver (14 to 17 weeks of gestation) contained a factor capable of increasing the DNA synthesis of GM-CFC. The stimulator is produced by an adherent population of human fetal liver cells and has a molecular weight of 30,000-50,000 D. It is not present in a thymus supernatant prepared in the same way.

The significance of stem cell inhibitors in the control of hemopoiesis is not clear. They are present both in adult marrow where the rate of CFU-S proliferation is low and in fetal liver where it is high. Also fetal liver is a good source of stem cells for transplantation. Moreover, the ability of stimulators to override the effect of inhibitors in adult marrow (Wright, Garland, Lord 1979) suggests that perhaps fetal liver also has large amounts of stimulator. The recent report of Labastie, Thiery, Le Douarin (1984) for the existence of an erythroid burst promoting factor in embryonic tissues would favour such an hypothesis and might provide a possible explanation for the intense erythrocytic activity of fetal liver.

BECKER AJ, McCULLOCH EA, SIMINOVITCH L and TILL JE (1965).
The effect of differing demands for blood cell production on DNA synthesis by hemopoietic colony forming cells of mice. Blood 26:296.
BROXMEYER HE, BOGNACKI J, DORNER NH and SOUSA M (1981).
Identification of leukemia-associated inhibitory activity as acidic isoferritins. J Exp Med 153:1426.
COLE RJ and PAUL J (1966).
The effects of erythropoietin on haem synthesis in mouse yolk sac and cultured fetal liver. J Embryol Exptl Morph 15:245.
CORK M, ANDERSON I, THOMAS DB and RICHES A (1981).
Regulation of the growth fraction of CFU-S by an inhibitor produced by bone marrow. Leukemia Res 5:101.

CORK MJ, WRIGHT EG and RICHES AC (1982).
Regulation of murine granulocyte-macrophage progenitor cell and haematopoietic stem cell proliferation by factors produced in human fetal liver. Leukemia Res 6:553.

FRINDEL E, CROIZAT H and VASSORT F (1976).
Stimulating factors liberated by treated bone marrow : in vitro effects on CFU-S kinetics. Exp Hematol 4:56.

GALLIEN-LARTIGUE O (1966).
Action du facteur érythropoiétique du plasma sur l'hématopoïèse in vitro du foie de souris embryonnaire. Exp Cell Res 41:109.

FRINDEL E and GUIGON M (1977).
Inhibition of CFU-S entry into cycle by a bone marrow extract. Exp Hematol 5:74.

GUIGON M, ENOUF J and FRINDEL E (1980).
Effects of CFU-S inhibitors on murine bone marrow during Ara-C treatment. Leukemia Res 4:385.

GUIGON M and FRINDEL E (1978).
Inhibition of CFU-S entry into cycle after irradiation and drug treatment. Biomedicine 29:176.

GUIGON M, MARY JY, ENOUF J and FRINDEL E (1982).
Protection of mice against lethal doses of $1-\beta$-D-arabino-furanosylcytosine by pluripotent stem cell inhibitors. Cancer Res 42:638.

GUIGON M, WDZIECZAK-BAKALA J, MARY JY and LENFANT M (1984).
A convenient source of CFU-S inhibitors : the fetal calf liver. Cell Tissue Kinet 17:49.

HORIUCHI M and ICHIKAWA (1977).
Control of macrophage and granulocyte colony formation by two different factors. Exp Cell Res 110:79.

JOHNSON GR, METCALF D (1977).
Pure and mixed erythroid colony formation in vitro stimulated by spleen conditioned medium with no detectable erythropoietin. Proc Natl Acad Sci 74:3879.

KURLAND JI, BROXMEYER HE, PELUS LM, BOCKMAN RS, MOORE MAS (1978).
Role for monocyte-macrophage derived colony-stimulating factor and prostaglandin in the positive and negative feedback control of myeloid stem cell proliferation. Blood 52:388.

KURLAND JI and MOORE MAS (1977).
Modulation of hemopoiesis by prostaglandins. Exp Hematol 5:357.

LABASTIE MC, THIERY JP and LE DOUARIN N (1984).
Mouse yolk sac and intraembryonic tissues produce factors able to elicit differentiation of erythroid burst-forming units and colony-forming units, respectively. Proc Natl Acad Sci 81:1453.

LAERUM OD, PAUKOVITS WR (1984).
Inhibitory effects of a synthetic pentapeptide on hemopoietic stem cells in vitro and in vivo. Exp Hematol 12:7.

LORD BI, MORI KJ and WRIGHT (1977).
A stimulator of stem cell proliferation in regenerating bone marrow. Biomedicine 27:223.

LORD BI, MORI KJ, WRIGHT EG and LAJTHA LG (1976).
An inhibitor of stem cell proliferation in normal marrow. Brit J Haematol:34, 441.

METCALF D and MOORE MAS (1971).
Embryonic aspects of haemopoiesis. In Haemopoietic Cells. North Holland Publishing Company, Amsterdam-London, p. 195.

MOORE MAS and WILLIAMS N (1973)
Analysis of proliferation and differentiation of foetal granulomacrophage progenitor cells in haemopoietic tissue. Cell Tissue Kinet 6:461.

NICOLA NA, METCALF D, VON MELCHNER H, BURGESS AW (1981).
Isolation of murine fetal hemopoietic progenitor cells and selective fractionation of various erythroid precursors. Blood 58:376.

OLOFSSON T and OLSSON I (1980a).
Suppression of normal granulopoiesis in vitro by a leukemia-associated inhibitor (LAI) of acute and chronic leukemia. Blood, 53:975.

OLOFSSON T and OLSSON FG (1980b).
Biochemical characterization of a leukemia associated inhibitor (LAI) suppressing normal granulopoiesis in vitro. Blood 55:983.

PAUKOVITS WR and LAERUM OD (1982).
Isolation and synthesis of a hemoregulatory peptide. Z. Naturforsch 37:1297.

PAUKOVITS WR, PAUKOVITS JB, LAERUM OD and HINTERBERGER W (1980).
Granulopoiesis inhibiting factor (Chalone) : purification and chemical composition. IRCS Int Res Commun Med Sci Libr Compend 8:305.

RICH IN and KUBANEK B (1976).
Erythroid colony formation (CFUe) in fetal liver and

adult bone marrow and spleen from the mouse. Blut 33:171.
SAINTENY F and FRINDEL E (1981).
Modulators of CFU-S kinetics in spleen and serum of Ara-C treated animals. Exp Hematol 9 Suppl 9:1314.
SINCLAIR UK (1967).
Hydroxyurea : effects on chinese hamster cells grown in culture. Cancer Res 27:297.
TARBUTT RG and COLE RJ (1970).
Cell population kinetics of erythroid tissue in the liver of fetal mice. J Embryol Exptl Morph 2412:429.
TILL JE and Mc CULLOCH EA (1961).
A direct measurement of the radiation sensitivity of normal mouse cells. Radiat Res 14:213.
VAINCHENKER W, GUICHARD J and BRETON-GORIUS J (1979).
Growth of human megakaryocyte colonies in culture from fetal, neonatal and adult peripheral blood cells : ultrastructural analysis. Blood cells 5:25.
WDZIECZAK-BAKALA J, GUIGON M, LENFANT M and FRINDEL E (1983).
Further purification of a CFU-S inhibitor : in vivo effects after cytosine arabinoside treatment. Biomedicine Pharmacoth 37:467.
WDZIECZAK-BAKALA J, LENFANT M and GUIGON M (1984).
Purification and biomedical characterization of a CFU-S proliferation inhibitor : preliminary results. IRCS Med Sci Biochem 12:868.
WORTON RG, Mc CULLOCH EA and TILL JE (1969).
Physical separation of hemopoietic stem cells from cells forming colonies in culture. J Cell Physiol 2:171.
WRIGHT EG, GARLAND JM and LORD BI (1980).
Specific inhibition of haemopoietic stem cell proliferation : characteristics of the inhibitor producing cells. Leukemia Res 4:537.
WRIGHT EG, SHERIDAN P and MOORE MAS (1980).
An inhibitor of murine stem cell proliferation produced by normal human bone marrow. Leukemia Res 4:309.
ZANJANI ED, MANN LI, BURLINGTON H, GORDON AS and WASSERMAN LR (1974).
Evidence for a physiological role of erythropoietin in fetal erythropoiesis. Blood, 44:285.
ZUCALI JR, ULATOWSKI JA and MIRAND EA (1980).
Erythroid progenitor cells and cells capable of producing erythropoietic activity from fetal mouse liver. Exp Hematol 8:971.

CHANGES IN THE GROWTH REQUIREMENTS OF BABOON LIVER HEMATO-POIETIC PROGENITORS DURING ONTOGENY

G. David Roodman, M.D., Ph.D.

Research Service
Audie Murphy Veterans Administration Hospital
San Antonio, Texas 78284

INTRODUCTION

During ontogeny the site of hematopoiesis changes in mammalian species. The yolk sac is the initial site of blood development, but is supplanted by the liver in humans and mice (Schwartz, Gill 1977; Moore, Metcalf 1970). Studies in mice have shown that the liver remains the primary site of blood formation for the majority of fetal life (Rifkind, Chui, Epler 1969; Tarbutt, Cole 1970). The marrow becomes the major hematopoietic organ about the twenty-fifth week of gestation in man and is essentially the only site of hematopoiesis in normal adult primates. The basis for the change in the site of hematopoiesis during development is unknown. Changes in the hematopoietic potential of an organ such as liver may result from intrinsic changes in the microenvironment of an organ during development, changes in the growth requirements of hematopoietic progenitor cells during development, or a combination of these possibilities.

Fetal and adult erythroid progenitor cells differ in several aspects besides the types of hemoglobins they produce. Fetal erythroid progenitors appear to be more sensitive to erythropoietin than are adult cells. For example, fetal and neonatal sheep and human fetal liver contain a subpopulation of erythroid colony forming cells (CFU-E) which can grow in the absence of added erythropoietin in vitro (eCFU-E) (Roodman, Zanjani 1979; Roodman, Lee, Gidari 1983). In contrast normal human adult marrow does not contain eCFU-E. Furthermore, erythropoietin dose-response curves and plating efficiency of fetal erythroid progenitors differ from adult erythroid progenitors in both human and murine species (Rich, Kubanek 1980; Linch, Knott, Rodeck 1982). These differences in Ep responsiveness appear to be due to intrinsic differences in fetal and adult erythroid progenitors. It is possible that an organ may lose its hematopoietic potential because of changes in the growth requirements of hematopoietic progenitor cells during development. Therefore, the growth characteristics of erythroid progenitors (CFU-E and BFU-E) in baboon fetal liver and marrow, newborn liver and marrow, and adult liver and marrow were compared to determine if the growth requirements for these cells differ. Adherent cells, which are predominantly monocyte-macrophages, from these organs were also cocultured with nonadherent cells, which contain hematopoietic progenitor cells, from these organs to determine the role monocyte-macrophages may play in modulating hematopoietic progenitor cell growth during development.

METHODS

Marrow and liver samples from twenty-six fetal baboons of 140 ± 3 days gestational age (normal gestation 180 days) were used in these studies. Liver cell suspensions were prepared by passing livers through #40 SS wire mesh and allowing the cell suspension to sediment for 10 minutes at unit gravity to remove debris. The cells above the sediment were collected and used in these studies. Fetal marrow was obtained by flushing the femurs with medium containing 100 units/ml preservative free heparin. Marrow mononuclear cells were then prepared using ficoll-Hypaque gradients (Boyum, 1968). Liver and marrow samples from 8 newborn baboons were also obtained and processed in a similar manner.

Marrow mononuclear cells were prepared from marrow obtained by sternal or posterior superior iliac crest aspirations from twenty-three adult baboons. Adult liver biopsy samples were obtained from 4 pregnant female baboons undergoing hysterotomy for delivery of 140 day gestational age fetuses.

Heparinized peripheral blood was collected from normal adult, pregnant adult, and newborn baboons. The mononuclear cells were prepared and used in these studies.

In selected experiments liver, marrow and peripheral blood cell suspensions were fractionated into cells adherent to plastic tissue culture dishes and nonadherent cells (Roodman, Horadam, Wright, 1983). The nonadherent cells were cultured for erythroid colony, burst and multipotent progenitor cell colonies (Tepperman, Curtin, McCulloch, 1974; Iscove, Sieber, Winterhalter, 1974; Ash, Detrick, Zanjani, 1981) and adherent cells used as feeder layers for assay of CFU-E, BFU-E and CFU-GEMM with nonadherent liver and marrow cell samples.

RESULTS

Baboon fetal liver, fetal marrow, and newborn marrow showed similar erythropoietin (Ep) dose response curves. The average concentration of Ep required for maximal colony formation for fetal, newborn, and adult CFU-E was 100-200 mu/ml for fetal and newborn and 300-400 mu/ml for adult marrow CFU-E. Newborn liver and adult liver did not form erythroid colonies regardless of the Ep concentration tested. Fetal liver and marrow BFU-E required lower concentrations of Ep (300 ± 67 mu/ml Ep) than newborn and adult marrow BFU-E (525 ± 188 mu/ml Ep) for maximal burst formation. No erythroid bursts were detected when newborn or adult liver unfractionated cells or nonadherent cells were cultured, regardless of the Ep concentration present in the cultures. Unfractionated and nonadherent cell fractions showed similar Ep sensitivity.

As seen in Table 1, fetal liver, fetal marrow, newborn marrow, and adult marrow formed colonies in the absence of added Ep in the cultures (eCFU-E). eCFU-E comprised $33\pm7\%$ of total CFU-E in fetal marrow and decreased to $15\pm7\%$ and $13\pm7\%$ in newborn and adult marrow respectively. Similarly, fetal liver and marrow contained endogenous BFU-E (eBFU-E) which comprised approximately $27\pm7\%$ of total BFU-E. Newborn marrow also contained eBFU-E in similar proportions as fetal marrow ($27\pm8\%$). eBFU-E were not detected in cultures of adult marrow cells. Similar results were seen in cultures of unfractionated or nonadherent fetal liver, fetal marrow, newborn marrow, and adult marrow.

Table 2 depicts the mean concentration of CFU-E and BFU-E present in cultures of unfractionated fetal, newborn, and adult liver and marrow from 20 fetal, 7 newborn, and 24 adult baboons. Fetal liver contained a lower concentration

TABLE 1
ERYTHROID COLONY AND BURST FORMATION IN CULTURES OF FETAL,
NEWBORN AND ADULT LIVER AND MARROW GROWN IN THE ABSENCE OF ERYTHROPOIETIN

Tissues Assayed	Experiments	Colonies/10^5 Cells Plated	Bursts/10^5 Cells Plated
Fetal Liver	10	32±20 (18±6%)	7±6 (25±14%)
Fetal Marrow	9	217±70 (33±7%)	10±3 (27±7%)
Newborn Liver	3	0	0
Newborn Marrow	3	35±21 (15±7%)	19±9 (27±8%)
Adult Liver	2	0	0
Adult Marrow	9	82±62 (13±7%)	0

Fetal, newborn and adult liver and marrow (1-2x10^5 cells/ml) were cultured with or without the addition of erythropoietin. Erythroid colonies and bursts were then counted using a Soret band filter after 5 days (colonies) or 10 days (bursts) in culture. All cultures were done in quadruplicate. The number of colonies or bursts/10^5 cells plated (mean ± SEM) formed in cultures lacking erythropoietin (endogenous colonies or bursts) are shown. Addition of erythropoietin to these cultures resulted in maximal colony or burst formation. The % of colonies or bursts which formed in the absence of erythropoietin compared to those formed in the presence of erythropoietin is shown in parenthesis.

TABLE 2
ERYTHROID COLONY (CFU-E), ERYTHROID BURST (BFU-E) AND MULTIPOTENT PROGENITOR CELL (CFU-GEMM) FORMATION IN FETAL, NEWBORN AND ADULT LIVER AND MARROW

	Fetal		Newborn		Adult	
	Liver	Marrow	Liver	Marrow	Liver	Marrow
CFU-E/10^5 Cells	129±50	731±175	0	278±53	0	242±34
Range	(10-381)	(214-1861)		(150-437)		(21-689)
BFU-E/10^5 Cells	80±45	116±33	0	88±20	0	54±23
Range	(8-298)	(40-268)		(31-158)		(5-235)
CFU-GEMM/10^5 Cells	2±1	19±7	0	9*	0	6±2
Range	(0-10)	(3-62)		(2-15)		(2-16)

Results are reported as the mean ± SEM for the number of experiments shown in the text. All experiments were done in quadruplicate. CFU-E, BFU-E, and CFU-GEMM were assayed in unfractionated liver and marrow cell cultures by standard techniques. The range of colony formation is given below each result.
*Mean of two experiments.

of progenitor cells than fetal marrow. No hematopoietic progenitor cell derived colonies were detected in newborn and adult liver. Newborn and adult marrow had similar concentrations of CFU-E and BFU-E and CFU-GEMM (CFU-E: 278 ± 53 vs 242 ± 34; BFU-E; 88 ± 20 vs 54 ± 23; CFU-GEMM: 9 vs 6 ± 2). Fetal hematopoietic tissues had higher concentrations of progenitor cells than their respective newborn or adult counterparts.

However latent erythroid progenitors present in newborn and adult baboon liver samples could be detected when newborn and adult liver cells were cocultured with an appropriate adherent cell feeder layer. As seen in Table 3 and 4 fetal, newborn or adult liver adherent cells did not stimulate expression of latent erythroid progenitors in newborn and adult liver samples.

However, these studies did not exclude the possibility that the erythroid progenitors assayed in newborn and adult liver cultures were derived from peripheral blood trapped in the liver. Therefore newborn liver cells were cocultured with autologous or adult peripheral blood cells in the presence or absence of a marrow adherent cell feeder layer. No erythroid colonies formed when peripheral blood cells were cultured in the absence or presence of a marrow adherent cell feeder layer (data not shown). As seen in table 5, culture of newborn liver nonadherent cells in the presence or absence of peripheral blood cells resulted in similar numbers of erythroid bursts being formed, even when 5×10^5 peripheral blood cells were added to the cultures. Few erythroid bursts were detected when peripheral blood was cultured alone under the culture conditions we employed.

DISCUSSION

These data show that during ontogeny hematopoietic progenitor cell concentration and Ep responsiveness decrease. Fetal liver and marrow erythroid progenitors had similar Ep responsiveness *in vitro* and were more responsive to Ep than adult CFU-E and BFU-E. Although the CFU-E in newborn marrow were more responsive to Ep than adult marrow CFU-E, newborn and adult marrow BFU-E had similar Ep sensitivity. As has been reported in murine and human systems (Rich, Kubanek 1980; Linch, Knott, Rodeck et al, 1982), baboon fetal liver and marrow formed colonies and bursts in the absence of ex-

TABLE 3
EFFECTS OF DIFFERENT ADHERENT CELL POPULATIONS
(AC) ON NEWBORN LIVER CFU-E AND BFU-E

	CFU-E			BFU-E		
Adherent Cells	Experiments	No AC	+AC	Experiments	No AC	+AC
Fetal Liver	(3)	0	0	(3)	0	0
Fetal Marrow	(4)	0	37+24	(3)	0	71+24
Newborn Liver	(7)	0	1+1	(7)	0	1+1
Newborn Marrow	(7)	0	34+16	(7)	0	10+3
Adult Liver	(2)	0	0	(2)	0	0
Adult Marrow	(5)	0	15+7	(5)	0	11+5

Results represent the mean $\pm$ SEM per 10^5 cells plated for the number of experiments shown in parentheses. Nonadherent liver cells were cultured in the absence or presence of various adherent cell feeder layers.

TABLE 4
EFFECTS OF DIFFERENT ADHERENT CELL POPULATION (AC)
ON ADULT LIVER CFU-E AND BFU-E

Adherent Cells	CFU-E			BFU-E		
	Experiments	No AC	+AC	Experiments	No AC	+AC
Fetal Liver	(4)	0	0	(2)	0	0
Fetal Marrow	–	ND*	ND	(1)	0	9+2
Newborn Liver	(2)	0	0	(2)	0	0
Newborn Marrow	–	ND	ND	–	ND	ND
Adult Liver	(4)	0	0	(2)	0	0
Adult Marrow	(4)	0	8+5	(2)	0	9

*ND – not done

Results represent the mean ± SEM per 10^5 cells plated for the number of experiments shown in parentheses. Nonadherent liver cells were cultured in the absence or presence of various adherent cell feeder layers.

TABLE 5
EFFECTS OF COCULTURING NEWBORN LIVER NONADHERENT CELLS WITH PERIPHERAL BLOOD MONONUCLEAR CELLS ON ERYTHROID BURST FORMATION

	Exp. 1		Exp. 2	
	No AC	+AC	No AC	+AC
	(bursts per 0.5 ml culture)			
Newborn Liver NAC	13±7	52±10	6±1	20±3
Newborn Liver NAC+1x10^5 PBC	14±9	41±9	ND*	21±7
Newborn Liver NAC+5x10^5 PBC	13±4	18±5	ND	21±3
1x10^5 PBC	2±2	0	ND	ND
5x10^5 PBC	3±3	4±4	2±2	2±2

1x10^5 newborn liver adherent cells (NAC) were cultured in 0.5 ml methylcellulose cultures in the presence (+AC) or absence (No AC) of a newborn marrow adherent cell feeder layer. In experiment 1 newborn liver cells were cocultured with autologous peripheral blood mononuclear cells (PBC), and in experiment two newborn liver cells were cocultured with adult peripheral blood nonadherent mononuclear cells. Unfractioned newborn peripheral blood cells were used in experiment one because of the difficulty in obtaining adequate numbers of newborn peripheral blood cells. Results represent the mean ± SEM for triplicate determinations and are reported as erythroid bursts per 0.5 ml culture.

*Not Done

ogenous Ep. These endogenous CFU-E and BFU-E comprised approximately 30% of total erythroid progenitors assayable. Unlike human marrow cultures, adult baboon marrow contains endogenous CFU-E, but like human marrow does not contain eBFU-E (Zanjani, Lutton, Hoffman, Wasserman 1977). Newborn marrow contains lower percentages of eCFU-E than fetal samples but still contains eBFU-E.

The concentration of CFU-E and BFU-E were greater in fetal samples than in corresponding newborn and adult liver and marrow. The concentration of progenitor cells in fetal liver was less than fetal marrow. This difference in progenitor cell concentration in fetal liver when compared to fetal marrow is consistent with the declining hematopoiesis seen morphologically in 140 day gestational age fetal baboon liver, but may also reflect differences in the cell preparations. Marrow progenitor cells were enriched by density gradient centrifugation, while liver progenitors were not. However, such density gradient techniques only enrich progenitor cells 2-3 fold (unpublished results), and do not account entirely for the differences in progenitor cell concentrations in fetal liver and marrow. Therefore, during development both progenitor cell concentration and Ep sensitivity decrease.

Other growth requirements for hematopoietic progenitor cells change during ontogeny. Fetal liver erythroid progenitor cells formed colonies in absence of any adherent cell feeder layer (Table 2), while newborn and adult liver progenitors were only detectable in the vast majority of experiments when these cells were cocultured with a marrow adherent cell feeder layer (Table 3,4). Similarly, in preliminary experiments multipotent progenitors from newborn and adult liver formed colonies only in the presence of a marrow adherent cell feeder layer. The absence of colony formation in cultures of newborn and adult liver cells does not appear to be due to suppression of progenitor cell growth by liver adherent cells. Newborn or adult liver nonadherent cells cultured in the absence of adherent cells failed to form erythroid or multipotent colonies. In other experiments, we have shown that fetal liver and marrow, newborn marrow and adult marrow CFU-E and BFU-E growth was not suppresed by newborn liver or adult liver adherent cells (Roodman, Vandeberg, Kuehl, 1985). More likely, newborn and adult liver progenitors require a factor produced by marrow monocyte-macrophages but not by liver macrophages for growth. This factor is probably not Ep because unfractionated or nonadherent liver cell cultures failed to form erythroid colonies or bursts in the presence of very high concentrations of Ep (3000 mu/ml). The stimulatory effect of marrow adherent cells on newborn and adult liver progenitors did not result from higher concentrations of macrophages in marrow adherent cell preparations than in liver adherent cell preparations. The percentage of monocytemacrophage were greater in liver (89-90%) than marrow adherent cell preparations (70-72%). Furthermore, the percentage of adherent cells present in unfractionated liver was approximately 50% while in marrow it was 25-30%, which would result in more cells being present in a liver adherent cell feeder layer than in a marrow adherent cell feeder layer. These data suggest that liver progenitor cells are normally not detected in newborn and adult liver in part because of a change in their growth requirements during development. The low number of progenitor cells detected in newborn and adult liver may result from suboptimal culture conditions or may reflect decline of progenitor cells in a nonsupportive microenvironment. Alternatively changes in the liver adherent cells during development resulting in an inability to support hematopoiesis may be responsible for the loss of hematopoietic function in the neonatal and adult liver. Marrow progenitor cells and fetal liver progenitor cells may not require an adherent cell feeder layer for growth in vitro because they differ intrinsically from newborn and adult liver progenitors. Alternatively, having been exposed to a supportive microenvironment in vivo, fetal liver and marrow progenitors only require Ep for growth in vitro. Changes in the intrinsic properties of progenitor cells seem a more likely explanation for our data, because fetal liver adherent cells did not stimulate the growth of latent erythroid and multipotent progenitor cells in newborn and adult liver.

ACKNOWLEDGEMENTS

Supported by funds from Veterans Administration Research Service and by Grant AM 28639 from the National Institutes of Arthritis, Diabetes, Digestive and Kidney Diseases.

REFERENCES

Ash RC, Detrick RA, Zanjani ED (1981). Studies on human pluripotential hemopoietic stem cells in vitro. Blood 58:309.

Boyum A (1968). Isolation of mononuclear cells and granulocytes from human blood. Scan J Clin Lab Invest (Suppl 97) 21:77.

Iscove NN, Sieber F, Winterhalter KH (1974). Erythroid colony formation in cultures of mouse and human marrow: Analyses of the requirement of erythropoietin by gel filtration and affinity chromatography on agarose concanavalin A. J Cell Physiol 83:309.

Linch DC, Knott LS, Rodeck CH et al (1982). Studies on circulating hemopoietic progenitor cells in human fetal blood. Blood 59:976.

Moore MAS, Metcalf D (1970). Ontogeny of the haemopoietic system: yolk sac origin of in vivo and in vitro colony forming cells in the developing mouse embryo. Br J Haematol 18:279.

Rich IN, Kubanek B (1980). The ontogeny of erythropoiesis in mouse detected by the erythroid colony-forming technique II. Transition of erythropoietin sensitivity during development. J Embryol Exp Morphol 58:143.

Rifkind RA, Chui D, Epler E (1983). An ultrastructural study of early morphogenetic events during the establishment of fetal hepatic erythropoiesis. J Cell Biol 40:343.

Roodman GD, Zanjani ED (1979). Endogenous erythroid colony forming cells in fetal and newborn sheep. J Lab Clin Med 44:699.

Roodman GD, Lee JL, Gidari AS (1983). Effects of dexamethasone on erythroid colony and burst formation from human fetal liver and adult marrow. Br J Haematol 53:621.

Roodman GD, Horadam VW, Wright TL (1983). Inhibition of erythroid colony formation by autologous bone marrow adherent cells from patients with the anemia of chronic disease. Blood 62:406.

Roodman GD, VandeBerg JL, Kuehl TJ (in press). Expression of latent hematopoietic progenitor cells in cultures of newborn and adult baboon liver. Blood.

Schwartz E, Gill FM (1977). Hematology of the newborn in Williams WJ, Beutler E, Erslev AJ Rundles RW (eds): Hematology, New York, McGraw-Hill Co p38.

Tarbutt RG, Cole EJ (1970). Cell population kinetics of erythroid tissue in liver of foetal mice. J Embryo Exp Morphol 24:429.

Tepperman AD, Curtin JE, McCulloch EA (1974). Erythrocytic colonies of human marrow. Blood 44:659.

Zanjani ED, Lutton JD, Hoffman R, Wasserman LR (1977). Erythroid colony formation by polycythemia bone marrow in vitro. J Clin Invest 59:841.

SECTION II
EXPERIMENTAL HEMATOPOIESIS AND IMMUNE DEVELOPMENT–MAN

EMBRYONIC HEMOPOIESIS IN HUMAN LIVER: MORPHOLOGIC ASPECTS AT SEQUENTIAL STAGES OF ONTOGENIC DEVELOPMENT

S. Petti[1], U. Testa[1], A.R. Migliaccio[1], F. Mavilio[1], M. Marinucci[1], D. Lazzaro[2], G. Russo[4], G. Mastroberardino[3], C. Peschle[1].
From: (1) Department of Hematology, Istituto Superiore di Sanità, Rome; (2) Istituto Patologia Generale, University of Rome "La Sapienza", Rome; (3) Division of Obstetrics and Gynecology, Ospedale Generale, Avellino; (4) Istituto di Patologia Medica VI, University of Rome "La Sapienza", Rome, Italy.

In mammalian embryos hemopoietic islands initially develop in yolk sac (YS) mesoderm (Browder 1984). These give rise to the first generation of hemopoietic stem cells and "primitive" erythroblasts, which are typically of megaloblastic type. The second generation of "definitive" erythroblasts derives from the liver (L), and gradually replaces the primitive lineage in the fetal bloodstream.

Morphological aspects of embryonic and fetal hemopoiesis in humans have been extensively described (Kelemen et al 1979). However, a satisfactory analysis of the early ontogenic stages has been hampered so far by a number of biases. Thus, human embryos in the 4-8-wk postconception have been scarcely available, particularly within a few hr from the abortion. This clearly precluded physiological studies. Furthermore, it rendered difficult systematic morphological observations, which were also prone to artefacts, particularly at the ultrastructural level. Finally, the analyzed embryos were rarely intact, and hence could not be accurately dated. This hampered the comparative analysis of hemopoiesis at precisely sequential stages of development.

We have established a large collection of hemopoietic tissues (i.e., YS, L and circulating blood) from virtually intact embryos and fetuses obtained by legal curettage abortions at 5-8- and 9-12-wk postconception respectively.

We report here morphological observations on embryonic L hemopoiesis at 5-8-wk. These studies include a detailed analysis of both blast cells and differentiated elements of the erythroid, granulo-macrophage (GM) and megakariocytic lineage, which were evaluated by conventional or electron microscopy as well as cytochemical reactions.

MATERIALS and METHODS

Hemopoietic tissues

Virtually intact embryos and fetuses, obtained from legal curettage abortions, were maintained in Iscove's modified Dulbecco's medium (Gibco, Co., USA). Their fertilization age was carefully established by crown-rump length measurement, as well as morphological staging according to unequivocal criteria (Moore 1982, England 1983). The integrity of the examined embryos allowed a dating error as little as $\pm$ 2 days (Moore 1982). All samples were processed within 4-6 hr from the abortion, thus minimizing the possibility of artefacts. Single cell suspensions were prepared from YS or L as previously described (Peschle et al. 1981, Peschle et al. 1985 a). Embryonic blood was obtained from heart or umbilical vein virtually free of maternal blood contamination (Peschle et al. 1985a).

Morphology studies

Cellular suspensions obtained from embryonic L were cytocentrifuged and stained by the May-Grünwald+Giemsa (MGG) method. Cytochemical ractions included periodic acid Schiff (PAS), naphtol-AS-D chloroacetate esterase (NASDCA) and Graham-Knoll peroxidase.

Histologic preparations of freshly dissected L were embedded in Epon Resin 812 (Fisher, USA) for light and transmission electron microscopy according to standard procedures.

RESULTS

At the end of the 4th week, the columnar epithelium of the diverticulum invades the ventral portion of the septum transversum. Cordonal formations of epithelial cells develop into the mesenchymal tissue of the septum (Fig. 1). In the contact areas the mesenchime gives rise to the primitive system of sinusoids, while epithelial cords develop around them in an interdigitating pattern (Fig. 1).

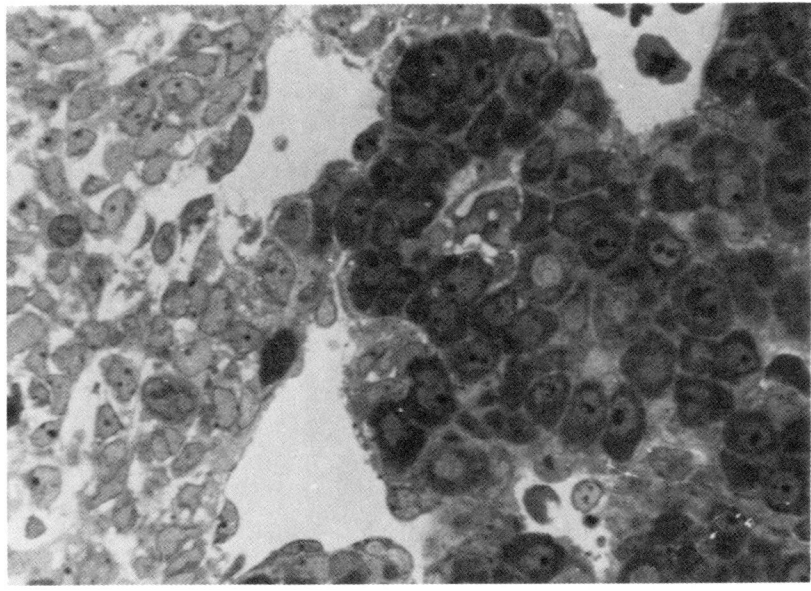

Fig. 1. 4-5-wk L: endodermal cords (right side) invade the mesenchymal tissue of the septum transversum (left side). The columnar epithelium of the cords progressively lines the primitive sinusoids, which are exclusively formed by mesenchymal cells (x300).

In 5-wk L numerous megaloblasts, at all stages of maturation (type I, II, III), were observed only in sinusoids (Fig. 2). This suggests that the megaloblasts are derived from YS. Rare number of undifferentiated blast cells were also observed in L sinusoids. Finally, an active phagocytic activity is suggested by presence of histyocytes in the sinusoidal wall (Fig. 2).

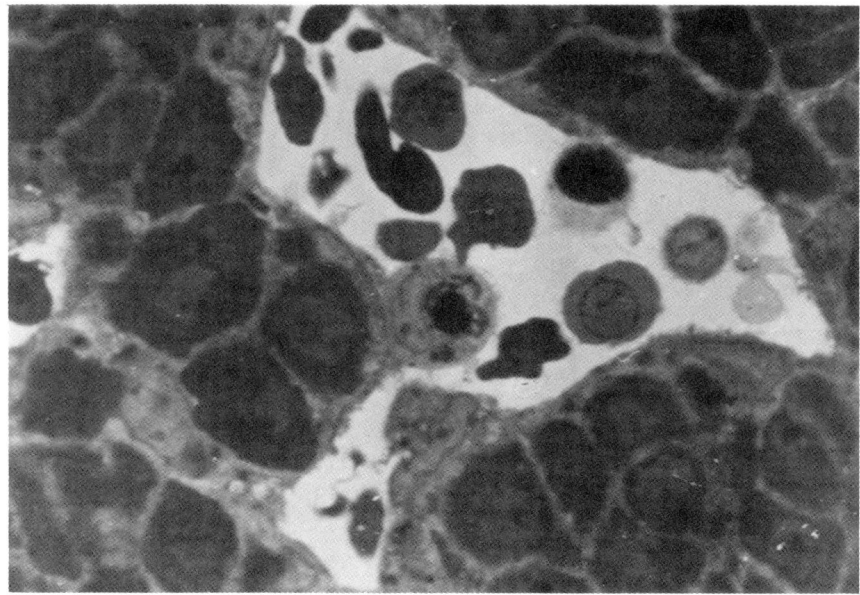

Fig. 2. 5-wk-L: the circulating erythroid cells in sinusoids are exclusively constituted by YS- derived megaloblasts, mostly of type I and II. A luminal histiocyte is observed in the endothelial wall (x500).

Although intra-parenchimal megaloblasts are not observed, discrete numbers of differentiated GM cells (Fig. 3) are present between the hepatic epithelial cords. A discrete number of mononuclear blast cells are randomly dispersed between the epithelial cords. Rare megakaryocytes can be observed (Fig. 4).

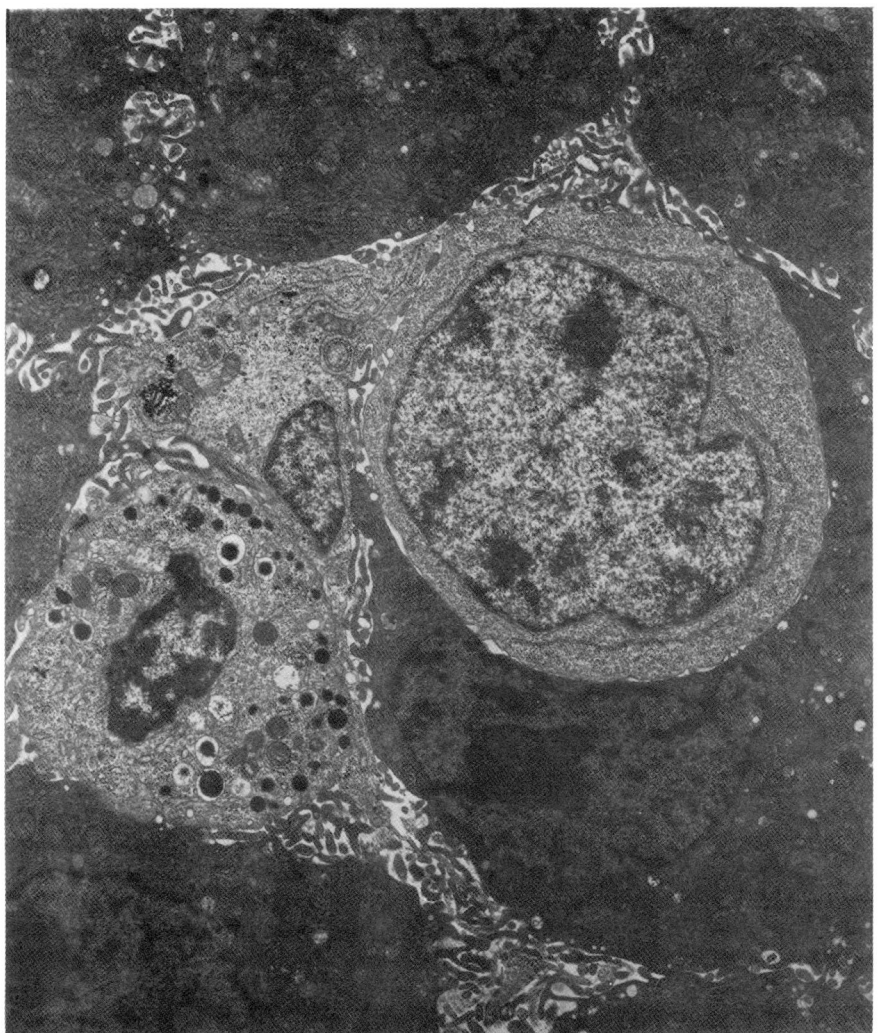

Fig. 3. 5-wk L: a granulocytic precursor (left side) close to a blast element (right side) within L parenchima (x 13,000).

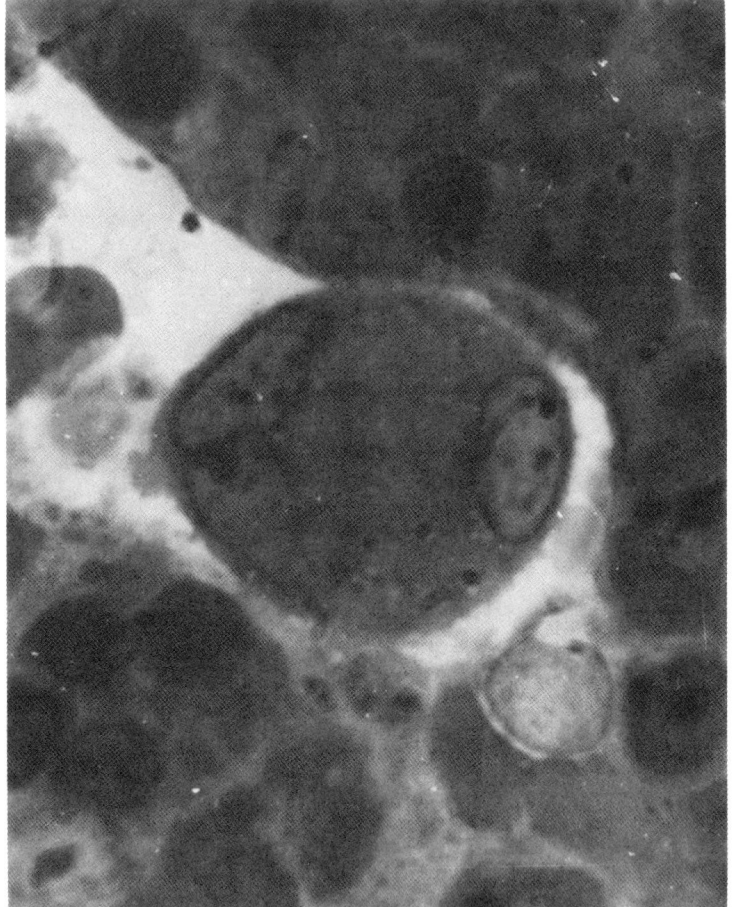

Fig. 4. A mature megakaryocyte within a L sinusoid.

In <u>cytocentrifuged smears</u> of 5-wk L cells, ~ 15% of megaloblasts exhibit various degrees of PAS positivity. Blast cells are fairly frequent (6-8% of non-hepatocytic elements). When tested with the Graham-Knoll peroxidase reaction, ~ 10% of them is slightly positive in the Golgi area. The monocytic-macrophagic series is well represented, and constitutes ~30% of non-hepatocytic cells (Table I). Granulocytic elements are markedly less frequent (~ 4%): their identification is rendered unequivocal by observations with MGG, NASDCA and peroxidase reactions (Table I). Furthermore, electron microscopy studies confirm that both neutrophilic and eosinophilic mature granulocytes are interspersed among hepatocytes. Rarely, basophilic and granular megakaryocytes are also observed.

Table I. Morphological analysis of GM elements in 5-8-wk L (mean values, expressed in terms of % of total hemopoietic cells)

	5-wk	6-wk	8-wk
Granulocytic lineage*	4	2	0,5-1
Monocytes and macrophages*	30	20	< 5
NASDCA positive cells	3,5	1,3	1
Peroxidase positive cells	7	5	3

* Identified by MGG staining.

The morphological pattern observed at 4-5-wk undergoes a rapid development: the number of L cells increases by a factor of 40 in the 6- through 12-wk period (not shown here).

At 6-7-wk definitive erythropoiesis is well represented at all stages of maturation in the L parenchina. It consists of macrocytic erythroblasts, which generate enucleated red cell entering into the circulation from 8-wk onward. A typical erythroid maturation "nest", is shown in Fig. 5. We have also confirmed the presence of cells pertaining to other hemopoietic lineages, although in very small number. However, lymphocytes and plasma cells are not apparently observed.

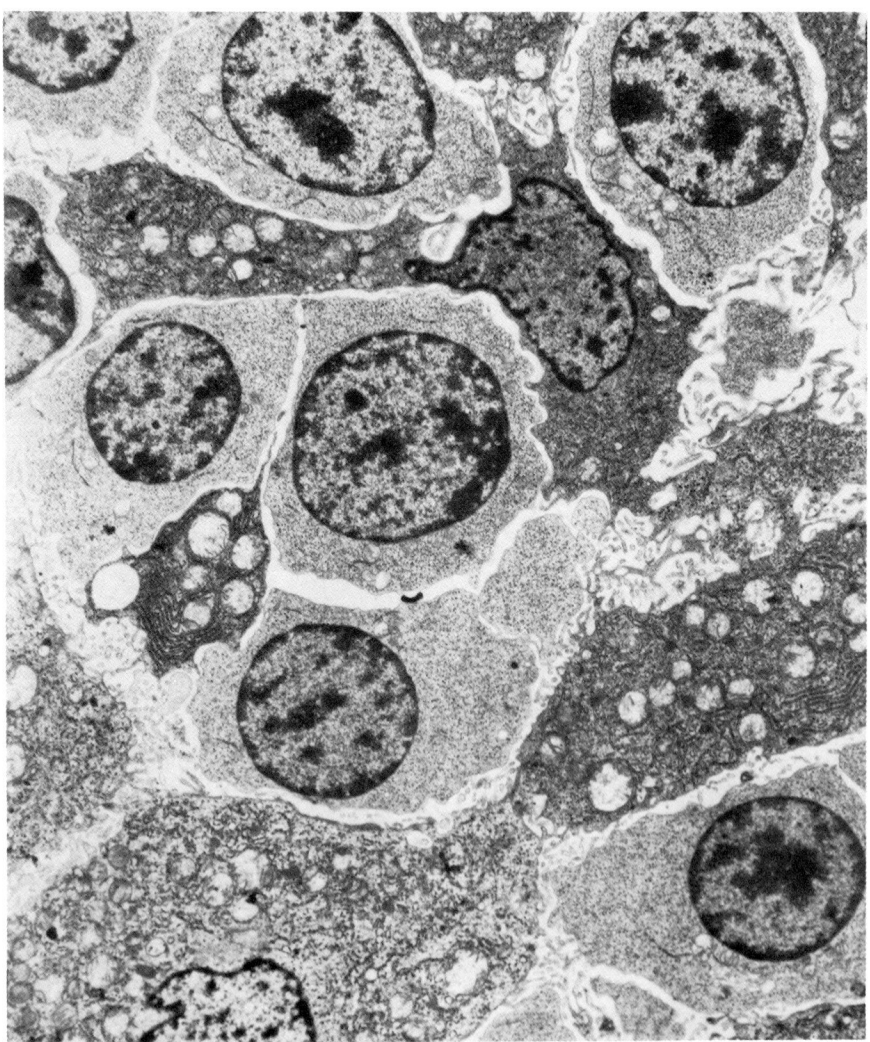

Fig. 5. 6-7-wk L: a maturative erythroid nest within the L parenchima (x3,000).

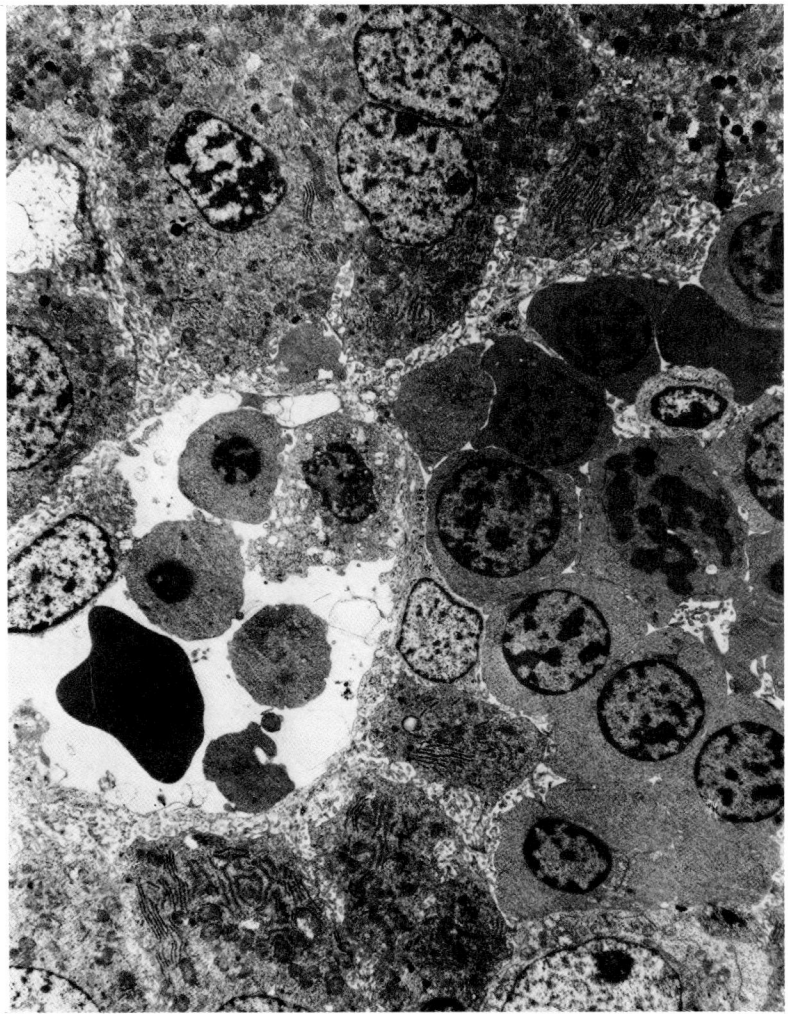

Fig. 6 — 8-wk-L: definitive erythroblasts invade the sinusoidal lumen after destroying the endothelial wall (x2,500).

A more detailed analysis at the ultrastructural level showed intimate contacts (desmosome-like structures) between erythroblasts and hepatocytes, particularly for proerythroblasts and basophilic elements, less frequently for more differentiated ones (not shown here). These contacts often revealed presence of micropinocytic coated vescicles, or coated pits. Interestingly, molecules of ferritin (reopheocytosis) were rarely observed in these vesicles.

In 8-9-wk L the maturation nests show a dramatic increase of the number of more differentiated (i.e., poly- and orthochromatic) erythroblasts, and hence undergo a rapid expansion. Thereby, the nests reach the sinusoidal wall, which is finally destroyed. This allows entrance of definitive erythroid cells into the sinusoidal blood from 8-wk onward (Fig. 6).

DISCUSSION

The morphologic pattern described here in 5-8-wk L may be considered in the framework of our observations on hemopoietic progenitors and precursors, as well as Hb synthesis, in embryonic YS, L and blood (Peschle et al. 1984, 1985a, 1985b).

(a) In 5-wk human embryos (Peschle et al. 1985b), early erythroid (BFU-E) and GM (CFU-GM) progenitors are present in both YS, L and blood, but are markedly more abundant in L. Conversely, late erythroid progenitors (CFU-E) are present in YS, but not in blood and L (Peschle et al. 1985b). Megaloblasts are observed in YS and blood, but not in L parenchima (see below). These findings may suggest that early progenitors (and presumably stem cells) originate in YS, enter into the bloodstream and colonize the L parenchima. Therein, they intensively proliferate but not differentiate, thus leading to rapid amplification of their pool. CFU-E are generated in YS, but are not present in circulating blood, as observed for the corrisponding adult progenitors (Peschle et al. 1983). Furthermore, they are not detected in L parenchima, in line with absence therein of differentiated erythroid precursors (see below).

b) The Hb synthesis program of YS and L BFU-E derived from the same embryo is virtually identical, thus suggesting but not proving that both pertain to a single pool (Peschle et al. 1984).

c) Embryonic (ζ, ε) and fetal (α, γ) chains are simultaneously produced in both late megaloblasts and early macrocytic erythroblasts (Peschle et al. 1985a).

d) Strong evidence suggests that stem cell migration from YS to L via blood may occur in murine embryos (Moore et al. 1970, Johnson et al. 1975).

Altogether, these studies are compatible with a monoclonal model, whereby a single stem cell pool originates in the YS, migrates into the bloodstream and finally colonizes the L parenchima. In the course of this phenomenon, the genetic program of stem cells undergoes a gradual development. This is expressed at the level of the erythroid progeny, which undergoes parallel switches of both morphology (megaloblasts $\rightarrow$ macrocytes) and globin synthesis ($\zeta \rightarrow \alpha$, $\varepsilon \rightarrow \gamma$). The primitive erythroblasts generated by YS stem cells are "megaloblasts", synthesizing initially only embryonic globin. Later on, the progeny of L stem cells is composed of definitive erythroblasts of macrocytic type, which finally produce only fetal chains.

An alternative biclonal hypothesis may be considered, with particular respect to a sophisticated model postulated for the avian system (Martin et al. 1978). Accordingly, two independent differentiation events would generate two distinct erythropoietic lineages, one deriving from YS and the other from intraembryonic tissues. Both lineages, endowed with an identical Hb synthesis program, may undergo a time-related embryonic adult Hb switch, independently from the site of erythropoietic differentiation. However, YS-derived cells would have a limited proliferative potential, while intra-embryonic elements may give rise to a permanent pool of hemopoietic stem cells. In contrast with this model, primitive and definitive lineages in humans are endowed with different Hb synthesis programs (Peschle et al. 1985a). Furthermore, it is difficult to postulate that in humans early embryonic vessels do not allow cross-circulation of stem cells and early progenitors between YS and L via blood (see also above and below). In order to reconcile this cross-circulation with the biclonal hypothesis, it is necessary to postulate that YS-derived stem cells migrated in L undergo massive death therein, and are replaced by a new generation of stem elements indipendently produced by L cells. In mammals, this hypothetical concept is not supported so far by any piece of evidence. Altogether, this biclonal model is not easily reconciled with our findings in humans (Peschle et al. 1985a,b) and previous observations in mice (Peschle et al. 1970).

The monoclonal model postulated above is compatible with and may shed light on the morphological observations reported here.

At 5-wk, primitive YS-derived erythroblasts are present in L sinusoidal spaces, but not in hepatic parenchima. Conversely, L blast cells are located in both sinusoids and parenchima: this is compatible with their migration from the former to the latter site. Indeed, detailed morphologic studies (not presented here) allowed to observe all the sequential stages of this putative migration (i.e., adhesion of blast cells to the endothelial wall, gradual passage of them through this barrier, location of blasts onto the sinusoidal wall, and finally within the epithelial cords). It may be suggested that at least some of the blast cells observed in L represent stem and early progenitor elements, originally deriving from YS.

At 6-wk erythroid cells of the definitive lineage appear in the L parenchima, and rapidly proliferate. At 7-8-wk "maturative nests" of definitive erythropoiesis develop in the L parenchima, thus compressing and deforming the hepatocytes, and finally destroying the sinusoidal wall from 8-wk onward.

It is emphasized that at 5-wk a discrete number of both immature and mature granulocytic cells are present in L parenchima, together with abundant macrophages. The origin of these GM elements is intriguing. It seems unlikely that they may derive from YS via blood. Indeed, the granulocytic series is virtually absent in YS (Kelemen et al. 1979, and our observations). Furthermore, GM elements are not observed in the circulating sinusoidal blood. Finally, cells at all stages of granulocytic maturation are observed within the L parenchima, distant from the sinusoidal spaces. These observations imply that, at this stage, L stem cells (originally derived from YS) may undergo GM differentiation, while generation of erythroid elements is suppressed. This is obviously in sharp contrast with the massive erythroid differentiation observed in L from 6-7-wk onward.

It is conceivable that this dramatic switch from GM to erythroid differentiation is under the control of an extrinsic mechanism(s), presumably represented by ontogenic maturation of the L microenvironment. In this regard, recent studies on mouse YS and embryonic L strongly suggest that the microenvironment may play a crucial role in the transition from primitive to definitive erythropoiesis (Cedennec et al. 1981, Ripoche et al. 1983, Labastie et al. 1984). In fact YS organ cultures, in the presence of medium supplemented only with fetal calf serum, produced exclusively primitive erythrocytes (Cedennec et al. 1981). However, if stimulated by a diffusible factor originating from various embryonic tissues (including the L rudiment), a second wave of erythropoiesis of adult type was elicited (Cudennec et al. 1981). The first wave of erythropoiesis may be under the control of a "burst-promoting activity" (BPA), released by YS cells. The second one would depend upon presence of both BPA and erythropoietin (Ep) (Ripoche et al. 1983, Labastie et al. 1984), the latter being selectively produced by L cells.

These murine studies are in line with our clonogenic findings (Peschle et al. 1985b) and morphologic observations mentioned above. At 5-wk CFU-E and definitive erythroblasts are virtually absent in L parenchima. However, early progenitors (BFU-E and CFU-GM) are demonstrable, and may be tentatively identified as a small part of the blast-like elements. Simultaneously, a discrete number of both immature and terminal granulocytic cells are present, together with abundant macrophages, rare megakaryocytes and even more rare definitive erythroblasts. It may be hence postulated that at 5-wk stem and early progenitor cells are preferentially triggered by microenvironment stimuli into GM differentiation. At 6-7-wk, CFU-E and definitive erythroblasts become present in the L parenchima, and their number undergoes an exponential rise. GM differentiation is still observed, but becomes markedly less prominent, if compared to the massive erythroid differentiation. It may be postulated that this morphological (i.e., GM→ erythroid) switch is modulated via release in the hepatic microenvironment of a factor(s) stimulating selectively erythroid differentiation. This putative hormone may be obviously identified with Ep, which is produced by fetal L cells (Zucali et al. 1975, Labastie et al. 1984), thus also in line with the murine studies mentioned above.

Acknowledgements This work was supported by CNR, Rome: Progetti Finalizzati "Ingegneria Genetica" (84.00902.51), "Oncologia" (84.00730440), and Gruppo Nazionale Ematoogia (84.00861.04).

REFERENCES

Browder L.W. (1984). "Developmental biology". Philadelphia: Saunders, p. 689.
Beaupin D., Martin C., Dieterlain-Liévre (1981). In Stamatoyannopoulos G., Nienhuis A.W. (eds.): "Hemoglobins in development and differentiation", New York, Alan R. Liss, p. 161.
Cudennec C.A., Thiery J.P., Le Douarin N. (1981). In vitro induction of adult erythropoiesis in early mouse in yolk sac. Proc. Natl. Acad. Sci. USA, 78: 2412.
England M.A. (1983). "Color atlas of life before borth". Chicago. Year book medical publishers Inc.
Johnson G.R., Moore M.A.S. (1975). Role of stem cell migration initiation of mouse liver hemopoiesis. Nature, 258: 726.
Kelemen E., Calvo W., Fliedner T.M. (1979). "Atlas of human hemopoietic development". New York, Springer Verlag.
Labastie M.C., Thiery J.P., Le Douarin N.M. (1984). Mouse yolk sac and intraembryonic tissues produce factors able to elicit differentiation of erythroid burst-forming units and colony-forming units, respectively. Proc. Natl. Acad. Sci. USA, 81: 1453.
Martin C., Beaupain D., Dieterlen-Liévre F. (1978). Developmental relationship between vitelline and intra-embryonic haemopoiesis studied in avian "yolk sac chimaeras". Cell Differentiation, 7: 115.

Moore K.L. (1982). "The developping human" (3rd edn.) Philadelphia Saunders.

Moore M.A.S., Metcalf D. (1970). Ontogeny of the hemopoietic system yolk sac origin in vivo and in vitro colony forming cells in the developing mouse embryo. Brit. J. Haemat., 18: 279.

Peschle C., Migliaccio G., Migliaccio A.R., Ciccariello R., Lettieri F., Quattrin S., Russo G., Mastroberardino G. (1981). Identification and characterization of three classes of erythroid progenitors in human fetal liver. Blood 58: 565.

Peschle C., Migliaccio G., Migliaccio A.R., Covelli A., Giuliani A., Mavilio F., Mastroberardino G. (1983). Hemoglobin switching in humans. In Dunn C.D.R. (ed.) "Current Concepts in Erythropoiesis", New York, Wiley and Sons, p. 339.

Peschle C., Migliaccio G., Migliaccio A.R., Petrini M., Calandrini, M., Russo G., Mastroberardino G., Presta M., Gianni A.M., Comi P., Giglioni B., Ottolenghi S. (1984). Embryonic fetal Hb switch in humans: studies on erythroid bursts generated by embryonic progenitors from yolk sac and liver. Proc. Natl. Acad. Sci. USA, 81: 2416.

Peschle C., Mavilio F., Carè A., Migliaccio G., Migliaccio A.R., Salvo G., Samoggia P., Petti S., Guerriero R., Marinucci M., Lazzaro D., Russo G., Mastroberardino G. (1985a). Hemoglobin switching in human embryos: asynchrony of and globin switches in primitive and definitive erythropoietic lineage. Nature 313: 235.

Peschle C., Migliaccio G., Lazzaro D., Petti S., Mancini G., Carè A., Russo G., Mastroberardino G., Migliaccio A.R., Testa U. (1985b). Hemopoietic development in human embryos, transition from yolk sac to liver erythropoiesis and Hb switching. Blood Cells, in press.

Ripoche M.A., Cudennec C.A. (1983). Adult hemoglobins are synthesized in yolk sac microenvironment obtained from murine cultured blastocysts. Cell Differentiation, 13: 125.

Zucali J.R., Stevens V., Mirand E.A. (1975). In vitro production of erythropoietin by mouse fetal liver. Blood, 46: 85.

Immune Development in Human Fetal Liver

Robert Peter Gale, M.D., Ph.D.

Department of Medicine
Division of Hematology and Oncology
UCLA School of Medicine,
Los Angeles, California 90024

INTRODUCTION

In man, embryonic hematopoiesis is initiated in the yolk sac during 2-7 weeks of gestation (for review see Keleman 1979; Immunol Rev 1981). In mice, early B-lymphocyte progenitors have been identified in the yolk sac and placenta (Melchers 1979). Although other hamtopoietic cells including immature erythroid cells, granulocytes, megakaryocytes and macrophages are present in the yolk sac in man, lymphocytes have not been identified convincingly. During this period the yolk sac contains a high proportion of immature mononuclear cells and it is possible that some of these are lymphoid cells. Detailed analyses of yolk sac cells using monoclonal antibodies or functional or clonogenic assays of lymphocytes have not been reported. One patient with severe combined immune deficiency (SCID) received a transplant of yolk sac and fetal liver cells and partial immune reconstitution (Keleman 1973). Although she improved, there was no evidence of engraftment and it is not possible to critically analyze the contribution of the yolk sac cells.

The fetal liver is a major site of immune development in man (for review see Keleman 1979; Immunol Rev 1981; Lowenberg 19875; Lucarelli 1980; Prindull 1974; Stites 1975). Lymphocytes are identifiable in human fetal liver at 6-7 weeks of gestation. The proportion of lymphoid cells are highly variable ranging between < 5% to 15% of the mononuclear, non-hepatic parenchymal cells. At this time the fetal liver also contains substantial "blast" cells some of which may be immature lymphoid cells or their progenitors. The proportion of lymphoid cells is relatively constant until 20-24 weeks when lymphoid cells constitute > 20% of the mononuclear cells. The proportion of unidentifiable immature cells gradually decreases during this period from 10% to < 2%. A current scheme of human hematopoietic development is shown in Figure 1.

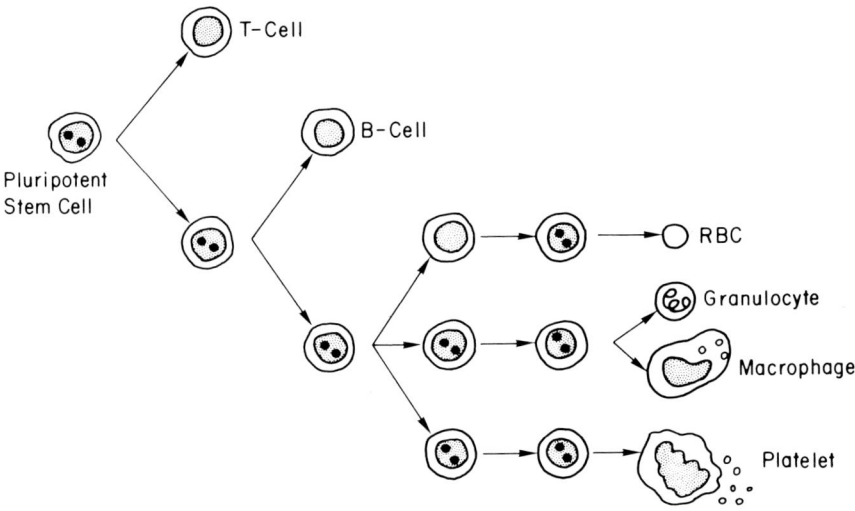

B-Lymphocyte Development

Hematopoietic stem cells, probably arising from yolk sac progenitors and possibly from other sites, migrate to the fetal liver after approximately 5 weeks of gestation. Under appropriate microenvironmental and probably growth factor control, these cells differentiate into B-lymphocyte progenitors (Gathings 1981; Calvert 1984; LeDouarin 1975; Owen 1977; Kamps 1982)) and eventually into mature

B-cells. Pre-B cells, cells with identifiable cytoplastic heavy μ-chain ($c\mu^+$), are the first readily detectable B-lymphocytes in mammals (Gathings 1981). Expression of C_μ results from the productive rearrangement of heavy chain V_H, D_H, J_H, $C\mu$ heavy chain genes from their germ-line configuration on one parental allele. This μ-chain probably has no hydrophobic tail (secreted type) explaining the absence of surface IgM. Next V_L, D_L, C_L light chain genes are rearranged with synthesis of κ or λ. μ-heavy chains of the membrane type are now produced; these combine with K or λ chains into monomeric IgM which is displayed on the cell surface. δ chains are also synthesized at this time, possibly because of alternate splicing of a $\mu\delta$ mRNA and IgD appears on the cell surface. Switching to γ, ϵ and α heavy chain synthesis occurs via further genomic rearrangements with deletion of the $C\mu S$ segment with resultant expression of IgG, IgE or IgA. Because persistence of μS mRNA, triplet cells with surface IgM, IgD and IgG or IgA are occasionally observed. Finally, mature B-cells differentiate into a plasma cell with subsequent loss of SMIg and secretion of large amounts of Ig as a result of alternate processing of the heavy chain mRNA. A model of B-cell development is indicated in Figure 2.

In birds, B-lymphocyte development occurs in discrete follicles within the bursa of Fabricius (Owen 1977). In mammals, the first recognizable cells of the B-lymphocyte lineage are found in the fetal liver and later in bone marrow. Generation of pre-B and B-cells has also been demonstrated in cultures of fetal liver cells in mice and man (Owen 1977). In this model of B-cell development, large dividing pre-B cells evolve from less mature hematopoietic stem cells. These immature pre-B cells give rise to small, non-dividing pre-B cells and ultimately into immature B-cells which express SMIgM (Calvert 1984). In the mouse these SMIgM$^+$ cells appear to be uniquely susceptible to clonal deletion or functional inactivation by treatment with antigen or anti-isotype or anti-idiotype antibodies.

Kamps and Cooper have reported detailed studies of B-cell development in human fetal liver (Kamps 1982). They found 3-4% pre-B and B-cells in fetal livers of 12-15 weeks gestation. Pre-B cells had a immune phenotype of $\mu^+ \kappa^- \lambda^-$ whereas B-cells were $\mu^+ \kappa^+ \lambda^-$ or $\mu^+ \kappa^- \lambda^+$ cells. The ratio of K to μ cells was similar to that observed in the adult, 2 to 1. Pre-B and B-cells were found to be randomly distributed throughout the fetal liver and are not observed in relation to other hematopoietic cells or in clusters as occurs in the germinal centers of the avian bursa. Kamps and Cooper found that these B-cells tended to occur singly but occasional doublets or triplets were identified (Kamps 1982). These multi-cell clusters contained both pre-B and B-cells but were restricted to a single isotype either $\mu^+ \kappa^+$ or $\mu^+ \lambda^+$. These data are consistent with a model of in-situ development of B-cells in human fetal liver.

It is also possible to study B-cell development in fetal liver using monoclonal antibodies to B-cell related antigens (Rosenthal 1983; Budger 1983). Some of the relevant antibodies are summarized in Table 1. The most useful are antibodies to the common acute lymphoblastic leukemia antigen (CALLA) which reacts with early and mature B-cells, B1 which reacts with a wide range of immature and mature B-cells, B2 which reacts with more mature B-cells, RFB-1, which reacts with terminal deoxynucleotidyl transferase (TdT) positive cells but not pre-B or B-cells, and BA-1 which also reacts with TdT+ cells. BA-1 has a pattern of reactivity similar to B1; it differs from RFB-1 by reacting with pre-B and B-cells. The relationship between B-cell development and antigen expression is shown schematically in Figure 2.

Table 1: Monoclonal Antibodies Reactive with Fetal Liver Cells

Antigen	Normal Expression
CALLA	Early B granulocytes
B 1	pan-B
B 2	mature B
BA-1	TdT+, pan B
RFB-1	TdT+, not pre B or B
TdT	immature cells, pan B

Rosenthal and coworkers have reported detailed analyses of fetal liver cells using the CALLA, B1 and B2 monoclonal antibodies (14). These data are summarized in Table 2. They found approximately 3-7% CALLA+ and/or B1+ cells in fetal livers of 11-26 weeks gestation. The highest numbers of positive cells were found in fetal livers of 22-26 weeks. B2+ cells were less common occuring at a frequency of approximately 1% from 11-26 weeks. Budger and colleagues studied BA-1 and RFB-1 expression on fetal liver cells of 12-21 weeks gestation (15). BA-1+ cells constituted 3-5% of fetal liver cells of 13 weeks gestation but only 1% of more mature fetal livers. RFB-1+ cells occurred at a slightly lower frequency. Both the BA-1+ RFB-1+ and BA-1- RFB-1+ phenotypes were observed; many of the BA-1+ and/or RFB-1+ cells were also CALLA+. These investigators studied the relationship between TdT activity and surface antigens. TdT+ was identified in 4-6% of early fetal liver cells and in 1% of more mature fetal liver cells. In 13 week fetal livers, 80% of TdT+ cells were BA-1+ and RFB-1+; the remaining 20% were BA-1-, RFB-1+. BA-1+ cells were more frequent than TdT+ cells and were SMIgM+ suggesting that they were more mature B-cells. RFB-1+ cells also occurred more frequently then TdT+ cells. These cells were SMIgM- and were probably immature hematopoietic cells rather than lymphoid cells. Additional studies have also been performed using OKB1,2,4 and 7 monoclonal antibodies (Knowles 1984). In most instances fetal liver cells are OKB2+ but unreactive with other OKB antibodies.

Table 2: Reactivity of Monoclonal Anti-B-Cell Antibodies in Fetal Liver

Antibody	Gestation Age (wk)			
	11-14	15-17	18-22	22-26
CALLA	3	4	4	6
B 1	1	2	2	7
B 2	1	1	1	1
BA-1	4	-	-	1
RFB-1	3	-	-	< 1
TdT	5	4	1	< 1

When multiple B-cell specifications are studied simultaneously, it appears that most immature B cells are TdT+, B1-, RFB-1-, and $C\lambda$-. These cells are probably progenitors of B1+ fetal liver cells most of which are also RFB1+, CALLA+, and OKB2+. Approximately 15% of these cells contain $C\mu$ and are probably best regarded as pre-B cells. Pre-B cells also express HLA-D, β_2-microglobulin, and HLA-heavy chain but lack SMIgM and TdT. As these cells mature to B cells they acquire SMIgM, and possibly SMIgD, and lose reactivity with RFB-1, CALLA, and OKB2; B1 and histocompatibility antigen reactivity is retained. These data are summarized in Table 2.

In summary, detailed analyses of human fetal liver B-lymphocytes using monoclonal antibodies are consistent with studies in other mammals. These indicate an orderly progression from hematopoietic stem cell progenitors to pre-B cells to B-cells and ultimately to mature B-lymphocytes. Most fetal liver cells are pre-B but several intermediate cell types can be identified.

Functional studies of B- and T-lymphocytes in human and murine fetal liver cells have also been reported (Lowenberg 1985; Lucarelli 1980; Prindull 1974; Stites 1975; Mukopadhyay 1978; Delfini 1980). Transplantation results in a variable reconstitution of the B-lymphocyte axis in irradiated, fetal liver reconstituted mice (Doria 1962; Tyan 1967; Umiel 1974; Rosenberg 1977; Rabinowich 1983). Reconstitution is more complete in recipients of syngeneic transplants. Allograft recipients have less complete recovery of B-cell function (Doria 1962; Gengozian 1965; Gengozian 1973). These mice have decreased to low-normal levels of circulating Ig; antibody responses are present but decreased and IgM to IgG switching is impaired or absent. Analysis of fetal liver transplants in man, predominantly in patients with severe combined immune deficiency (SCID), indicate a low rate of permanent B-cell engraftment (O'Reilly 1978). The reason for this is unknown. In dogs, we observed consistent B-cell engraftment with functional Ig and antibody responses after 6 months-1 year (Champlin, this volume)). Similar data by Prummer and coworkers is reported in this volume (Prummer 1985). In contrast to patients with SCID, these dogs are irradiated and achieve both lymphoid and hematopoietic engraftment. It is therefore conceivable that the functional B-cells in these animals arise from relatively uncommitted hematopoietic stem cells or B-cell progenitors rather than from pre-B or B-lymphocytes present in fetal liver. Irradiation of the recipient may also be a factor by providing "space" in the lymphoid compartment for B-cell engraftment. Alternatively the unirradiated recipient may have cells or factors which inhibit the engraftment of immature B-cells.

In vitro studies of B-cells derived from fetal liver indicate the presence of functional B-cells responsive to polyclonal mitogens such as pokeweed mitogen (PWM).

Specific antibody responses to sheep red blood cells
following in vivo immunization in mice indicate present but
decreased SRBC directed plaque-forming cells (PFC). Normal
responses to dextran and lipopolysaccharide have been
reported in mice (Rabinowich 1983). Detailed studies using
other antigens following in vivo or in vitro have not been
reported nor have in vitro studies in man.

Hannam-Harris and Smith analyzed Ig synthesis by human
fetal liver cells by biosynthetic labeling (Hannam-Harris
1981). They found that fetal liver cells synthesized and
secreted free Ig light-chain; some cells also secreted
free μ-heavy chain. This imbalance in Ig light chain
synthesis is thought to be typical of immature B cells
(pre-B) and is also found in B-cells from patients with
chronic lymphocytic leukemia. The specificity of
antibodies produced in cultures of fetal liver cells is
unknown in most instances. Some data indicate the presence
of anti-idiotype antibodies specific for autoantigens.
Interestingly, several dogs transplanted with fetal liver
cells have developed autoantibodies and occasionally
autoimmune diseases such as myasthenia gravis (Cain 1985).
The frequency of autoimmune diseases appears increased
compared to canine recipients of bone marrow transplants,
this may be related to the relative immaturity of B-cells
in fetal liver.

In summary, fetal liver is the major site of
B-lymphocyte development in the human fetus. Mature
B-cells that can synthesize Ig and probably antibody arise
from B-cell progenitors. B-lymphocytes derived from fetal
liver stem cells or their progeny are capable of restoring
B-cell immunity in mice and dogs; data in man are less
convincing but this may be related to factors other than
the immune competence of the stem cells transplanted.

T-Lymphocyte Development

In contrast to B-lymphocyte development which occurs
primarily in the fetal liver, T-lymphocyte development
occurs primarily in the thymus. Nevertheless, most if not
all T-cells arise from fetal liver progenitors. In mice,
rats, dogs, horses, monkeys and man, transplantation of
fetal liver cells alone or in combination with thymus cells
results in restoration of T-cell immunity (Lowenberg 1975;
Lucarelli 1980; Rabinowich 1983; Gengozian 1965; Gengozian
1973; O'Reilly RJ 1978; Champlin this volume; Prummer 1981;

Hannam-Harris 1981; Cain 1985; Gale 1980; Touraine 1980; Izzi 1985; Bortin 1971; Putten 1968; Lucarelli 1980; Perryman 1980; Stutman 1978; Umiel 1968; Hunt 1981). T-cell recovery is impaired if the recipient is thymectomized suggesting that most of the fetal liver cells responsibe for T-cell reconstitution are pre-thymic (Rabinowich 1983).

Attempts to demonstrate mature T-lymphocytes in human fetal liver have been unsuccessful (Prindull 1974; Stites 1975; Mukopadhyay 1978; Delfini 1980; Champlin 1980). E-rosette forming cells, cells capable of binding sheep red blood cells, are present at < 1% frequency. Recent studies have used monoclonal anti-T cell antibodies including T1,3,4,6, and 5/8, Leu 1,2 and 3, and T101 (Rosenthal 1983). In all instances, < 2% of positive cells are found suggesting the absence of mature T-cells.

Functional analyses of T-cells in human fetal liver include studies of reactivity to alloantigens in mixed leukocyte culture (MLC), and to mitogens including phytohemagglutinin A (PHA) and conconavalin A (conA). We and others studied MLC reactivity of fetal liver cells (Prindull 1974; Mukopadhyay 1978; Champlin 1980; August 1971; Carr 1973; Stites 1974). Most studies indicate that these cells are unreactive or only slightly reactive in MLC. Studies which suggested strong MLC reactivity in all likelihood, measured the response of myeloid rather than lymphoid cells. There have been several studies of mitogen reactivity of fetal liver cells (Mukopadhyay 1978; Delfini 1980; Champlin 1980; August 1971; Carr 1973; Stites 1974; Toivanen 1981; Sirianni 1980). In most instances only weak reactivity to PHA and no response to conA was detected. This pattern of reactivity is consistent with other species in which acquisition of PHA reactivity preceeds conA reactivity. One possible exception may be sheep in whom fetal liver cells appear to be reactive in MLC; interestingly and in contrast to mature T-cells, cytotoxic lymphocytes could not be demonstrated (Granberg 1980). Irradiated dogs reconstituted with fetal liver cells recovery mitogen responsiveness within 3 months; MLC reactivity recovered less rapidly but relatively few animals have been studied (Champlin this volume; Prummer 1985). Data in dogs from ourselves and Prummer and coworkers suggest that B-cell recovery precedes T-cell recovery. This was unanticipated since, in man, T-cell rather then B-cell engraftment is more easily achieved (Gale 1980; O'Reilly this volume). These differences may be species specific or may be related to either DLA-matching between donor and recipient or to the fact that recipients were irradiated and therefore achieved complete hematopoietic rather than only lymphoid grafts. Several investigators have evaluated T-cell content of human fetal livers by histochemical tehnics, such as reactivity with acid alpha-naphthyl acetate esterase (ANAE). ANAE reactive cells were undetectable in fetal livers < 14 weeks; 1-3% were detectable thereafter increasing to 5-7% by 24 weeks and then declining (Toivanen 1981). These data are in agreement with the previously cited monoclonal antibody studies.

Despite the relative absence of mature T-cells in fetal liver, T-cell progenitors are clearly present. We studied the presence of T-lymphocyte colony forming cells (CFU-TL) in semisolid agar in 15 fetal livers of 10 to 24 weeks gestation (Champlin 1980). CFU-TL were present at a frequency similar to that observed in adult bone marrow. In these instances there was no correlation between CFU-TL and the presence of E-rosette forming cells or reactivity to PHA. These data suggest that the CFU-TL, under these circumstances, are indicative of T-cell progenitors rather than mature T-cells. Cells recovered from CFU-TL colonies had the phenotype of mature T-cells and were alloantigen and mitogen reactive. Similarly Pyke and Gelfand and Lowenberg have reported T-cell progenitors in human fetal liver (Pyke 1976; Lowenberg 1980).

Rabinowich and coworkers have studied T-cell progenitors in murine fetal liver (Rabinowich 1983). They reported that irradiated mice reconsitituted with fetal liver cells were similar to bone marrow chimeras in their ability to reject thyroid allografts, and in reactivity to alloantigens, PHA and conA. In general these responses recovered less rapidly following fetal liver than bone marrow transplantation and were markedly impaired or absent in thymectomized recipients. Interestingly, these investigators also reported that B-cell responses recovered more rapidly than T-cell responses similar to the aforementioned results in dogs and in contrast to results in patients with SCID receiving fetal liver grafts.

Natural Killer Cells

Recently there has been interest in natural killer (NK) cells which are capable of reactivity with selected target cells without prior sensitization (for review see Herberman 1981). The origin of NK cells is controversial and it is uncertain whether they are a form of T-cells or of monocyte/macrophages. NK cells appear to be distinct from K cells which are responsible for mediating antibody dependent cellular cytotoxicity (ADCC). NK cells are present in murine fetal liver cells (Koo 1982; Haller 1977). Toivanen and coworkers detected NK activity in most human fetal livers of 9-23 weeks gestation. This activity could be increased by incubation with interferon similar to NK cells from other sources (Toivanen 1981).

Regulation of Immunity by Fetal Liver Cells

There are considerable data, reviewed previously and elsewhere in this volume, indicating that transplantation of fetal liver cells is associated with a lower incidence and severity of graft-versus-host disease (GvHD) in animal models and man (for review see Lowenberg 1975; Lucarelli 1980). The most obvious explanation of decreased GvHD is the relative immune incompetance of fetal liver cells. This may arise from several factors: (1) absent or infrequent mature T-lymphocytes; (2) education of donor derived T-cell progenitors in the recipient thymus; or (3) the relative ease of tolerization or clonal deletion of alloantigen reactive fetal liver cells.

Another possible explanation of the decreased immune reactivity of fetal liver cells are possible immunoregulatory features of fetal liver cells. Several investigators have reported that suppressor T-cells in murine fetal liver (Globerson 1975; Globerson 1978; Umiel 1977; Bortin 1969; Bortin 1971). Recently, Muraoka and Miller demonstrated that murine fetal liver cells or cells from fetal liver CFU-TL colonies can specifically suppress reactivity of allogeneic lymphocytes to self (Muraoka 1983). This anti-self suppressor effect is mediated by fetal liver derived cells and appears to act by preventing differentiation of cytotoxic-T-cell precursors into cytotoxic effector cells. The suppressor cells are termed "veto" cells to distinguish them from other types of suppressor cells. These "veto" cells appear to be non-T, non-B cells and are relatiavely radioresistant. Sula and Nouza reported a similar observation in mice whereby addition of fetal liver cells syngeneic to the recipient decreased regional GvHD in irradiated recipients (Sula

1981).

In summary it appears that fetal liver contains cell(s) capable of regulating reactivity of immune competent cells either present in the fetal liver or syngeneic to the fetal liver cells. This regulatory aspect of fetal liver immune development may be important in the normal regulation of anti-self immunity as well as in the setting of fetal liver transplantation. In the latter, "veto" cells would tend to suppress the ability of the recipient to reject the graft.

Interactions of Fetal Liver and T-Cells

In addition to the subject of immune development in fetal liver, interesting observations have been made regarding the interaction of fetal liver cells with other immune cells, particularly thymocytes. Bortin and coworkers reported that addition of syngeneic thymocytes increased the likelihood of successful fetal liver transplantation in mice (Bortin 1969; Bortin 1975). Relatively small numbers of thymocytes were effective. These authors suggested that this activity was mediated by a soluable factor since thymuses transplanted within millipore filters had the same activity as intact thymocytes. The precise mechanism by which this effect occurs is unknown. Bortin and coworkers reported successful engraftment of an irradiated dog following multiple fetal liver and thymus grafts (Saltzstein 1974). Simultaneous controls were not performed so it is impossible to conclude whether engraftment was a consequence of the combined use of fetal liver and thymus. Perryman has reported similar data in horses (Perryman 1980). Touraine and coworkers and others have reported results of combined fetal liver and thymus transplants in man (Touraine 1980; Touraine this volume). Again critical analyses are not possible.

In summary, there are reasonably convincing data in rodents that thymocytes increase the probability of successful engraftment of fetal liver cells; data in other species are less clear. This effect may not require intact cells and therefore need not necessarily increase the risk of GVHD. Controlled trials of this approach in man are needed.

Conclusion

Human fetal liver contains progenitors of both B and T cells capable of restoring humoral and cellular immunity in irradiated, fetal liver reconstituted recipients. The fetal liver is the major site of B-cell development in man. Although maturation of T-cells occurs primarily in the thymus, the fetal liver contains T-cell progenitors and is therefore critical to T-cell development. Other immune functions of fetal liver cells, such as NK-activity, are probably also present but have not been studied in detail. Fetal liver cells appear to have relatively unique self-regulatory functions which may play an important role in the maintenance of tolerance to self and in the prevention of graft-rejection and GvHD following fetal liver transplantation. Transplantation of fetal liver cells and thymocytes appears to be more effective than fetal liver cells alone in rodents; controlled trials in large animals and man are needed.

August CS, Berkel AJ, Driscoll S, Marler E 1971. Onset of lymphocyte function in the developing human fetus. Pediatr Res 5:539.

Bortin MM, Rimm AA, Saltzstein EC 1971. Survival and immune competance of murine radiation chimeras. Fed Proc 30:652.

Bortin MM, Rimm AA, Saltzstein EC 1969. Graft-versus-host inhibition. I. Incubated parental strain spleen and liver cells administered to F_1 mice. J Immunol 102:1042.

Bortin MM, Rimm AA, Saltzstein EC 1971. Graft-versus-host inhibition. IV. Production of allogeneic radiation chimeras using incubated spleen and liver cell mmixtures. J Immunol 107:1063.

Bortin MM, Saltzstein EC 1969. Graft-versus-host inhibition. Fetal liver and thymus cells to minimize secondary disease. Science 164:316.

Bortin MM, Rimm AA, Saltzstein EC 1975. Potentiating effect of fetal thymus on fetal liver cells for the promotion of recovery from the radiation injury in murine allogeneic radiation chimeras or a little bit of thymus goes a long, long way. Birth Defects: original article series, 11:544.

Budger MP, Janossy G, Bollum FJ, Burford GD, Hoffbrand AV 1983. The ontogeny of terminal deoxynucleotidyl

transferase positive cells in the human fetus. Blood 61:1125.
Cain GR, Cardinett III GN, Cuddon PC, Gale RP, Champlin RE 1985. Myasthenia gravis and polymyositis in a dog following fetal hematopoietic cell transplantation. Transplantation, in press.
Calvert JE, Maruyama S, Tedder TF, Webb CF, Cooper MD 1984. Cellular events in the differentiation of antibody secreting cells. Sem Hematol 21:226.
Carr MC, Stites DP, Fudenberg HH 1973. Dissociation of response to phytohemaglutinin and adult allogeneic lymphocytes in human foetal tissues. Nature New Biol 241:279.
Champlin RE, Mitsuyasu RM, Gale RP, et al. Transplantation of T-lymphocyte depleted bone marrow to prevent graft-versus-host disease: its implications for fetal liver transplantation. This volume.
Champlin R, Niskanen E, Gale RP 1980. Hematopoiesis and immune reactivity of human fetal liver cells. In Lucarelli G, Fleidner TM, Gale RP (eds). Op Cit p. 117.
Delfini C, Izzi T, Porcellini A, Lucarelli G 1980. Immunologic features of human fetal liver, spleen and thymus of various gestational ages. In Lucarelli G, Fleidner TM, Gale RP (eds) op cite p. 126.
Doria G, Goodman JW, Gengozian N, Congdon CC 1962. Immunologic study of antibody-forming cells in mouse radiation chimeras. J Immunol 88:20.
Gale RP 1980. Fetal liver transplantation in man. In Lucarelli G, Fleidner TM, Gale RP (eds). op cite p. 268.
Gathings WE, Kubogawa H, Cooper MD 1981. A distinctive pattern of B-cell immaturity in perinatal humans. Immunol Rev 57:107-28.
Gengozian N, Rabette B, Congdon CC 1965. Abnormal immune mechanism in allogeneic radiation chimeras. Science 149:645.
Gengozian N, Congdon CC 1973. Immunologic memory in radiation chimeras. Transplantation 16:32.
Globerson A, Zinkernagel RM, Umiel T 1975. Immunosuppression by embryonic liver cells. Transplantation 20:480.
Globerson A, Rabinowich H, Umiel T 1977. Ontogeny of suppressor cells. IN Solomon JB, Horton JD (eds). Developmental Immunobiology. Elsevier, Amsterdam p. 331.
Globerson A, Umiel T 1978. Ontogeny of suppressor cells. II. Suppression of graft-versus-host disease and mixed leukocyte cultures by embryonic cells. Transplantation

26:438.
Granberg C, Hirvonen T 1980. Cell-mediated lympholysis by fetal and neonatal lymphocytes in sheep and man. Cell Immunol 51:13.
Haller O, Kiessling R, Orn A, Wigzell H 1977. Generation of natural killer cells: an autonomous function of the bone marrow. J Exp Med 145:1411.
Hannam-Harris AC, Smith JL 1981. Free immunoglobulin light chain synthesis by human fetal liver and cord blood lymphocytes. Immunol 43:417.
Herberman RB, Ortaldo JR 1981. Science 214:24.
Hunt SV, Fowler MH 1981. A repopulation assay for B and T lymphocyte stem cells employing radiation chimeras. Cell Tissue Kinetics 14:445.
Immunol Rev 1981; 57.
Izzi T, Polchi P, Galimberti M, et al 1985. Fetal liver transplantation in aplastic anemia and acute leukemia. This volume.
Kamps WA, Cooper MD 1982. Microenvironmental studies of pre-B and B cell development in human and mouse fetuses. J Immunol 129:526.
Keleman E, Calvo W, Fleidner TM 1979. Atlas of Human Hematopoietic Development. Srpinger-Verlag, Berlin.
Keleman E 1973. Recovery from chronic idiopathic bone marrow aplasia of a young mother aftter intravenous injection of unprocessed cells from the liver (and yolk sac) of her 22mm CR-length embryo. A preliminary report. Scand J Hematol 10:305.
Knowles DM, II, Tolidjian B, Marboe CC, et al 1984. Distribution of antigens defined by OKB monoclonal antibodies on benign and malignant lymphoid cells and on nonlymphoid tissue. Blood 63:886-896.
Koo GC, Peppard JR, Hatzfeld A 1982. Ontogeny of NK-1+ natural killer cells. 1. Proportion of NK-1+ cells in fetal, baby and old mice. J Immunol 129:867.
LeDouarin NM, Houssaint E, Joterean FV, Belo M 1975. Origin of hematopoietic stem cells in the embryonic bursa of Fabricius and bone marrow studied through inter-specific chimeras. Proc Natl Acad Sci U.S.A. 72:2701.
Lowenberg B 1975. Fetal liver transplantation. Radiobiological Institute of the Organization for Health Research TNO, Rijswijk, The Netherlands.
Lowenberg B 1980. Lymphocyte maturation and graft versus host disease following fetal liver transplantation. IN Lucarelli G, Fleidner TM, Gale RP (eds). Op cite p. 198.

Lucarelli G, Fleidner TM, Gale RP 1980. Fetal Liver Transplantation. Excerpta Medica, Amsterdam.

Lucarelli G, Andreani M, Agostinelli F 1980. Fetal liver transplantation in rats. In Lucarelli G, Fleidner TM, Gale RP (eds). Op cite p. 175.

Melchers F 1979 Murine embryonic B lymphocyte development in the placenta. Nature 277:219.

Mukopadhyay N, Fernbach DJ, Mumford DM, South MA 1978. T and B cells and immune competance in human fetal liver cells. Clin Immunol Immunopath 10:59.

Muraoka S, Miller RG 1983. Cells in murine fetal liver and in lymphoid colonies grown from fetal liver can suppress generation of cytotoxic T lymphocytes directed against their self antigen. J Immunol 131:45.

O'Reilly RJ, Pahwa R, Sorrell M, et al 1978. Transplantation Transplantation of fetal liver and thymus in patients with severe combined immunedeficiencies. In The Immune System: Functions and Therapy of Dysfunctions. Academic Press.

O'Reilly – this volume.

Owen JJ, Weight DE, Habu S, Raff MC, Cooper MD 1977. Studies on the generation of B lymphocytes in fetal liver and bone marrow. J Immunol 118:2067.

Perryman LE 1980. Use of fetal tissues for immunoreconstitution in horses iwth severe combined immunodeficiency. In Lucarelli G, Fleidner TM, Gale RP (eds) Ibid p. 183.

Prindull G 1974. Maturation of cellular and humoral immunity during human embryonic development. Acta Pediatr Scand 63:607.

Prummer O, Calvo W, Werner C, Carbonell F, Fliedner TM 1985. Hemopoiesis and immune function in dogs following fetal liver transplantation. This volume.

Putten LM van, Bekkum DW van, Vries MJ de 1968. Transplantation of fetal hematopoietic cells in irradiated rhesus monkeys. IN Radiation and the Control of the Immune Response. Internat Atomic Energy Comm, Vienna p. 41.

Pyke KW, Gelfand EW 1976. Detection of T precursor cells in human bone marrow and foetal liver. Differentiation 5:189-191.

Rabinowich H, Uniel T, Globerson A 1983. T cell progenitors in the mouse fetal liver. Transplantation 35:40.

Rosenberg YJ, Cunningham AJ 1977. Ontogeny of the antibody-forming cell line in mice. III The generation

of mature antisheep red blood cell-specific B cells is antigen dependent. Eur J Immunol 7:257.
Rosenthal P, Rimm IJ, Umiel T, et al 1983. Ontogeny of human hematopoietic cells: Analysis using monoclonal antibodies. J Immunol 131:232.
Saltzstein EC, Bortin MM, Rimm AA, Hussey JL 1974. Long lived canine allogeneic radiation chimera produced with combined fetal liver and thymus cells. Transplantation 18:461.
Sirianni MC, Fiorilli M, Casadei AM, Auiti F 1980. Response to B and T cell mitogens and surface markers in human fetal lymphoid tissues. Thymus 1:257.
Stites DP, Caldwell J, Carr MC, Fudenberg HH 1975. Ontogeny of immunity in humans. Clin Immunol Immunopath 4:519.
Stites DP, Carr MC, Fudenberg HH 1974. Cell Immunol 11:257.
Stutman O 1978. Intrathymic and extrathymic T cell maturation. Immunol Rev 42:138.
Sula K, Nouza K 1981. Immunogenetic requirements for regulatory effects of fetal cells. IN Hraba T, Hasek M (eds) Cellular and Molecular Mechanisms of Immunologic Tolerance. Marcel Dekker, New York, p. 161.
Toivanen P, Uksila J, Leino A, Lassila O, Hirvonen T, Ruuskanen O 1981. Development of mitogen responding T-cells and natural killer cells in the human fetus. Immunol Rev 57:89-105.
Touraine J-L 1980. Transplantation of both fetal liver and thymus in severe combined immunodeficiencies. Interaction between donor and recipient cells. In Lucarelli G, Fleidner TM, Gale RP (eds). Ibid p. 276.
Touraine JL. This volume.
Tyan ML, Cole LJ, Herzenberg LA 1967. Fetal liver: a source of immunoglobulin producing cells in the mouse. Proc Soc Exp Biol Med 124:161.
Umiel T, Globerson A 1974. Analysis of lymphoid cell types developing in the mouse fetal liver. Differentiation 2:169.
Umiel T, Globerson A, Auerbach R 1968. Role of the thymus in the development of immunocompetence of embryonic liver cells in vitro. Proc Soc Exp Biol Med 129:598.
Umiel T 1977. Development of specific suppressor cells of embryonic or neonatal fetal liver origin and their possible role in immunological tolerance. IN Solomon JB, Horton JD (eds). Op cit p. 323.

IMMUNE CHARACTERIZATION OF HUMAN FETAL TISSUES WITH MONOCLONAL ANTIBODIES

M. DeBiagi, M. Andreani, F. Centis

Division of Hematology
Pesaro Hospital
Pesaro, Italy

We studied the immune phenotype of thymus, spleen and liver of human fetuses of several gestational ages using monoclonal antibodies. The data indicate a correlation between some antigens and the functional role of the organs during development. In fact, fetal thymus consists of cells whose phentype is similar to that of mature thymocytes. These cells express T cell-associated antigens, but not CALLA, DR, or B cell-associated antigens. Moreover, there are a substantial number of cells with OKT 10. Fetal spleen, like thymus, shows lymphoid characteristics at early stages of development including $CALLA^+$ cells. Fetal liver had a small number of cells with pan T cell antigens, but contained antigens associated with early progentiors of B cells.

INTRODUCTION

Several studies have determined sites and stages of lymphopoiesis in the human fetus. These studies utilize cytology, histochemistry and immunofluorescent techniques (Toivanen 1981). In addition, attempts have been made to define the functional activity of the immunocompetent fetal cells during vertebrate ontogeny. The phenotype and the functional role of adult lymphoid cells has also been studied to understand human hematopoietic differentiation. Development of monoclonal antibodies (MoAb) has enabled analysis and characterization of cells in fetal lymphoid organs. We characterized the immune phenotype of thymus, spleen and liver cells from human fetuses of various gestational ages with a panel of MoAb.

MATERIAL AND METHODS

Fetal Tissues

Tissues were removed from human fetuses of different gestational ages, obtained from patients undergoing therapeutic abortion. Age was determined by crown-rump and foot length measurements as correlated with the last menstrual period.

Preparation of Cells

Liver, spleen and thymus tissues were cut into pieces while in RPMI Medium 1640 (GIBCO) and passed through a syringe until no lcusters of cells were observed. Cell suspensions were filtered through a wire mesh to remove remaining pieces of tissue. In some instances, lymphocytes were isolated by Ficoll-Hypaque density separation gradient (Pharmacia Fine Chemicals AB, Uppsala, Sweden) and washed twice in RPMI Medium 1640 (Boyum 1968). Cell viability was evaluated by trypan blue dye exclusion.

Monoclonal Antibodies

We used the following MoAb: OKT3, OKT4, OKT8 and OKT10 (Ortho Diagnostic Systems); LEU7, HLA-DR and CALLA (Becton Dickinson Laboratory Systems); B1 (Coulter Electronics Limited, Luton, England) (Kung 1979). Antign expression on normal cells using these MoAb is indicated in Table 1.

Table 1: MOAB Used to Evaluate Antigen Expression on Normal Cells

Antigen	Antigenic Distrubution
T Lineage	
OKT 3	Pan T
OKT 4	Helper/Inducer T
OKT 8	Suppressor/Cytotoxic T
B Lineage	
B 1	Pan B
DR	B, Macrophage, Activated T
CALLA	Early B
Multilineage	
OKT 10	Early hematopoietic and rapidly dividing cells.

Indirect Immunofluorescence Technique

Mononuclear cells were suspended at 5×10^6 cells/mo in RPMI Medium 1640 with 10% of FCS 200 1 of cell suspension was added to 5 1 of each MoAb and incubated at 4°C for 30', cells were washed three times with RPMI 1640 and stained with 100 1 of fluorescein-conjugated goat antimouse IgG (dilution 1/40, 1/50) (Becton Dickinson Laboratory System) for 30' at 4°C. Cells were washed three times resuspended in 50% RPMI 1640 and 50% of Glycerol for microscopic analysis. Cells were examined with a fluorescence microscope with epifluorescence (Karl Zeizz, West Germany) with fluorescence filter. Two hundred cells per sample were counted and the percent of immunofluo-rescent-positive cells determined.

RESULTS AND DISCUSSION

T Cell-Associated Antigens

Fetal thymus contained a high percent of cells positive for T cell associated antigens; 79-90% were stained by the OKT3 (Pan T) MoAb, 68-79% by OKT4 (helper/inducer), and 68-73% by OKT8 (suppressor/cytotoxic). The proportion of positive cells with the OKT4/OKT8 ratio is approximately 1 (Rosenthal 1983). The spleen contained 40% T cells at 18-21 weeks of gestation decreasing to 33% at 22-25 weeks. The percentage of OKT8 positive cells as constant through fetal spleen development; in contrast, there was a slight decrease in OKT4 positive cells in later stages of development. Fetal liver contained a small proportion of T cells throughout gestation.

Table 2: Expression of T Cell-Associated Antigens on Human Fetal Tissues

Gestational Age –		15-17 Wks	18-21 Wks	22-25 Wks
Organ	Antigen	%	%	%
Thymus	OKT 3	79 ± 3	89 ± 7	99 ± 6
	OKT 4	68 ± 2	79 ± 6	74 ± 7
	OKT 8	68 ± 2	73 ± 3	71 ± 4
Spleen	OKT 3	N.D.	40 ± 2	33 ± 2
	OKT 4	N.D.	28 ± 3	23 ± 2
	OKT 8	N.D.	15 ± 2	14 ± 2
Liver	OKT 3	N.D.	1 ± 1	6 ± 1
	OKT 4	N.D.	2 ± 2	2 ± 2
	OKT 8	N.D.	2 ± 1	3 ± 1

N.D. = Not Determined
Values as ± S.E. of the mean of positive cells

B Cell-Associated Antigens

B1 A pan B cell antigen, was present on fetal liver and spleen cells, but was not expressed on fetal thymus (Gathings 1977; Cooper 1981). B1 positive cells were present in fetal liver at a small percent that was constant throughout development. In contrast, the number of B1 positive cells in fetal spleen increased with advancing gestational age. We observed more mature B-cells in spleen than liver; this is consistent with the hypothesis of migration of cells from liver to lymphoid organs Rosenthal 1983). CALLA positive cells have been found in fetal liver and spleen cells; these cells were not found in fetal thymus.

Table 3:   Expression of B Cell-Associated Antigens on Human Fetal Tissues

Gestational Age -		15-17 Wks	18-21 Wks	22-25 Wks
Organ	Antigen	%	%	%
Thymus	B1	N.D.	NEG.	NEG.
	DR	N.D.	NEG.	NEG.
	CALLA	N.D.	NEG.	NEG.
Spleen	B1	N.D.	16 ± 2	29 ± 3
	DR	N.D.	24 ± 3	32 ± 4
	CALLA	N.D.	5 ± 1	4 ± 2
Liver	B1	N.D.	4 ± 1	6 ± 2
	DR	N.D.	55 ± 8	42 ± 3
	CALLA	N.D.	16 ± 4	6 ± 1

N.D. = Not Determined
Values as $\pm$ S.E. of the mean of positive cells

The highest progenitor of CALLA positive cells were detected at 18-21 weeks of gestation in the fetal liver; this decreased in the second part of intrauterine life. The observation that CALLA positive cells could be demonstrated in normal fetal tissues suggests that the CALLA antigen might be expressed on lymphoid progenitor cells (Hokland 1983). DR antigens were not detected in thymus although this antigen was expressed by a high proportion of cells in fetal liver and spleen.

Multilineage Antigens

OKT10 MoAb recognizes an antigen associated with early hematopoietic stem cells and rapidly dividing cells. OKT10 was found on cells of all three fetal tissues studied, the highest proportion of OKT10 positive was found in fetal thymus. We found no cells with the HNKI antigen using the LEU7 MoAb in liver, spleen or thymus cells at any stage of fetal development.

Table 4: Expression of Multilineage Antigen on Human Fetal Tissues

Gestational Age –		15-17 Wks	18-21 Wks	22-25 Wks
Organ	Antigen	%	%	%
Thymus	OKT 10	82 ± 7	80 ± 5	73 ± 5
Spleen	OKT 10	N.D.	12 ± 3	15 ± 2
Liver	OKT 10	N.D.	26 ± 3	17 ± 3

N.D. = Not Determined
Values as ± S.E. of the mean of positive cells

REFERENCES

Toivanen P, Uksila J, Leion A (1981). Development of mitogen responding T cells and Natural killer cells in the human fetus. Immunol Rev 57:89.
Boyum A (1968). Separation of leucocytes from blood and bone marrow. Scand J Clin Lab Invest 21(Suppl. 97):77.
Kung PC, Goldstein G, Reinherz EL, Schlossman SF (1979). Monoclonal antibodies defining distinctive human T-cell surface antigens. Science 206:347.
Rosenthal P, Rimm J, Uniel T, Griffin JD, et al (1983). Ontogeny of human hematopoietic cells: analysis utilizing monoclonal antibodies. J Immunol 31:232.
Gathings WE, Lawton AR, Cooper MD (1977). Immunological studies of the development of the Pre-B cells, B lymphocytes and immunoglobulin isotype diversity in humans. Eur J Immunol 7:804.
Cooper MD (1981). Pre-B cells: normal and abnormal development. J Clin Immunol 1:81.
Hokland P, Rosenthal P, Griffin JD, et al (1983). Purification of fetal hematopoietic cells which express the common acute lymphoblastic leukemia antigen (CALLA). J Exp Med 157:114.

EXPERIMENTAL STUDIES ON HEMOPOIETIC STEM CELLS OF FETAL LIVER ORIGIN AND ITS CLINICAL APPLICATION

Wu, Chu-tse

Department of Experimental Hematology,
Institute of Radiation Medicine, P.O. Box 130,
Beijing, China

In the recent twenty years bone marrow transplantation has become an important measure in the treatment of severe hematological disorders including combined immunodeficient disease, aplastic anemia, leukemia and radiation sickness. Owing to the extreme complexity of histocompatibility of immunological significance, there is very rare chance in the unrelated population to find a histocompatibly matched donor to meet the need of a patient requiring bone marrow transplantation. Because of the unavoidable occurrence of immunological reaction, particularly the graft versus host disease (GVHD), the bone marrow transplantation is only applicable in a very limited scale. With the recent development of HLA typing, improvement of irradiation method in the patient and the development of different ways of cell separation to eliminate immunocompetent cells from hemopoietic stem cell population, a trend to cross the histoincompatibility barrier in allogeneic bone marrow transplantation has become feasible.

Hemopoiesis in the embryonic stages of development first appears in yolk sac, then gradually shifts to the liver and bone marrow. Therefore, the fetal liver can be considered as a source of hemopoietic stem cells.

Uphoff (Uphoff 1958) in 1958 first demonstrated that fetal liver cells possess the function to promote the recovery of hemopoiesis in lethally irradiated mice. Yunis et al (Yunis 1976) provided evidence that GVHD following fetal liver transplantation is somewhat weaker than that caused by allogeneic bone marrow transplantation. Hence, the application of fetal liver in place of bone marrow transplantation would be of great value to patients when the histocompatible match is not available (Gale 1979; Lucarelli 1982).

We have carried out some experimental work on the hemopoietic stem cells from fetal liver and revealed some problems of interest which form the subject of discussion in this paper.

BIOLOGICAL STUDIES OF HEMOPOIETIC STEM CELLS OF FETAL LIVER ORIGIN

It has long been known that a certain amount of hemopoietic stem cells was consistently present in the hemopoietic organs, and through their proliferation and differentiation the blood cells are maintained at a constant level. It was until 1961 that Till and McCulloch (Till 1961) developed the spleen colony technique which provided a semi-quantitative method for the estimation of hemopoietic stem cells from different sources including bone marrow and fetal liver.

By adopting the sex chromosome as a cytogenetic marker and c-band staining technique we have observed the behavior of a single spleen colony forming cell from adult bone marrow or fetal liver as depicted in Figure 1.

The intravenous injection of 1.5×10^4 normal bone marrow cells or 3×10^4 fetal liver cells derived from pregnant mice 15-18 days of gestation to a 8.0Gy gamma ray irradiated syngeneic mouse of LACA or C57 strain produced a few gross colonies in the recipient spleen 13 days later. A single spleen colony was randomly dissected and dispersed in 0.8ml culture medium and transfused into a 7.5-8.0Gy gamma irradiated secondary recipient. Seven to 8 weeks later, the sex chromosome was identified in the secondary recipient which involves the bone marrow cells and its CFU-S, T and B-lymphocytes of the spleen and lymph nodes after in vitro transformation under the stimulation of mitogens. Since we used opposite sex of donor and recipient in paired experiments as described above, it provided a reliable and nature technique to follow up a single spleen colony forming cell in their pathway of proliferation and differentiation (Wu 1984).

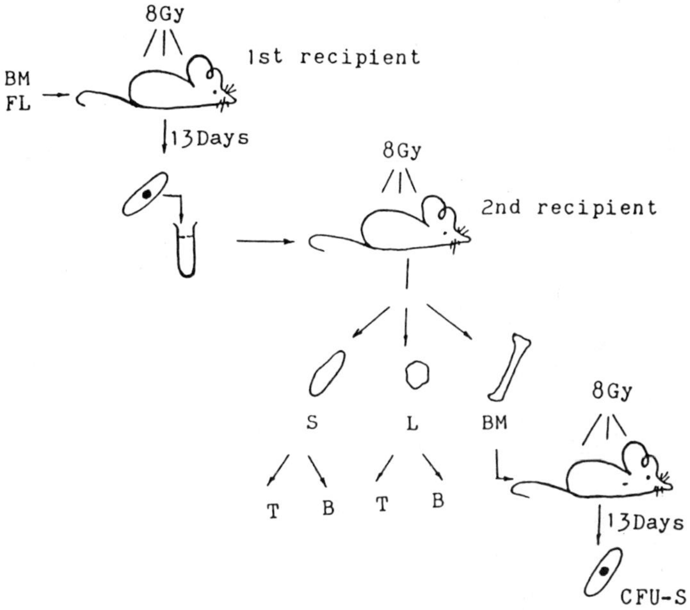

Fig.1 Experimental design for the observation of proliferation
and differentiation of a single spleen colony forming cell
    BM: Bone marrow   FL: Fetal liver
    L: Lymph nodes   S: Spleen
    T: T-lymphocyte   B: B-lymphocyte

Table 1 The ability of spleen colony forming cells(CFC_S) from adult bone marrow and fetal liver in re-establishment of lymphoid and myeloid lines of cells in 7.5-8.0Gy irradiated mice

Strain of mice	Origin of CFC_S and Exp.No.	Radiation dose for 2nd recipient (Gy)	Interval after spleen colony transfusion (weeks)	Donor cells in 2nd recipient %					Spleen colonies Donor karyotype Total
				ST	LT	SB	LB	BM	
C57	Bone marrow	7.5							
	42-1		12	77	87	77	70	93	—
	42-3		12	27	—	17	—	33	—
	42-4		12	43	37	47	30	40	—
	42-5		12	—	—	13	20	13	—
	42-8		14	—	—	40	40	47	—
	42-9		14	50	57	57	47	53	—
	42-10		14	40	—	27	—	40	—
	42-13		16	—	17	—	20	17	—
LACA	Bone marrow	8.0							
	3-5		12	77	73	80	53	—	2/5
	1-2		8	54	—	—	—	19	2/9
	13-1		7	97	—	93	93	100	10/10
	13-2		7	13	13	20	—	—	0/9
	13-3		8	8	21	7	13	3	2/12
	A		6	38	33	28	36	40	—
LACA	Fetal liver	7.5							
	40-3		9	42	40	63	43	37	—
	40-4		9	50	57	57	71	60	—
	40-5		9	69	67	67	70	60	—
	40-6		9	70	75	70	77	33	—
	40-7		10	60	60	70	67	53	—
	40-8		10	20	22	27	30	53	—
	40-10		11	27	14	20	25	33	—
	40-11		11	13	—	17	—	20	—
	40-12		11	—	33	—	40	37	—
	40-13		11	44	—	40	—	50	—

ST: T-lymphocyte in spleen SB: B-lymphocyte in spleen BM: Bone marrow
LT: T-lymphocyte in lymph nodes LB: B-lymphocyte in lymph nodes CFU-S: Spleen colony

The results in Table 1 show that spleen colony forming cells from adult LACA mice bone marrow or C57 fetal liver possess the same property of re-establishment of myeloid and lymphoid systems in lethally irradiated recipients. Thus, spleen colony forming cells of both adult bone marrow and fetal liver are endowed with the fundamental properties of pluripotent hemopoietic stem cells or lymphoid-myeloid stem cells.

KINETIC STUDIES OF HEMOPOIETIC STEM CELLS IN FETAL LIVER DURING THE DEVELOPMENT OF HUMAN FETUS

Up to the present the assay method of hemopoietic stem cells, except in rodents, remained unsolved. But the accumulated facts as provided in kinetic studies in mice incline to the view that hemopoietic stem cells are closely related to the granuloid progenitor cells. Therefore, it is reasonable to use the assay method of GM-CFU$_C$ as a means to elucidate the behavior of hemopoietic stem cells.

During the development of the fetus the weight of the liver and its cellularity are steadily increasing. We have determined the GM-CFU$_C$ yiels, total number of GM-CFU$_C$ and T-lymphocytes in liver from 22 fetuses of different ages and found that the GM-CFU$_C$ yield is very low at 1.5 months of gestation, it increases rapidly with the increase in time of gestation and the maximum yield as well as the total number of GM-CFU$_C$ in fetal liver appears at 4-5 months of gestation. Thereafter, although the liver is continuously increasing in weight, the GM-CFU$_C$ yield and the total number of GM-CFU$_C$ tend to decline and at about the 7th month of gestation the fetal hepatic GM-CFU$_C$ has dropped to nadir value. The kinetic changes of GM-CFU$_C$ content in fetal liver constitute typical bell shaped curves as shonw in Figure 2 and 3 (Wu 1982).

During the course of fetal development the total number and the percentage of lymphocytes in fetal liver are gradually increasing. We have studied the kinetic changes of T-lymphocytes in the fetal liver. The cytochemical staining method of acid-estarase and measurement of E-rosette formation are adopted for the estimation of T-lymphocytes. Table 2 indicates that within 6 months of gestation the number of T-lymphocytes in fetal liver almost keeps a constant level of about 1-2% (Wu 1982). The increase in liver weight and its cellularity does not seem

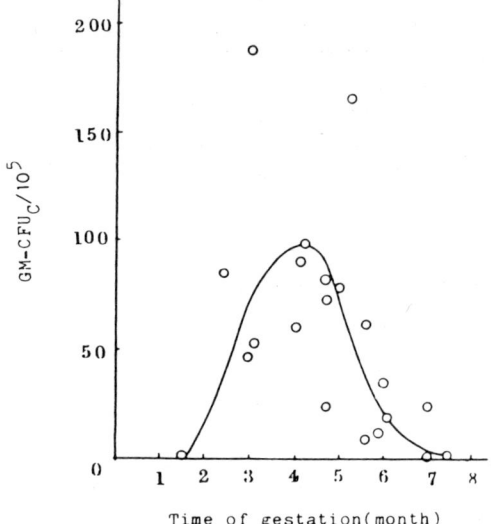

Fig. 2 The kinetic changes in yield of GM-CFU$_C$ in fetal liver during the course of gestation

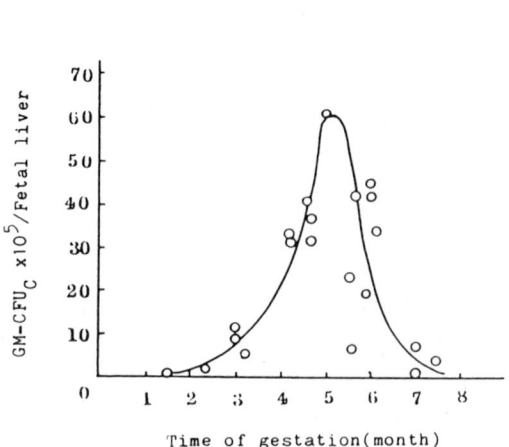

Fig. 3 The changes of total number of GM-CFU$_C$ in fetal liver with fetal age

Table 2 Percentage of T-lymphocytes in fetal liver during the first 7 months of gestation

Months of gestation	Acid-esterase staining method(%)	E-rosette formation (%)
2.5	0.42	
3	0.23,0.56,0.30	
4	1.06,0.29	0.5
4.5	0.34,0.20	
5	1.12,0.96,0.53	1.5,0.8
5.5	0.92	2.8
6	0.50,0.63	
7		4.0

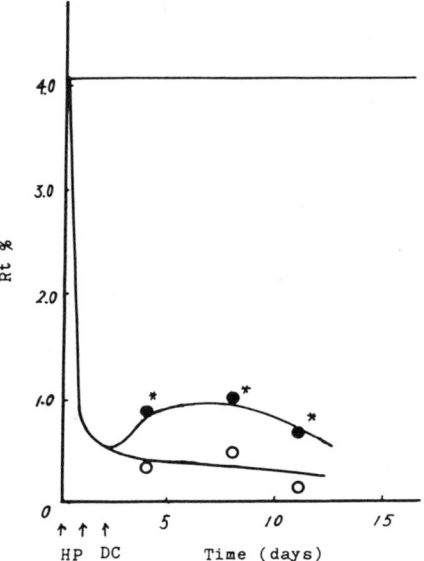

Fig.4 The effect of fetal liver cells in diffusion chamber on the peripheral reticulocyte count of normal mice
o normal plethoric mice implanted intraperitoneally with DC containing culture medium
● normal plethoric mice implanted intraperitoneally with DC containing fetal liver cells
HP: hypertransfusion of 0.8ml concentrated red blood cells for two successive days
*$p < 0.05$

to affect the percentage of T-lymphocytes in any significant degree, showing that the content of T-lymphocytes in fetal liver is relatively low in comparison with other hemopoietic organs.

CLINICAL TRANSFUSION OF FETAL LIVER CELLS

Since 1980 we have given 61 patients with aplastic anemia and some other hematooogical disorders the transfusion of fresh fetal liver cell suspension containing 1.8-12.4x10^9 nucleated cells from 4-5 months old fetus intravenously or by iliac post crest route (Ye 1983; Ji 1984).

Among them 26 cases of aplastic anemia received 28 transfusions of fetal liver cell suspension, about 30% of them showed effective result in the reconstitution of hemopoiesis. Meanwhile, the improvement of immunological function as evidenced by the increase of peripheral lymphocyte transformation under the stimulation of phytohemagglutinin and the number of T-lymphocytes in peripheral blood was observed (Li 1984; Xao 1984).

Fetal liver cell transfusion was given to a group of 14 patients with aplastic anemia. Among them 11 cases showed increase in the number of E-RFC and ANAE positive cells in peripheral blood, but no changes were observed in the other 3 cases. The possibility of fetal liver cell transfusion in stimulation of non-specific immunological function was assumed that the transfused fetal liver cells, as an allogeneic antigen, may activate T-lymphocyte and enhance the proliferation of T-lymphocyte in vivo by the lymphocyte proliferating factors released from the activated T-lymphocytes. This assumption is supported by the fact that giant E-rosette formation is always observed in the peripheral lymphocyte of patients after transfusion of fetal liver cells.

Another patient received three successive transfusions of fetal liver cell suspension within a period of 10 days, the symptomatic improvement was very marked.

Since the complexicity of etiology of hematological disorders, we adopted self-control method to evaluate the therapeutic effect of fetal liver transfusion in a group of leukemia patients. The protocol of the treatment was similar in two successive courses of chemotherapy with an interval of one month off. After first course of chemotherapy the blood picture including hemoglobin (Hb), red blood cell (RBC), white blood cell (WBC) and platelet (Pt) declined and recovered slowly. However, a dose of fetal liver cell suspension was transfused within 4 days after the end of the second course of chemotherapy, the recovery of blood pictures, particularly Rt, WBC and Pt, was markedly accelerated as shwon in Table 3. These results may provide evidence to show that fetal liver cells are efficacious in promoting the recovery of hemopoiesis in case of functional deficiency of the bone marrow.

We have given 11 patients with aplastic anemia or leukemia after chemotherapy the transfusion of fetal liver cells from opposite sex of fetus, but none of them showed chimera formation as evidenced by karyotype examination of bone marrow or peripheral lymphocytes.

For elucidating the underlying mechanism of the stimulating effect of fetal liver transfusion on hemopoiesis, the following experiments were performed. 0.12ml fetal liver cell suspension containing 5×10^6 nucleated cells were inoculated into a diffusion chamber. Two diffusion chambers were implanted into the peritoneal cavity of a normal plethoric mouse. At intervals of in vivo culture the peripheral reticulocyte count was markedly increased as shown in Figure 4.

Fetal liver cells at the concentration of $4-8 \times 10^7$/ml were destroyed by ultrasonic wave and the cell-free supernatant was separated. A group of 5 normal mice or plethoric mice received intraperitoneal injection of 0.5ml cell-free supernatant of fetal liver separately. It shows that fetal liver cells contain erythropoietin-like substance which could stimulate and speed up erythropoiesis in both normal and plethoric mice (Figures 5 and 6).

Normal mice received successive injections of cell-free supernatant of fetal liver cells for 5 days, 24 hours later, the mice were killed and cell differentiation of bone marrow from sterum was determined. From Table 4 it is clear that mitotic index of erythroid cells is obviously increased from the normal value of 3.57% to 5.04%, and the ratio of granuloid to erythroid elements in the bone marrow tends to decrease, indicating that cell-free supernatant of fetal liver activates in the main the erythropoiesis.

Table 3 Comparison of the blood pictures of leukemic patients after first course of chemotherapy and the second course of chemotherapy with transfusion of fetal liver cells

Case no.	Hb(g%) 7 Days 1st	Hb(g%) 7 Days 2nd	Hb(g%) 14 Days 1st	Hb(g%) 14 Days 2nd	Rt(%) 7 Days 1st	Rt(%) 7 Days 2nd	Rt(%) 14 Days 1st	Rt(%) 14 Days 2nd	WBC(/mm³) 7 Days 1st	WBC(/mm³) 7 Days 2nd	WBC(/mm³) 14 Days 1st	WBC(/mm³) 14 Days 2nd	Pt(x10⁴/mm³) 7 Days 1st	Pt(x10⁴/mm³) 7 Days 2nd	Pt(x10⁴/mm³) 14 Days 1st	Pt(x10⁴/mm³) 14 Days 2nd
1	8.0	4.1	7.0	5.0	0.1	0.2	0.1	2.4	2200	1050	1900	1850	6.5	8.9	6.7	22.9
2	4.6	4.3	4.1	3.0	0.1	1.2	0.0	6.6	2700	8300	2100	11000	4.3	1.3	1.8	8.6
3	9.0	9.5	10.0	11.2	0.1	1.2	0.4	1.4	2300	7450	4000	6500	5.4	7.9	2.3	15.8
4	9.3	8.7	8.0	9.0	0.0	0.7	0.1	1.4	2100	5500	3200	4700	12.0	16.8	–	22.6
5	10.0	8.0	11.0	9.5	0.2	–	0.6	3.4	4500	3800	3200	10600	10.7	17.0	8.3	13.2
6	4.8	10.2	5.1	12.0	0.7	0.4	0.2	0.2	1900	3000	2900	4300	10.3	17.8	5.0	12.3
7	4.7	5.0	3.6	5.5	0.1	0	0.1	0.2	2300	7000	3400	4500	7.5	17.4	2.1	22.0
8	4.7	8.5	8.0	9.0	0.2	–	1.0	2.4	4600	900	1600	3600	3.3	3.3	13.0	7.9
x̄	6.6	7.3	7.1	8.0	0.2	0.5	0.3	2.3	2825	4625	2785	5881	7.5	9.7	5.6	15.7
±S.D	2.2	2.4	2.7	3.2	0.2	0.5	0.3	2.0	1089	2875	834	3297	3.2	6.6	4.1	6.2
							p<0.05				p<0.05				p<0.05	

Table 4 Comparison of the mitotic index(I_M) of erythroid cells and the ratio of granuloid to erythroid elements(G/E) in bone marrow of normal mice after injections of cell-free extract of human fetal liver or saline solution as control

	Control group			Experimental group		
Animal No.	G/E	I_M(%)	Animal No.	G/E	I_M(%)
1	2.85	3.75	1	2.53	5.60
2	3.15	3.20	2	2.31	5.45
3	3.35	3.70	3	2.22	5.40
4	1.82	3.50	4	2.61	6.35
5	3.18	3.35	5	2.61	4.10
6	3.09	3.90	6	2.97	4.10
Mean±S.D.	2.91±0.56	3.57±0.26	Mean±S.D.	2.42±0.35	5.04±0.88*

*p<0.001

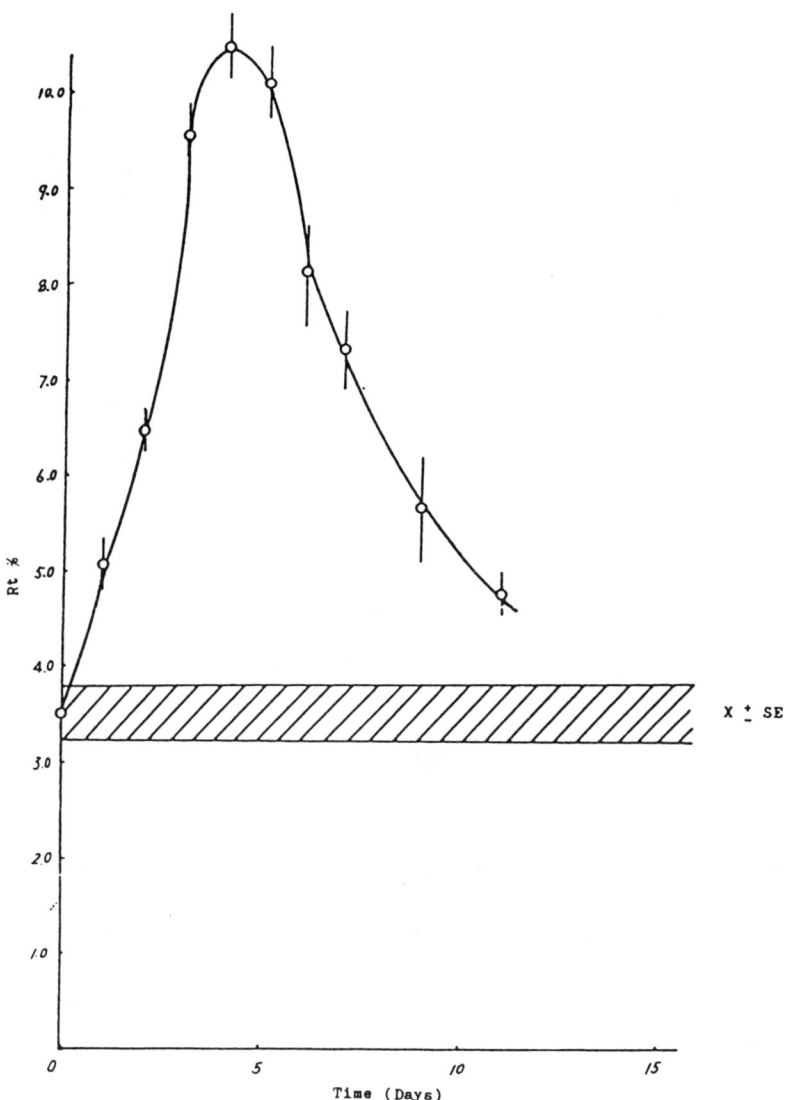

Fig. 5 The effect of cell-free supernatant of human fetal liver on the peripheral reticulocyte count of normal mice

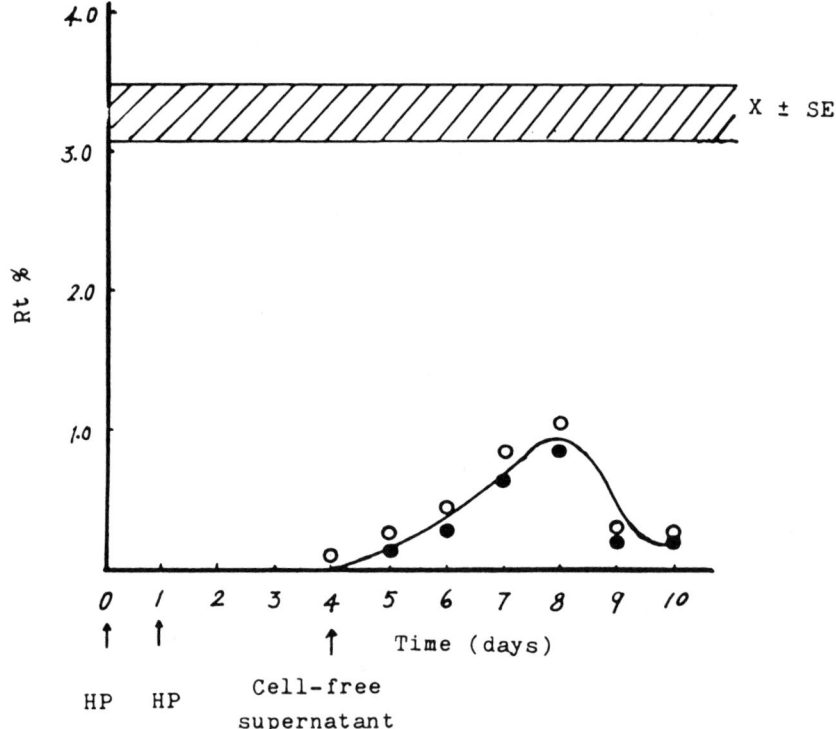

Fig.6 The effect of cell-free supernatant of human fetal liver on the peripheral reticulocyte count of normal plethoric mice in duplicated experiments

Similarly, normal mice received injections of cell-free supernatant of fetal liver every other day, 24 hours after the fourth injection the phagocytic index of intra-peritoneal phagocytes (the average number of cock red cells phagocytized by an intra-peritoneal phagocyte) was increased from 2.48 ± 0.12 to 4.81 ± 0.57 and the reticulocytes count in the peripheral blood increased from $4.12 \pm 0.61\%$ to $6.26 \pm 1.1\%$ (Wu 1984).

These facts demonstrated that fetal liver transfusion is effective in promoting erythropoiesis and non-specific immunological function in vivo. This effect is strengthened when the administration is prolonged. These are consistant with the clinical observation.

CLINICAL TRANSPLANTATION OF HEMOPOIETIC STEM CELLS FROM THE FETAL LIVER

So far there were 7 patients with acute leukemia in our cooperation group who received fetal liver transplantation after being pre-conditioned with cyclophosphamide and total body gamma irradiation (Meng 1984; Qian 1984; Yao 1984; Liu 1984).

Among them three cases which have been reported in a separate paper at this symposium were given with a single fetal liver respectively from 4-5 month old fetus. Another four cases, as shown in Table 5, were transfused with multiple fetal livers, three of them showed temporary engraftment as evidenced by karyotype analysis of bone marrow or peripheral lymphocytes, i.e. 2-5% of cells of donor origin on day 30, which gradually disappeared afterwards, none of them showing permenant engraftment after transplantation of multiple fetal livers. One patient (case 1 in Table 5) at terminal phase of acute lymphoblastic leukemia died due to relapse at 133 days after transplantation. The other three patients were performed at the first complete remission. No MTX prophylaxis was given. Mild syndromes of GVHD were observed only in case 3 with transient skin rashes and abnormal liver functions and further proved by skin biopsies on day 45 after fetal liver transplantation. (Liu 1984).

DISCUSSION

When patients were treated with large doses of chemo-

Table 5 Results of transplantation of multiple fetal livers in the patients after being pre-conditioned with cyclophosphamide (Cy) and total body irradiation (TBI) (Qian 1984; Yao 1984; Liu 1984)

	Patient				Fetus			Results			
case	age sex	diagnosis	status	pre-conditioning	number	age (month)	sex	engraftment %	GVHD	post FLT survival(days)	outcome
1	7m	ALL	4PR	day-3 Cy 40mg/Kg -2 Cy 40mg/Kg 0 TBI 5.5Gy (4.3 rad/min)	5	4-5	3f 2m	day30,3%in PB day45,0%in PB	no	133	relapse
2	12m	ALL	1CR	day-6 Cy 40mg/Kg -5 Cy 40mg/Kg -3 DNR 20mg -2 DNR 20mg 0 TBI 5.0Gy (4.3 rad/min)	6	3.5-5	3f 3m	day15,2%in PB day30,0%in PB	no	>330	living
3	21m	AML	1CR	day-7 Cy 40mg/Kg -6 Cy 40mg/Kg -4 Ara-C 3mg/Kg -3 Ara-C 3mg/Kg 0 TBI 5.0Gy (12.5 r/min)	5	3.5-4.5	5f	day30,5%in BM day45,0%in BM	mild	>180	living
4	10m	AML	1CR	day-5 Cy 60mg/Kg -4 Cy 60mg/Kg -3 DNR 20mg -2 DNR 20mg 0 TBI 5.5Gy (12.5 r/min)	6	3.5-4.5	3f 3m	day14,0 in PB day21,0%in PB day43,0%in PB	no	>80	living

* DNR:daunorubicin   ** % of donor karyotype in bone marrow or peripheral blood
CR:complete remission   PR:partial remission   m:male   f:female

therapy or received large doses of ionizing irradiation in some accidental events, the normal hemopoiesis is usually severely damaged. In such cases transplantation of 2.7×10^6 GM-CFUc from an identical twin bone marrow is sufficient to restore normal hemopoiesis. From the study of kinetic changes of total GM-CFUc in fetal liver, we have provided some evidence to show that whole fetal liver at 4-5 months of gestation contains about $3-6 \times 10^6$ GM-CFUc. It is, therefore, that fetal liver can be considered as an important source of hemopoietic stem cells. However, transplantation of fetal liver is of allogeneic nature, and the hemopoietic stem cells from fetal liver are gradually expelled or unable to graft in adult bone marrow, thus the nature of such histoincompatibility and ontogenetic barriers remain to be elucidated.

In the experiments by using inbred animals as donor and recipient, the lower seeding efficiency of hemopoietic stem cells from fetal liver in recipient spleen or bone marrow of adult mice cannot be attributed to the presence of some barrier of histoincompatibility, but rather to some barrier belonging to the ontogenetic stages of development which may hamper the premature CFU-S passing through from the fetal liver to the adult bone marrow.

In our preliminary experiment two dogs were given 10.0 Gy gamma irradiation and transfused with 5.9×10^9 fetal liver cells from 5.5-6.0 week old fetuses of two unrelated pregnant dogs. The yield of granuloid progenitors as assayed by in vivo agar diffusion chamber culture method was 15.0 GM-CFUc/10^5 on the average. During the observational period of 9-11 days after irradiation and transfusion of fetal liver cells, none of them showed any sign of recovery of hemopoiesis. Nevertheless, a dog in a parallel experiment given 10.0Gy gamma irradiation and transfused with 10×10^9 bone marrow cells from a normal sibling, showed a marked increase of peripheral white blood cells from 6th day after irradiation and transplantation.

Fliedner, et al (Fliedner 1980) reported that beagle dogs were given 1200 roentgens x-ray irradiation and transfused with fetal liver cells at a dose of $5-10 \times 10^4$ GM-CFUc per kilogram body weight. An engraftment was observed.

It is therefore, in case of allogeneic transplantation with fetal liver, both ontogenetic barrier and histoincompatibility barriers may play an important role. The failure of fetal liver transplantation in different animals as revealed by expulsion of the transplant is probably due to the cytotoxic effect of lymphocyte or natural killer cells in recipient which are particularly harmful to the fetal liver cells (Gale 1979).

From the above described characteristics of hemotopoietic stem cells we propose that as a possible measure to overcome the ontogenetic barrier or the lower seeding efficiency of hemopoietic stem cells of fetal liver origin is by increasing the number of transfused fetal liver cells.

In order to overcome the histoincompatibility barrier in allogeneic hemopoietic stem cell transplantation of fetal liver origin, more intensive immunosuppression of the recipient is likely necessary. From clinical observations it is obvious that no chimera was found in the fetal liver transfused recipients. Nevertheless, preconditioning the recipients with special immunosuppression before transfusion of fetal liver cells, the chimera containing both donor and recipient karyotypes in the bone marrow and peripheral blood was proved existing.

In the course of gestation, the development of fetus includes the migration of hemopoietic stem cells from yolk sac to fetal liver, and to bone marrow. This is accompanied with the changes of hemopoietic stem cell itself. Therefore, through further extensive studies on the properties of hemopoietic stem cells and the immune development of fetuses, the difficulties of histoincompatibility in the case of transplantation of fetal liver stem cells may be hopefully overcome.

Uphoff DE (1958). Preclusion of secondary phase of irradiation syndroms by inoculation of fetal hemopoietic tissue following lethal total-body x-irradiation. J Nat Cancer Inst 20:625.

Yunis EJ, Fernandes G, Smith J and Good RA (1976). Long survival and immunological reconstitution following transplantation with syngeneic or allogeneic fetal liver and neonatal spleen cells. Transpl. Proc 8:521

Gale RP (1979). Fetal liver transplantation in man. In "Proceedings of the First International Symposium on Fetal Liver Transplantation. p. 268.

Lucarelli G, Izzi T, Porcellin A, Delfini G, Galimberti M, Moretti L, Polchi P. Agostinelli F, Andreani M, Manna M and Dallapiccola B (1982). Fetal liver transplantation in 2 patients with acute leukemia after total body irradiation. Scand J Haemat 28:65.

Till JE and McCulloch FA (1961). A direct measurement of the radiation sessitivity of normal mouse bone marrow. Radiat Res 14:213.

Wu C-T and Lie M-P (1984). Characteristics of proliferation and differentiation of spleen colony forming cells from bone marrow. Int J Cell Cloning 2:68

Wu C-T, Fei R-G, Zhou S-Z, Shi F-M, Li C-H, and Wang B-Z (1982). Kinetic studies of haemopoietic progenitors (CFU-C) and T-lymphocytes in the liver of human foetus. Scientia Sinica 25:168.

Ye G-Y, Wu C-T, Qian F-W, Yu W-Y, Fei R-G, Jiang B-Y, Cheng X-Y, Li Y-Q, and Xao P (1983). Fetal liver transfusion in the treatment of aplastic anemia. Chinese J of Int Med 22:71.

Ji S-Q, Zhu M, Li Z-M, Ke Z-M, Ding X-Y, Wu C-T, Zhang Y-H, Zhou S-Z, Tian H-B, and Lie X-L (1984). The effectiveness of fetal liver transfusion in the treatment of aplastic anemia and leukemia after chemotherapy. Beijing Med J 6:6.

Li C-H, Ye G-Y, Wu C-T, and Mu X-W (1984). Changes of T-lymphocytes in patients with aplastic anemia after transfusion of fetal liver cells. submitted to publish.

Xao P, Si F-W, and Wu C-T (1984). Effect of transfusion of fetal liver cells on the peripheral lymphocyte transformation in patients with aplastic anemia. submitted to publish.

Wu C-T, Chen J-P, Xue H-H, Tian H-B, Zhou S-Z, and Liu X-Y (1984). Studies on the mechanism of fetal liver transfusion or whole embryoic extract injections in the treatment of aplastic anemia. Chinese J of Applied Physiology. 1:5.

Meng P-L, Ye W-Z, Fei R-G, Gu D-W, Wang X-H, Man Z-G, Zhu L-X, Chen B-Z, and Yu Y-Y (1984). Allogeneic fetal liver transplantation of acute lymphotic leukemia: report of one case. Chinese J of Organ Transplantation 5:24.

Qian F-W, Cheng X-Y, Sun H-P, Tan H-J, Peng J-Y, Zhong Y-G, Jiang B-R, Li X, Hu L-R, Ye G-Y and Wu C-T (1984). The clinical report of allogeneic fetal liver transplantation in a case of acute lymphoblastic leukemia. submitted to publish.

Yao S-Q, Lui H-C, Meng F-Y, Zhang P, Qian F-W, Cheng X-Y and Zeng T-Q. Fetal liver transplantation in a case of lymphoblastic leukemia. submitted to publish.

Liu H-C (1984). Personal communication

Fliedner TM, Grilli G, Calvo W, Nothdurft W, Haen M and Carbonell F (1980). Fetal liver as an alternative source of stem cells for hemopoietic reconstitution: A canine model. Exp Hemat 8 suppl No. 7:23.

Gale RP (1979). Concepts of fetal liver transplantation in man. In "Proceedings of First International Symposium on Fetal Liver Transplantation". p 246.

FETAL LIVER: ERYTHROPOIESIS IN VIVO, SUSTAINED GRANULOPOIESIS IN VITRO

M.D. CAPPELLINI, C.G. POTTER and W.G. WOOD

MRC Molecular Haematology Unit,
and the Nuffield Department of Clinical Medicine,
University of Oxford, John Radcliffe Hospital,
Headington, Oxford, OX3 9DU, U.K.

Attempts to adapt the Dexter-type long-term marrow culture system (Dexter et al 1977) for human hemopoietic cells have been rather disappointing; granulocyte production can be maintained for a few months under the best of conditions but there is considerable variability between individual samples (Moore and Sheridan 1979; Hocking and Golde 1979; Toogood et al 1980; Gartner and Kaplan 1980; Potter et al 1981). In all species that have been examined, the standard conditions do not promote erythroid differentiation although survival of erythroid progenitor cells (BFU-E) has been demonstrated in murine marrow cultures and differentiation has been triggered by shaking the cultures in the presence of erythropoietin (Eliason et al 1979) or by the addition of anemic mouse serum (Dexter et al 1982). Limited BFU-E survival has been reported in human marrow cultures but their differentiation has required removal to semisolid medium (Coulombel et al 1983).

In fetal life, the liver is the major site of erythropoiesis and hemopoietic differentiation is largely restricted to this lineage, suggesting that the hepatic microenvironment is specifically suited to erythroid cell development. We have attempted, therefore, to develop long-term cultures of human fetal liver hemopoietic cells in the hope that erythropoiesis might be maintained and with the possibility that a better understanding of what makes this a preferred site of erythropoiesis might emerge. However, in culture, a dramatic shift from erythroid to granulocytic cell production occurred in the first week. Furthermore, prolonged survival of in vitro granulopoiesis, up to one year, was obtained using fetal hemopoietic cells seeded on adult marrow stromal layers (Cappellini et al 1984).

Culture Conditions

Fetal liver cells were obtained from prostaglandin-induced abortuses of 13-18 weeks gestation. A cell suspension was made by scraping the liver with a scalpel blade and serial passage through 19-25 gauge needles. These cells were either cultured directly or after depletion of hepatocytes using a Ca^{++}-induced agglutination technique. Cultures were initiated at a concentration of 10^6/ml in α medium containing 20% horse serum, 10% fetal calf serum, 10^{-6} M hydrocortisone and antibiotics (Potter et al 1981; Cappellini et al 1984). Cells were gassed with 5% CO_2 in air and incubated at 37°C. Refeeding was carried out weekly, usually by replacement of half the medium, the supernatant cells obtained being used for cell counts and morphological assessment.

Fetal Liver Cell Cultures

An adherent stromal layer developed in the fetal liver cell cultures, similar to that seen in adult marrow cultures with the exception that fat cells were rare, even in the presence of hydrocortisone. The stroma was generally confluent by 3 weeks but took a little longer in the hepatocyte-depleted cultures, and tended to retract and detach more easily than in marrow cultures. The cells in suspension showed a gradual decline in number with time and, not taking into account the weekly demidepopulation, reached 10^4 cells/ml after ~ 10 weeks. However, a dramatic shift in the pattern of hemopoiesis occurred in culture, with erythroid cells disappearing over the first week to be replaced by an impressive wave of granulopoiesis, with myeloblasts comprising ~70% of the suspension cells after 7 days. Thereafter, granulocytic cells of all stages of maturation accounted for most of the recognizable suspension cells, with a gradual increase in the proportion of monocytes and macrophages occurring as the overall level of hemopoiesis declined beyond 10 weeks in culture. Neither human spleen conditioned medium, (2-10%) nor erythropoietin (0.5 u/ml), alone or together, could prevent the rapid replacement of erythropoiesis by myeloid cells and neither could the presence of severely anemic sheep serum (Cappellini et al 1984).

Fetal Liver Cells Cultured on Adult Marrow Stromas

Fetal liver cells, depleted of hepatocytes, were also used to recharge stromal layers derived from long-term adult marrow cultures in which hemopoietic cell production had long ceased. The fetal cells rapidly infiltrated the quiescent layer and foci of active hemopoiesis were visible within 1 week. Thereafter an increase in the number of cells in suspension was observed, with a plateau of ~10^5 cells/ml being maintained until week 15, declining gradually to ~10^4/ml by week 39 (Figure 1). The rapid replacement of erythroid cells by myeloid elements was as great under these conditions as in the direct liver cell cultures, with granulocytes accounting for up to 50% of the cells in suspension during the plateau phase but declining as the overall cell number declined, to be replaced by macrophages. Cells removed from the supernatant at week 13 (Figure 1, point a) were able to repopulate further 'burnt out' marrow stromas and continue hemopoietic cell production for a further 25+ weeks.

Altering the medium-changing procedure at week 39 (Figure 1, point b) to a complete medium change, plus the return of ~80% of the supernatant cells resulted in a rapid increase in the total number of cells in suspension (back to 10^5 cells/ml) and a return of granulopoiesis (back to 30-50% of the total cells).

After 48 weeks (Figure 1, point c) the stromal layer from this particular flask retracted and detached. It was treated with 0.1% collagenase and the resulting cell suspension was washed and used to generate a fresh layer. This formed readily, granulopoiesis recovered and the culture was finally discontinued more than one year after it was originally generated. This is a considerably longer period of continuous in vitro hemopoietic cell production than has previously been reported for human cells (Cappellini et al 1984).

Lack of Erythropoiesis

In order to assess the reasons for the rapid disappearance of erythropoiesis, BFU-E assays were carried out on the cultures weekly. From an initial input of ~4000 BFU-E/flask, the number of bursts recovered after the first week showed a > 50-fold reduction and in subsequent weeks only occasional BFU-E could be grown from the supernatant. The numbers of CFU-GM, however, which were high in the initial liver cell preparation, increased further in culture initially before declining slightly.

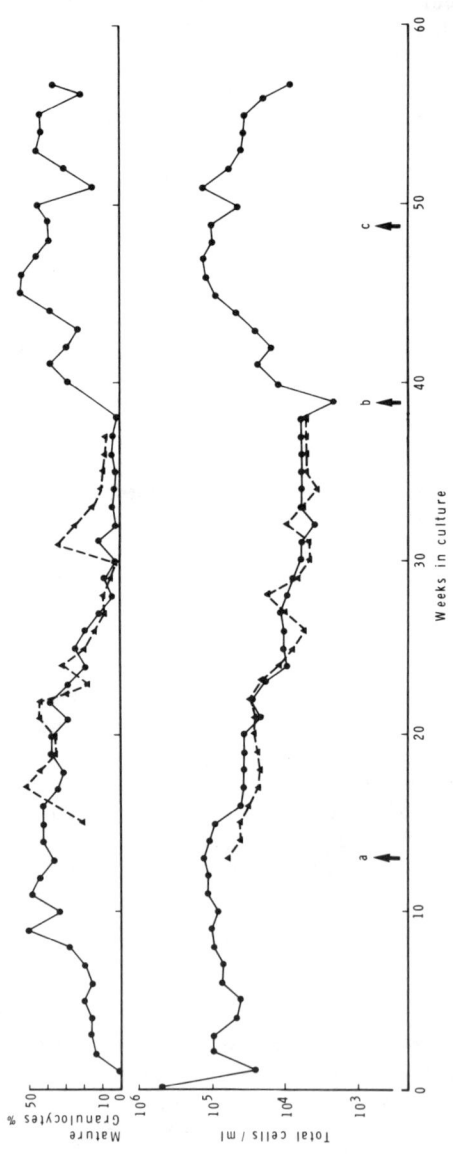

Figure 1. Cell concentration and granulocyte proportion in cultures of human fetal liver cells seeded onto an adult marrow stromal layer (see text for details).

Collagenase digestion of the stromal layer itself during the first few weeks in culture did not reveal a significant reservoir of progenitor cells but further investigation is necessary to determine whether the treatment itself might have resulted in progenitor cell damage or loss.

In order to assess whether the long-term cultures contained cellular or humoral inhibitors of erythropoiesis, normal adult peripheral blood BFU-E cultures were co-cultured with suspension cells from long-term cultures and the effect of conditioned medium from the long-term cultures was also examined. Co-culture of adult peripheral blood mononuclear cells (PBMC) with an increasing number of cultured fetal liver cells (CFLC) produced a moderate stimulation of the number of bursts obtained in a dose dependent manner (maximum stimulation ~50%). That this was not due to additional BFU-E in the CFLC was shown when this pattern remained unchanged when they were irradiated. Similarly, when the total cell number was kept constant but the ratio of PBMC to CFLC suspension cells was varied, no reduction in burst production was observed. These experiments, therefore, provided no evidence for cellular inhibition of erythropoiesis; similar experiments with dissociated stromal cells are now required. No humoral inhibitors of BFU-E growth were seen when PBMC were cultured with 2-20% spent medium from the CFLC at any time from the beginning of the culture out to more than 20 weeks.

Discussion

Fetal liver is the major site of erythropoiesis for much of gestation and although the presence of high concentrations of myeloid progenitor cells is well documented, there is little if any granulopoiesis in this organ, implying that the microenvironment is particularly suited to erythroid differentiation in vivo. The dramatic shift in vitro to myelopoiesis, sustainable for long periods, suggests that all the information necessary for granulocyte production is present in the cells of the fetal liver, and that the culture conditions allow their production, either by the selective survival or proliferation of cells producing the necessary 'factors' or by altering the regulatory pathways of the hemopoietic or accessory cells to suppress erythropoiesis and promote granulopoiesis. The experiments reported here do not provide any evidence for the level of cellular differentiation at which regulation is occurring. The sustained production of granulocytes, particularly when the fetal liver cells are seeded onto an adult stromal layer, could be the result of differentiation from a pluripotent progenitor cell, with restriction to the myeloid lineage being dictated by the culture conditions; alternatively the conditions may allow the proliferation of a committed myeloid progenitor cell with a high proliferation potential (Cappellini et al 1984).

The lack of erythropoiesis in vitro is disappointing and again presumably reflects a deficiency in the culture conditions, which have been shown to favour myelopoiesis in a variety of species. Although we were unable to demonstrate the presence of cellular or humoral inhibitors of erythropoiesis in our cultures, this aspect probably warrants further attention, particularly in light of experiments suggesting that stromal fibroblasts inhibit human BFU-E development in vitro (Gordon et al 1983) and that the stroma is inhibitory to erythropoiesis in a hamster system (Eastment and Ruscetti 1982). Previous studies have shown that human fetal liver cultures can sustain the presence of BFU-E for up to 7 weeks in vitro but no details of culture conditions or cell numbers were provided to enable assessment of the significance of this observation (Stamatoyannopoulos et al 1981). Thus, while not solving the problem of long-term in vitro erythropoiesis, this system, with its rapid shift from erythroid to granulocytic cell production in vitro, may be of great value in dissecting the influence of the accessory cell microenvironment on the direction of hemopoietic cell differentiation.

References

Cappellini MD, Potter CG, Wood WG (1984). Long term haemopoiesis in fetal liver cultures. Brit J Haematol **57**:61.
Coulombel L, Eaves AC, Eaves CJ (1983). Enzymatic treatment of long-term human marrow cultures reveals the preferential location of primitive hemopoietic progenitors in the adherent layer. Blood **62**:291.
Dexter TM, Allen TD, Lajtha LG (1977). Conditions controlling the proliferation of hemopoietic stem cells in vitro. J Cell Physiol **91**:335.
Dexter TM, Testa NG, Allen TD, Rutherford T, Scolnick E (1982). Molecular and cell biologic aspects of erythropoiesis in long term bone marrow cultures. Blood **58**:699.

Eastment CE, Ruscetti FW (1982). Evaluation of erythropoiesis in long-term hamster bone marrow suspension cultures: absence of a requirement for adherent monolayer cells. Blood **60**:999.

Eliason JF, Testa NG, Dexter TM (1979). Erythropoietin-stimulated erythropoiesis in long term marrow culture. Nature **281**:382.

Gartner S, Kaplan HS (1980). Long-term culture of human bone marrow cells. Proc Natl Acad Sci USA **77**:4756.

Gordon MY, Kearney L, Hibbin JA (1983). Effects of human marrow stromal cells on proliferation by human granulocyte (GM-CFC), erythroid (BFU-E) and mixed (MIX-CFC) colony forming cells. Brit J Haematol **53**:317.

Hocking WG, Golde DW (1979). Long term human bone marrow cultures. Blood **56**:118.

Moore MAS, Sheridan APC (1979). Pluripotential stem cell replication in continuous human prosimian and murine bone marrow cultures. Blood Cells **5**:297.

Potter CG, Rowell AC, Weatherall DJ (1981). Continuous long term culture of human bone marrow. Clin Lab Haematol **3**:245.

Stamatoyannopoulos G, Papayannopoulou T, Brice M, Kurachi S, Nakamoto B, Lim G, Farquhar M (1981). Cell biology of hemoglobin switching. In Stamatoyannopoulos G and Nienhuis AW: 'Hemoglobins in Development and Differentiation', New York: AR Liss, p 287.

Toogood IRG, Dexter TM, Allen TD, Suda T, Lajtha LG (1980). The development of a liquid culture system for the growth of human bone marrow. Leuk Res **4**:449.

CRYOPRESERVATION OF HUMAN FETAL LIVER: FACTORS INFLUENCING GRANULOCYTE-MACROPHAGE COLONY (CFU-GM) SURVIVAL AFTER CRYO-PRESERVATION

Moretti L., Stramigioli S., Talevi N., Bartolucci M., Marchetti-Rossi M.T., Polchi P., Porcellini A., Lucarelli G..

Divisione di Ematologia, Ospedale di Pesaro. U.S.L. N. 3 , Pesaro, Italy.

Bone marrow transplantation has emerged as an effective therapy in several diseases including immunodeficiency disease, aplastic anemia and acute leukemia. Unfortunately, most patients lack an H.L.A.-identical donor.

There are considerable data in animals suggesting a potential role of fetal liver as an alternative source of hematopoietic stem cells for transplantation, with low frequence of severe graft-versus-host disease (G.V.H.D.) Uphoff 1958. Van Putten 1968. Lowenberg 1975. Lucarelli 1981.

Recently the possibility of using human fetal liver cell suspension to restore hemopoiesis in aplastic anemia and acute leukemia has been reported by the Group of Pesaro, confirming previous observations of other authors. Thomas 1959. Scott 1961. Kelemen 1973. Kansal 1979. Lucarelli 1979, 1983.

In order to propose the use of human fetal liver transplantation, a correct and reproduceable tecnique of cryopreservation of fetal liver cells is urgently required.

We have examined the effects of different important variables namely the effect of cryoprotective agent, rate of cooling and various thawing manipulations.

The present studies were undertaken to examine and compare these important variables in cryopreservation of human fetal liver cells.

MATERIALS AND METHODS

1) PREPARATION OF HUMAN FETAL LIVER CELLS SUSPENSION.

Human fetuses were provided by various Institutions in Italy following spontaneous abortions of hysterectomy procedures. Fetuses were obtained from dead abortuses after informed maternal consent. The age of fetus was estimated by the last menstrual period. Fetal livers were minced with scissors and suspended in Hank's balanced salt solution (H.B.S.S.). The fragments were dispersed mechanically by vigorous pipetting and passed twice through a stainless steel mesh and a 21 and a 25 gauge needle to produce a single cell suspension.

2) FREEZING METHOD.

Fetal liver cells suspended in HBSS for the freezing experiments were mixed at +10° C, with an equal volume of the cryopreservation medium, containing 20% of dimethyl sulphoxide (D.M.S.O.), 80% or 40% A.B.Rh negative serum. The final concentration of D.M.S.O. in the suspension was 10%. The cellular suspension was transfered into polyolefin freezing bags (UCAR) and 2 ml polypropylene vials (NUNC). The bags were trasferred, pressed between aluminum holders in the freezing chamber of an electronic freezer (NICOOL 416. SIO, Italy), with a programmed freezer rate.

The cooling rate in degrees centigrade per minute was recorded by inserting a thermocouple into bags which contained the freezing medium. The specimens were cooled from +10° C to -140° C at predetermined rates of 0,5°, 1°, 2°, 3°, 5° C/min. At the end of the freezing cycle the bags were rapidly placed into a liquid nitrogen container at -196° C. Moretti 1979, 1981.

3) THAWING PROCEDURE.

The specimens were removed from the storage container and

rapidly thawed in +37° C water bath without agitation. Using the thawed specimen, the effects of cooling rate, washing and storage on stem cell viability were examined, using the agar culture method.

4) IN VITRO STUDIES.

Nucleated cell counts were performed using an electronic blood cell counter. Slides were made and cell morphology was examined. Microbiological cultures were performed on all fetal liver cells after cryopreservation. Myeloid stem cell assays (CFU-GM) were performed in the semisolid agar system. Cell samples were plated at a concentration of 1×10^5 cells/plate in 0,3% Mc Coy's agar containing 10% fetal calf serum (F.C.S.). Colony stimulating activity was provided by human placenta conditioned medium (H.P.C.M.). Porcellini 1983. The samples were cultured in triplicate. Colonies of at least 50 cells were counted after 10 days of incubation in 7.5% CO_2 at +37° C. The results were expressed as number of colonies per 1×10^5 cells/plate or per total number of cells per organ (means ±1 SD). Student's "t" tests were used for analysis where appropriate.

RESULTS.

Data on fetal liver are summarized in Tab. 1. From January 1978 to August 1984, 98 fetuses at various gestational ages have been studied. The number of nucleated cells per organ varied from 0.04 to 7.4×10^9 cells. 58 fetal liver cells suspensions were thawed, the nucleated cells count ranged from values of 0.1 to 5.0×10^9, with a medium recovery of 74%. The CFU-GM content in the liver at varying gestational ages prior to cryopreservation is reported in Tab. 2.

Age (weeks)	Number of fetuses	N.N.C. $\times 10^9$	Number of fetuses thawed	N.N.C. $\times 10^9$	N.N.C. % recovery
8- 9	2	0.04	–	–	–
10-11	25	0.16	9	0.10	66.6
12-13	5	0.48	1	0.28	60.0
14-15	7	1.56	5	1.00	72.0
16-17	12	2.07	4	1.45	70.3
18-19	7	4.50	6	3.90	87.0
20-21	17	5.64	17	4.34	77.0
22-23	15	5.40	9	5.70	93.7
24-25	7	7.40	7	5.02	68.0
26-29	1	3.90	–	–	–

Tab. 1 – CRYOPRESERVATION OF FETAL LIVER CELLS. PESARO 1978-84.
Note: N.N.C. Number of Nucleated Cells; results are means.

Age (weeks)	Number of fetuses	CFU-GM/1×10^5	Total CFU-GM/organ $\times 10^4$
8- 9	2	45.5 ± 5.6	0.9
10-11	25	21.6 ± 4.2	4.5
12-13	5	26.2 ± 3.5	26.2
14-15	7	16.4 ± 2.2	25.7
16-17	12	25.1 ± 5.6	98.4
18-19	7	12.5 ± 1.7	108.3
20-21	17	15.7 ± 3.0	63.5
22-23	15	21.6 ± 9.4	120.8
24-25	7	37.3 ± 2.2	348.8
26-29	1	5.7	28.5

Tab. 2 – CFU-GM CONTENT AT VARIOUS GESTATIONAL AGES.
Note: results are means ± 1 S.D.

Effect of DMSO.

The CFU-GM assay performed immediately before and after the addition of dimethyl sulphoxide (D.M.S.O.) indicated that the addition in a final concentration of 10% significantly inibits the CFU-GM growth (Fig. 1).

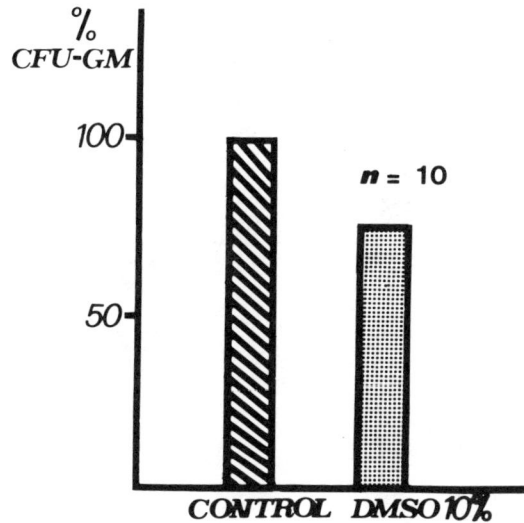

Fig. 1 - EFFECT OF DMSO ON CFU-GM RECOVERY.
Note: results are means; control = fresh suspension; n = number of samples studied.

Effect of cryopreservative medium.

The use of a culture medium with both 20% and 40% of A.B. Rh. negative serum, showed that the best protection is obtained with the lower serum concentration (20%) gave a CFU-GM recovery of 76,2%, as compared to 59,6% obtained with 40% of A.B. serum at 1° C/min.; using a higher cooling rate (2° C/min.), the presence of 20% concentration serum showed a recovery of 119.2% and 83.5 with 40% A.B. serum.

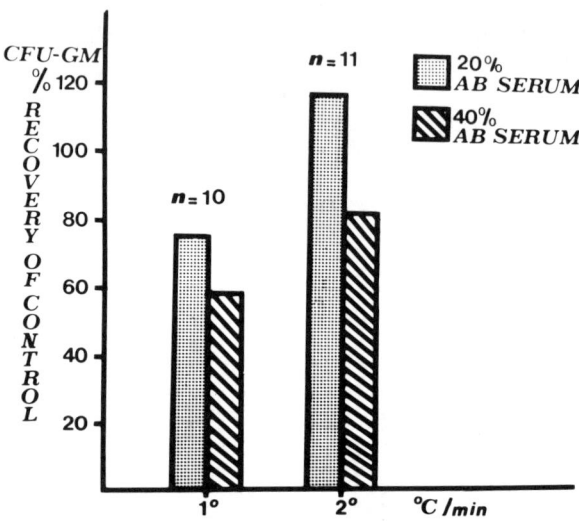

Fig. 2. — EFFECT OF CRYOPRESERVATIVE MEDIUM ON CFU-GM RECOVERY.
Note: see fig. 1.

Effect of cooling rate.

The CFU-GM recovery plotted against the cooling rate is showed in Fig. 3. The mean values of thawed samples, without washing out the DMSO were compared to the prefreezing values and expressed in percent recovery.

Maximum recovery was obtained at a cooling rate of 2º C/min. with peak values of 119.2 ± 10.0. Recovery of CFU-GM declined progressively with cooling rates higher or lower than 2º C/min.

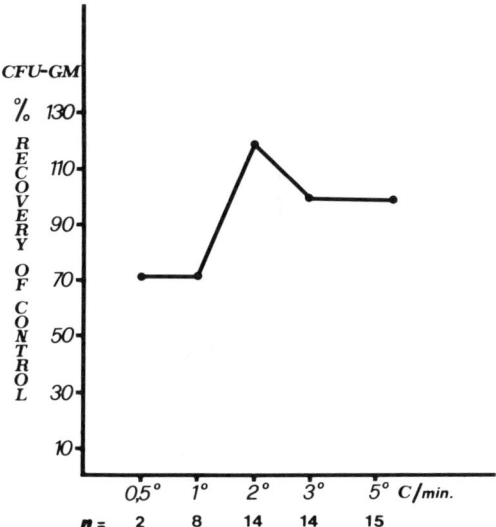

Fig. 3 — EFFECT OF COOLING RATE ON CFU-GM RECOVERY.
Note: see fig. 1.

Effect of washing on thawed cells.

After thawing aliquots of cryopreserved cells were centrifuged at 1000 rpm for 10 min., the cell pellet resuspended in HBSS with 10% A.B. serum and cells plated in semisolid agar for the CFU-GM assay as previously described. Porcellini 1983.
It was found that removing the DMSO caused a recovery of CFU-GM/per plate of 129% of the prefreezing values. However calculation of total CFU-GM per whole fetal liver, showed a reduction of 50%, as compared to values obtained with fresh fetal liver cells suspension (Fig. 4).

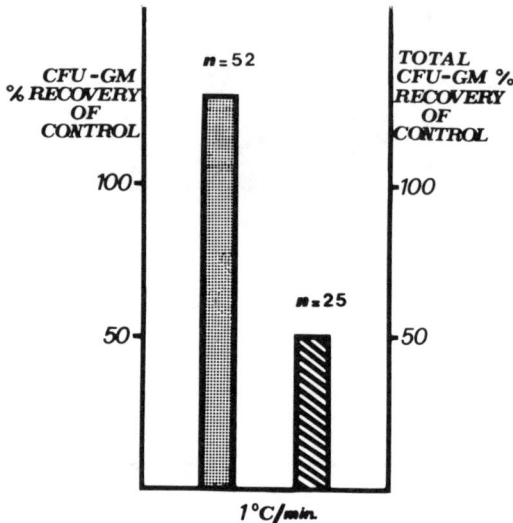

Fig. 4 — EFFECT OF WASHING ON CFU-GM RECOVERY.
Note: see fig. 1.

Effect of storage in ampoules versus bags.

To examine the effect of two different types of storage containers on CFU-GM recovery, cells from the same fetal liver were cryopreserved both in bags and in ampoules under the same freezing procedures. The recovery % of CFU-GM was calculated in these samples. As shown the results from both bags and ampoules, expressed as % of recovery were similar.
It was found that the recovery of CFU-GM in bags ranged from 85 to 39% and recovery of CFU-GM in ampoules ranged from 77 to 35%. Ampoules and bags were removed from liquid nitrogen at variables intervals up to a period of 4 years and the CFU-GM recovery remained reasonably constant over 48 months of storage (Fig. 5).

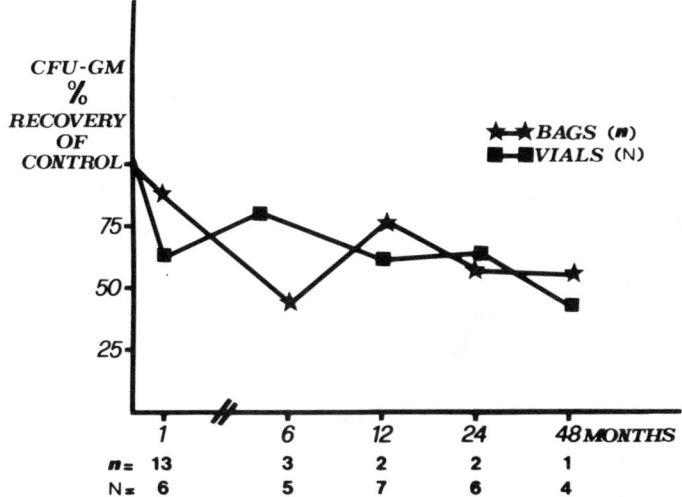

Fig. 5 — EFFECT OF STORAGE IN AMPOULES VERSUS BAGS.
Note: results are means; control = fresh suspension; n = number or bags studied; N = number of ampoules studied.

DISCUSSION

Preliminary studies in man have confirmed animal data indicating that fetal liver cells are source of hematopoietic stem cells with decreased immune reactivity. The success of fetal liver transplantation depends on the presence of sufficient hemopoietic stem cells to restore hematopoiesis in a recipient. Thereafter it has become urgent to adapt the technique of cryopreservation of bone marrow to the cryopreserved of fetal liver cells suspension.

During the last few years many experimental studies have been performed on the cryopreservation of fetal liver cells, but most of the experiences have been performed in animals, on the basis of data previously obtained from the cryopreservation of bone marrow cells. Fereebee 1959. Githens 1961. Polchi 1978. Prümmer 1983.

From our results it appears that the fetal liver cells are more resistent using higher cooling rates. These cells differ from bone marrow cells, in size, function and probably in physical-chemical characteristics (i.e. permeability to cryoprotective agents, concentration of intercellular electrolytes, toxicity to cryoprotective agents, etc.).

To the purpose of a more efficient cryopreservation of fetal liver cells this study was carried out, to determine the optimal cooling and thawing conditions for human fetal liver cells frozen in the presence of 10% of DMSO.

The DMSO at the concentration of 10% was found to be relatively toxic to the fetal liver cells shown by the in vitro CFU-GM studies, while usually it does not inhibit the CFU-GM growth of bone marrow cells. Ma 1982.

It was shown that the optimal cooling rate for fetal liver cells ranged between 2° C to 5° C/min.

In contrast to what happens on bone marrow where the survival of CFU-GM varies with cooling rates, according to the Mazur's hypotesis of freezing injury, that at cooling rates above the optimal cooling rate the cells are destroyed by events associated with intracellular freezing, while at cooling rates below the optimal cooling rates the cells succumb to the increased concentration of solute intra and extracellular solute. Mc Gaan 1981.

This difference can be found in the diverse capacity of fetal liver cells and bone marrow cells to resist osmotic variations of the extracellular medium. Perhaps the cellular membrane of fetal liver cells has a different capacity of adapting to the osmotic variations which resists more to the elevated rates which normally cause intercellular freezing. However further studies are necessary in order to better higlight the effect of cooling rate either below 0.5° C/min. or above 5° C/min. respectively.

The purpose of washing by centrifugation is to remove from the freezing solution the DMSO and free hemoglobin which may be harmful to humans. Because of this studies, infusion in vivo was performed without washing but only by dilution with HBSS and A.B. serum. Our clinical experience has demonstrated that infusion of up to 40 gr. of DMSO had no adverse effect on patients.

It was found that washing increased the recovery of CFU-GM per plate, but reduced the total numbers of CFU-GM per organ. In numerous cases the CFU-GM yeld after thawing was higher than that originally present in the fresh suspension. It may be due to the high numbers of granulocyte precursors and mature granulocyte that are selectively damaged by the cryopreservation procedures. Moretti 1983.

The results compared to those without washing, show that the optimal recovery of fetal liver cells, for clinical use, are without centrifugation.

CONCLUSION

At present the factor affecting the fetal liver survival after cryopreservation are:
1. - HBSS 80% and A.B. serum 20% as medium of suspension.
2. - DMSO 10% as cryoprotective agent.
3. - The use of electronical programmed freezer.
4. - The optimal cooling rate is 2° C/min.
5. - Removal of DMSO with centrifugation is not necessary.

REFERENCES

FEREEBEE J.W., LOCHTE H.L., SWANBER H., THOMAS E.D.
The collection and storage of viable human fetal hematopoietic tissue for intravenous use.
Blood 14: 1173. 1959.
GITHENS J.H., TSCHETTER P.N., MOSCOVICI G.M., HATHAWAY W.E.
Studies of irradiation protection effect of fetal liver in mince II. Storage by freezing.
Blood 10: 344-348. 1961
KANSAL V., SOOD S.K., BATRA A.K., ADHAR G., MALVIYA A.K., KUCHERIA K., BALAKRISHNAN K.
Fetal liver transplantation in aplastic anemia.
Acta Hemat. 62. 128-136. 1979.
KELEMEN E.
Recovery from chronic idiopathic bone marrow aplasia of young mother after intravenous injection of unprocessed cells

from liver of her 22 mm. lenght embryo.
Scand. J. Haemat. 11: 305-308. 1973.
LOWENBERG B.
Fetal liver cell transplantation role and nature of fetal haemopoietic stem cell.
Radiobiological Institute of O.H.R.T.N.O. Rijswijk. Netherlands. 1975.
LUCARELLI G., IZZI T., PORCELLINI A., DELFINI C., POLCHI P., MORETTI L., MANNA A., GRILLI G.
Fetal liver transplantation in aplastic anemia and acute leukemia in "Fetal Liver Transplantation" Eds. Lucarelli G., Fliedner T.M., Gale R.P.
Excerpta Medica p. 284-299. 1980.
LUCARELLI G., ANDREANI M., AGOSTINELLI F., MANNA M., MORETTI L., POLCHI P.
Transplantation of fetal liver at different ages in the rat.
Blut 42. 337. 1981.
LUCARELLI G., IZZI T., PORCELLINI A., DELFINI C., GALIMBERTI M., POLCHI P., MORETTI L., MANNA A., SPARAVENTI G.
Fetal liver transplantation in aplastic anemia and acute leukemia in "Recent Advances in Bone Marrow Transplantation" Alan L. Inc. N.Y. p. 865-874. 1983.
MA D.D.F., JOHNSON L.A., CHAMP. M., BIGGS J.C.
Factors influencing myeloid stem cell CFU-C survival after cryopreservation of human marrow and chronic granulocytic leukemia cells.
Cryobiology 19. 1-9. 1982.
MC GAAN L.E., TURNER A.R., ALLALUNIS M.J., TURC J.M.
Cryopreservation of human peripheral blood stem cells: optimal cooling and warming conditions.
Cryobiology 18. 469-472. 1981.
MORETTI L., POLCHI P., STRAMIGIOLI S., ANDREANI M., CORTIGLIONI P., MANNA M., IZZI T., LUCARELLI G.
Contributo allo studio della tecnica di criopreservazione di cellule di fegato fetale.
Proc. 3th Nat. Meeting of Exp. Hematology. p. 223-240. 1979.
MORETTI L., POLCHI P., MANNA M., TALEVI N., MANNA A., PORCELLINI A.
Cryopreservation of human fetal liver cells.

Proc. 4th Nat. Meeting of Exp. Hematology. p. 64-70. 1981.
MORETTI L., PORCELLINI A., TALEVI N., STRAMIGIOLI S., DONATI M., SPARAVENTI G.
Cryopreservation of human fetal liver.
Proc. 5th Nat. Meeting of Exp. Hematology. p. 150-152. 1983.
POLCHI P., MORETTI L., MANNA M., BENETTI P., AGOSTINELLI F., ANDREANI M., PROIETTI A., FONTEBUONI A., LUCARELLI G.
Trapianto di fegato fetale criopreservato nel ratto.
Haematologica 63. 265. 1978.
PORCELLINI A., MANNA A., MANNA M., TALEVI N., DELFINI C., MORETTI L., RIZZOLI V.
Ontogeny of granulocyte-macrophage progenitor cells in the human fetus.
Int. J. of Cell Cloning 1. 92-104. 1983.
PRÜMMER O., ARUNA R., CALVO W., CARBONELL F. FLIEDNER T.M.
Restoration of hemopoiesis by cryopreserved fetal liver cells in canine model.
Recent Advances in B.M. Transplantation. Alan L. Inc. N.Y. p. 857-863. 1983.
SCOTT R.B., MATTHIAS J.Q., CONSTANDOULAKIS M., KAY H.E.M., LUCAS P.F., WHITESIDE J.D.
Hipoplastic anemia treated by transfusion of foetal haemopoietic cells.
Brit. Med. J. 2. 1385-1388. 1961.
THOMAS E.D., YAFFEY J.M.
Human foetal haematopoiesis II.
Brit. J. Hematol. 10: 193. 1959.
THOMAS E.D., COLLINS Y.A., KASAKURA S., FEREEBEE J.W.
Lethally irradiated dogs given infusion of fetal and hematopoietic tissue.
Transplantation 1: 514-520. 1963.
UPHOFF D.E.
The preclusion of secondary phase of irradiation syndrome by inoculating of fetal hemopoietic tissue following total body irradiation.
J. Nat. Cancer Inst. 20. 625. 1958.
VAN PUTTEN L.M., VAN BEKKUM D.W., DE VRIES M.J.
Transplantation of foetal hemopoietic cells in irradiated rhesus monkeys.
In "Radiation and control of immune response". Vienna. International Atomic Energy Agency. p. 41. 1968.

ISOLATION OF ERYTHROID AND MYELOID HEMATOPOIETIC PROGENITORS FROM HUMAN FETAL LIVER

Stephen G. Emerson, M.D., Ph.D.

Division of Hematology, Brigham & Women's Hospital, Hematology/Oncology, Dana-Farber Cancer Institute and Children's Hospital, and the Departments of Medicine and Pediatrics, Harvard Medical School, Boston, MA 02115

While the physiologic regulation of hematopoiesis is believed to focus at the level of the progenitor cell, direct studies of such mechanisms have been hindered by the extreme rarity of these cells in the bone marrow and peripheral blood (1,2,3). Approaches to the purification of progenitor cells have included differential density centrifugation (4) and density gradient electrophoresis (5), immune selection utilizing rosetting (6) or fluorescence activated cell sorting (7,8), and various combinations of these physical and immunologic techniques (9). While these techniques have led to a significant progenitor enrichment, cell yields have been notably low, particularly when the prefractionation sample consists of normal, non-neoplastic human hematopoietic cells. This limitation has heretofore restricted biochemical analysis of the enriched progenitors, and has failed to permit detailed studies of the interactions of growth factor and accessory cells with the human progenitor cells.

We have therefore developed a simple and efficient procedure to purify large numbers of human erythroid and myeloid progenitors. Beginning with fetal liver cells, which are two-to-five fold enriched for progenitors compared with bone marrow (10,11,12), the technique utilizes negative selection by panning (13,14,15) to greatly enrich the progenitor cells. This preparative method recovers the majority of progenitors detectable in unfractionated fetal liver, and provides, for the first time, sufficient numbers of progenitors to allow direct morphological and biochemical studies of these cells. In this report, we describe this progenitor purification technique, present preliminary morphologic analysis of the progenitors, and employ fluorescence antibody labelling to measure directly the presence of class II histocompatibility antigen in these critical cells.

Methods

<u>Isolation of progenitor cells from fetal liver</u> (Figure 1). Abortuses induced by prostaglandin infusion were obtained within thirty minutes of delivery from patients who had previously signed consent forms for research studies, under a protocol approved by the Brigham and Women's Hospital Human Investigation Committee. Livers from 17 to 23 week fetuses were sterilely dissected and teased into IMDM containing 50 mg% collagenase Type IV (Sigma Pharmaceuticals, St. Louis, Mo) using forceps and scissors. Hepatic stroma was digested by incubating the collagenase rich cell suspension at 37° under 5% CO_2 for 15 to 30 minutes (16) and large clumps were allowed to settle out by standing the cell suspension in vertical 50 ml centrifuge tubes. A mononuclear cell preparation was prepared by centrifugation over Ficoll Hypaque SG 1.077, through which sedimented mature blood cells and hepatocytes. The cells at the interface were washed three times, and then subjected to a second buoyant density separation over Ficoll Hypaque SG 1.077. The cells at the interface were washed three times and then depleted of adherent cells by overnight adherence to 100 x 15 mm plastic tissue culture dishes (Lux, Miles Laboratories, Naperville, IL) in IMDM[1] with 20% FCS at 37° under 5% CO_2.

Non-adherent cells were incubated with saturating quantities of a panel of murine monoclonal antibodies recognizing determinants on maturing human lymphoid, myeloid, and erythroid cells (Table 1) for one hour at $4^{o}C$. Labelled cells were then washed three times to remove excess antibody prior to panning. Preparative separation of antibody-negative cells (panning) was performed by a modification of the method of Biddison et. al. (14). Anti-Ig plates were prepared by incubating 100 x 15 mm plastic culture plates (Lux) with 5 ml affinity purified rabbit

---

[1] Abbreviations used in this paper: Ad^-, nonadherent cells; Ab^- antibody negative cells after panning; BSA, bovine serum albumin; FCS, fetal calf serum; GM-CSF, granulocyte-macrophage colony stimulating factor; IMDM, Iscove's modified Dulbecco's Medium; PBS, phosphate-buffed saline.

Isolation of Hematopoietic Progenitors / 137

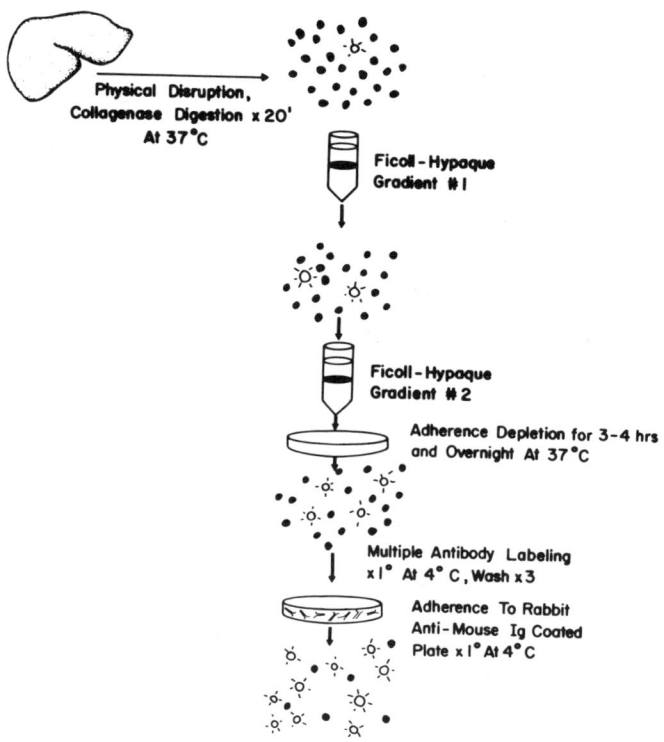

Figure 1. Purification protocol for fetal liver progenitors. Disruption and collagenase digestion followed by two Ficoll-hypaque gradients, adherence depletion, and multiple antibody panning.

anti-mouse Ig (100 ug/ml in PBS) overnight at 4°C and washing with cold PBS prior to use. Coating the plates with less than 250 ug antibody resulted in suboptimal cell binding. Murine antibody-labelled, washed cells were suspended in PBS with 5% heat inactivated FCS and incubated over the rabbit anti-mouse Ig coated plates for 1 hour at

TABLE 1

Monoclonal Antibodies Employed in Fetal Progenitor Purification

Antibody	Specificity	Source
Leu 1	Pan T	Becton Dickinson
Leu 5	Pan T, NK	Becton Dickinson
BA-1	B cell	Hybritech
CALLA	Pre-B cell	Hybritech
Leu 10	HLA-DC	Becton Dickinson
Leu M1	Monocytes, granulocytes	Becton Dickinson
TG-1	Granulocytes, myeloid precursors, some monocytes	P. Beverley (7)
R.18	Erythroid precursors (Glycophorin A)	P. Edwards (26)

$4^{\circ}C$, after which time the non-adherent antibody negative cells were recovered by gentle pipetting without disrupting the antibody coated cells bound to the plates. Incubation times of less than 40 minutes were ineffective at allowing maximal cell binding to the plates, while cells could be allowed to adhere to the plates for at least two hours without decreased binding or subsequent plating efficiency. <u>In vitro short term cultures</u>. Cells were cultured in 0.9% methyl cellulose in $IMDM$ plus 30% FCS, 0.9% deionized BSA (Sigma Fraction V), $10M^{-4}$-mercaptoethanol, 1 unit/ml erythropoietin (Terry Fox Laboratories, Vancouver, B.C.) (17), and 10% Mo cell conditioned medium (kindly provided by Dr. David Golde, UCLA). Red colonies containing at least 100 cells present on day 14 were scored as BFU-E; colonies containing non-hemoglobinized cells (primarily granulocytic precursors and macrophages) were scored as CFU-C, including CFM-M, CFU-G, or CFU-GM, while colonies containing both erythroid elements and one or more classes of non-erythroid

cells were scored as CFU-GEMM. Cultures were plated either in quadruplicate 250 ul volumes in 24 well tissue culture plates or in 10 replicates in 100 ul volumes in 96 well plates (Falcon). The cultures were established at sufficiently low density to clearly distinguish individual colonies, usually 5×10^4 cells/ml for cells after one Ficoll gradient, 10^4 cells/ml for cells obtained after the second gradient step and adherence depletion, and 10^3 cells/ml obtained after depletion by panning. No filler cells or irradiated feeder cells were added to the cultures.
Immunofluorescence staining. After immune depletion by panning, the presence of residual hematopoietic precursor cells was assessed morphologically and by indirect fluorescent labelling under three conditions: 1) Cells were immediately relabelled with fluoresceinated goat anti-mouse Ig to detect residual mouse antibody coated cells; 2) other aliquots of cells were immediately relabelled with the individual murine monoclonal antibodies, followed by fluoresceinated goat anti-mouse Ig to assay cells which had been ineffectively labelled; and 3) a final aliquot was cultured at 37^0 for 4 hours prior to relabelling, to identify cells which might have modulated surface antigens on exposure to the murine antibodies and so escaped the secondary antibody-coated plates. Fluorescent antibody-stained cells were quantitated by flow cytometric analysis (Becton Dickinson fluorescence analyzer).

Results
Cell recovery and analysis through the fractionation. The first ficoll step removed the mature erythrocytes, rare mature myeloid cells and hepatocytes. The cells at the interface were primarily mature erythroid precursors with scattered myeloid and mononuclear precursors. The second ficoll step further removed 70-90% of the cells, including the majority of the more mature hematopoietic precursors, including metamyelocytes, myelocytes, orthrochromatophilic and polychromatophilic normoblasts.

Following adherence depletion, the remaining cells were labelled with a panel of eight murine monoclonal antibodies (Table 1). These antibodies were selected to include at least two antibodies that would detect each major class of leukocyte and anti-glycophorin A to detect the predominant antigen on erythroid precursors. The use of several overlapping anti-leukocyte antibodies and a very potent anti-erythroid antibody allowed for excellent cell depletion after a single 1 hour pan at 4^0C. Under a variety of relabelling conditions, no more than 2% of the remaining

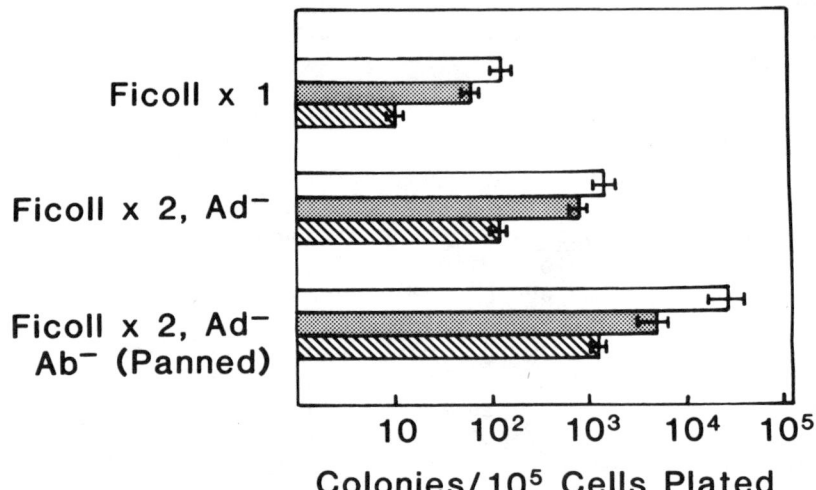

Figure 2. Progressive purification of fetal liver progenitors. Aliquots of cells were removed from three steps in the purification protocol and plated in methylcellulose in the presence of erythropoietin and Mo cell CM. (☐), BFU-E; (▒), CFU-C; (▨), CFU-GEMM. All data are means ± standard deviations, and are compiled from twelve experiments.

cells were stained with antibodies detecting known hemato-lymphoid subsets. The single pan removed 90-95% of the cells, and the remaining antibody-negative cells were at least 97% viable by trypan blue exclusion.

Progressive purification of hematopoietic progenitors. This sequential fractionation procedure resulted in marked enrichment of the progenitor cells (Figure 2). The mononuclear cells obtained after one Ficoll step contained approximately 0.3% progenitors. After the second gradient step and adherence depletion, over 3% of the remaining cells scored as progenitors in vitro. Following the panning step, the progenitors were greatly enriched with 22-75% of the cells scoring as progenitors in short term culture.

The majority of the progenitors present in the original fetal liver mononuclear cell suspension were recovered throughout the fractionation procedure. In the final

fraction, after double ficoll separation, adherence depletion and panning, 88 ± 10% of BFU-E, 62 ± 20% of CFU-GM and 98 ± 10% of CFU-GEMM were recovered. Thus the 2-60 x 10^6 cells obtained from each fractionation contained most of the progenitors present in the original fetal liver.
Linear plating efficiency to low cell concentration. This high degree of progenitor purity permitted short term in vitro culture at low cell density. Cells obtained following the first ficoll step were routinely cultured at 10^5 cells/ml, and could only be diluted to 10^4 cells/ml while still retaining normal growth characteristics. Below this concentration the colonies which began to develop disintegrated a few days into the culture. Cells obtained following a second gradient separation and adherence depletion could be cultured over a range from 10^3-10^5 cells/ml with linear plating characteristics.

The highly enriched progenitors isolated after panning could be cultured at 10^2-10^4 cell/ml while maintaining qualitatively normal colony growth and linear plating characteristics. When cultured at higher density, the colonies overlapped in the plates and could not be accurately enumerated. When the cells were plated at less than 10^2/ml (10-25 cells per well), colony growth was poor, with only small poorly differentiated colonies which disintegrated prematurely.
Initial characterization of the purified progenitors. Sufficient quantities of purified progenitors were thus obtained to permit direct morphological, biochemical and histochemical characterization of these cells. When stained with routine Wright-Giemsa, the cells appeared to be undifferentiated blasts of variable size with basophilic cytoplasm, prominent Golgi zones, and often containing multiple nucleoli. In addition, the cell membranes showed many small areas of extrusion suggesting uropod formation (Figure 3). There were no detectable cells resembling small lymphocytes, and as expected, only very rare contaminating recognizable erythroid or myeloid precursors. The panned progenitor cells did not stain with standard histochemical dyes, including myeloperoxidase, periodic acid-Schiff, nonspecific esterase, alkaline phosphatase, and acid phosphatase.

The purified progenitors were then directly analyzed for the presence of class II histocomptibility antigens. Labelling with murine anti-human HLA-DR demonstrated a biphasic pattern of fluorescence, with approximately 35% of the cells labelling brightly and the remainder showing dimmer fluorescence (Figure 4). Few if any of the cells were

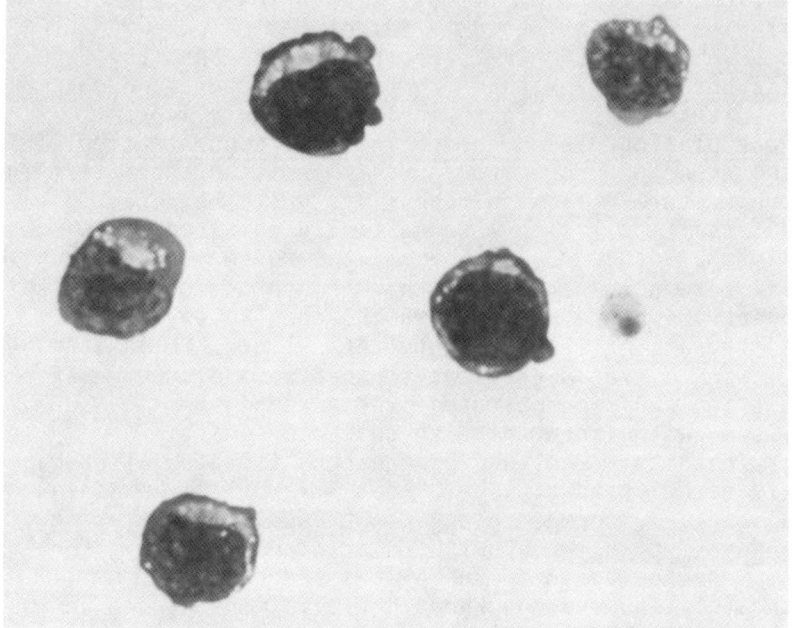

Figure 3. Wright-Giemsa stain of the panned progenitor cells. Note the prominent Golgi, nucleoli, and membrane exfoliation. Colony frequencies from this particular preparation were: BFU-E 39%, CFU-GM 9.5%, CFU-GEMM 1.5%.

truly DR$^-$, as the fluorocytogram for even the dimly staining cells was shifted in its entirety as compared with control staining. As anticipated, none of the cells labelled with mouse anti-human HLA-DC.

Discussion

Negative selection by panning provides a superior method for the isolation of large numbers of highly enriched, relatively unmanipulated progenitors. The calculated progenitor frequency of 22-75% may actually be an underestimate of the actual number of progenitors present in the final fraction. Visser et.al. have found that murine progenitor cells which they calculate to be 100% in vivo primary CFU-S have only a 25-30% plating efficiency in vitro (18). Ogawa and his colleagues (19) have found that the replating efficiency of observable, dividing colony

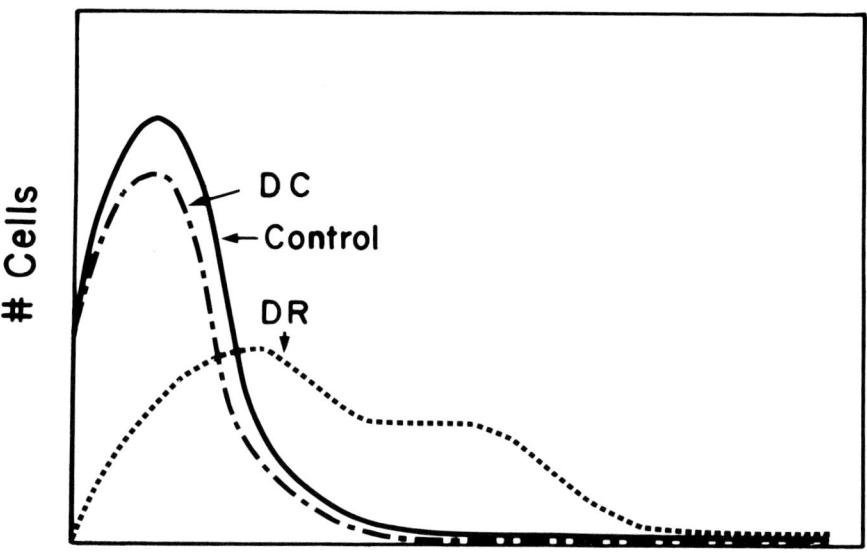

Figure 4. Class II histocompatibility antigens on the panned progenitor cells. Cells obtained following multiple antibody labelling and panning depletion were relabelled with mouse anti-human HLA-DR (Becton Dickinson) or mouse anti-human HLA-DC (Leu-10, Becton Dickinson) followed by fluoresceinated rabbit anti-mouse Ig. The spectrum of antigen density on the panned cells was measured by flow cytometry. (.....)-HLA-DR,(-.-.)HLA-DC,(-----) NMS control. Colony frequencies from this preparation were: BFU-E 55%, CFU-GM 11%, CFU-GEMM 3.5%.

progenitors is only 50-75%. Thus the actual frequency of progenitors in the post-panning fraction may be closer to 50-100%, with the lower observed frequency due to the imperfect plating efficiency of the methyl cellulose system itself.

This approach has several advantages over other techniques for progenitor purification. Unlike rosetting (20) or complement mediated lysis, panning involves no potential nonspecific toxins, such as $CrCl_3$ or complement, which can damage the progenitors. This is extremely important for normal progenitors, which we have found are quite sensitive to nonspecific damage by $CrCl_3$ coupled red cells used for rosetting, unlike leukemic progenitors which may be somewhat more resistant. Moreover, the panning procedure is based on the labelling of only undesired cells, without direct manipulation of the progenitors, themselves. Thus the in vitro behavior of the recovered progenitors is unlikely to be artifactually influenced by the antibody treatment per se. Finally, panning is very simple and easy to perform, and results in an extremely high yield of recovered progenitors. In these respects it is superior to multi-parameter fluorescence-activated cell sorting, for example, which requires sophisticated equipment and still results in typical cell yields of only 20-50%.

The isolated progenitors appear to be basophilic, undifferentiated blasts with prominent Golgi zones and frequent membranous extrusions. The active Golgi suggests that these cells are actively synthesizing membrane glycoproteins, likely including membrane receptors for hematopoietic growth factors. Thus these cells might be an excellent cell population for identification and study of such receptors. The unusual folded membrane may reflect submembranous cytoskeletal structures responsible for the immature progenitors' motility thought to be responsible for the multicentric nature of erythroid bursts and multilineage colonies.

The direct fluorescence labelling analysis of class II major histocompatibility antigens confirms previous reports of differential expression of DR versus DC antigens (21,22), and may further explain why initial experiments suggested that approximately one-half or the progenitor pool was found to be DR-negative (23). As the DR distribution is strongly bimodal, it is possible that the use of suboptimal antibody or complement concentrations may have obscured the presence of DR-dim progenitors, as has been recently demonstrated by Falkenburg et.al (24). Alternatively, it is possible that the two peaks of fluorescence are actually detecting distinct products of two different DR gene loci (25). Direct radiolabelling studies of these purified progenitors could indeed address this alternative possibility.

Ideally, one would like to be able to culture these progenitors at limiting dilution to address directly questions such as the role of soluble factor, and auxiliary cells in altering the stochastic program of differentiating progenitors. Thus far, however, we have only succeeded in routinely culturing these cells at 100 cells/ml (10-25 cells/well), despite trials of irradiated feeder layers, added progenitor conditioned culture medium, and a variety of added soluble factors. Whether fetal progenitors require a continuous supply of autocrine factors, or have stringent buffering requirements which we have not yet solved remains to be determined.

The method for progenitor purification should prove to be extremely valuable for the direct study of the regulation of hematopoiesis. The preparations provide, for the first time, sufficient normal cells for the direct biochemical isolation of human progenitor membrane proteins, including membrane receptors for such proteins as erythropoietin and GM-CSF. Likewise, these cells should be an excellent assay system for the evaluation of potential newly isolated hematopoietic growth factors such as human burst promoting activity or the human equivalent of interleukin-3. Similarly, the purified progenitors are an ideal immunogen and screening cell source for the generation and screening of antibodies truly specific for hematopoietic progenitors. Purification by panning is thus a simple, highly efficient technique for the isolation of fetal liver progenitors, and should prove to be a valuable tool for improving our understanding of the molecular and cellular regulation of human hematopoiesis.

Acknowledgements

Dr. Emerson is the recipient of a Clinical Investigator Award for the National Heart, Lung and Blood Institute. These studies were supported by U.S. Public Health Service grants, P01-CA18662 and K08-HL01378, and by a grant from the the Dyson Foundation.

References

1. Stephenson, J.R., A.A. Axelrad, D.L. McLeod, and M.M. Shreve. 1971. Induction of hemoglobin synthesizing cells by erythropoietin in vitro. Proc. Natl. Acad. Sci. USA 68:1542-1546.

2. Bradley, T.R. and D. Metcalf. 1966. The growth of mouse bone marrow cells in vitro. Austr. J. Exp. Biol. Med. Sci. 44:287-300.

3. Fauser, A.A. and H.A. Messner. 1978. Granuloerythropoietic colonies in human bone marrow, peripheral blood, and cord blood. Blood 52:1243-1248.

4. Wells, J.R., G. Opelz, and M.J. Cline. 1977. Characterization of functionally distinct lymphoid and myeloid cells from human blood and bone marrow. I. Separation by a buoyant density gradient technique. J. Immunol. Method. 18:63-78.

5. Platsoucas, C.D., J. D. Beck, N. Kapoor, R.A. Good, and S. Gupta. 1981. Separation of human bone marrow cell population by density gradient electrophoresis: Differential mobilities of myeloid (CFU-C), monocytoid and lymphoid cells. Cell Immunol. 59:345-354.

6. Griffin, J.D., R.P. Beveridge, and S.F. Schlossman. 1982. Isolation of myeloid progenitor cells from peripheral blood of chronic myelogenous leukemia patients. Blood 60:30-37.

7. Beverley, P.C.L., D. Linch, and D. Delia. 1980. Isolation of human haematopoietic progenitor cells using monoclonal antibodies. Nature 287:332-333.

8. Bodger, M.P., G.E. Francis, D. Delia, S.M. Granger and G. Janassy. 1981. A monoclonal antibody specific for immature human hemopoietic cells and T lineage cells. J. Immunol. 127:2269-2274.

9. Nicola, N.A, D. Metcalf, H. von Melchner, and A.W. Burgess. 1981. Isolation of murine fetal hemopoetin progenitor cells and selective fractionation of various erythroid precursors. Blood. 58:376-386.

10. Rowley, P.T., B.M. Ohlsson-Wilhelm and B.A. Farley. 1978. Erythroid colony formation from human fetal liver. Proc. Natl. Acad. Sci. USA. 75:984-988.

11. Hassan, M.W., J.D. Lutton, R.D. Levere, R.F. Reider and L.L. Cederquist. 1979. In vitro culture of erythroid colonies from human fetal liver and umbilical cord blood. Br. J. Haemotol. 41:477-484.

12. Hann, I.M., M.P. Bodgen, and A.V. Hoffbrand. 1983. Development of pluripotent hematopoietic progenitor cells in the human fetus. Blood 62:118-123.

13. Wysocki, L.J. and V.L. Sato. 1978. Panning for lymphocytes: A method for cell selection. Proc. Natl. Acad. Sci. USA. 75:2844-2848.

14. Biddison, W.E., S.O. Sharrow and G.M. Shearer. 1981. T cell subpopulations required for the human cytolytic T lymphocyte response to influenza virus: Evidence for T cell help. J. Immunol. 127:487-491.

15. Greenberg, P.L., S. Baker, M. Link and J. Minowada.

1985. Immunologic selection of hemopoietic precursor cells utilizing antibody-mediated plate binding ("Panning"). Blood 65:190-197.

16. Schwartz, A.L., D. Rupp, and H.F. Lodish. 1980. Difficulties in the quantification of the ASGP receptor on the rat hepatocyte. J. Biol. Chem. 255. 19:9033-9036.

17. Iscove, N.N., F. Sider, and K.N. Winterbalten. 1974. Erythroid colony formation in cultures of mouse and human bone marrow: Analysis of the requirement for erythropoietin by gel filtration and affinity chromatography on agarose-Con-concanavalin A.J. Cell Physiol. 83:309-320.

18. Visser, J.W.M., J.G.J. Bauman, A.H. Mulder, J.F. Eliason and A.M. de Leeuw. 1984. Isolation of murine pheripotent hemopoietic stem cells. J. Exp. Med. 59:1576-1590.

19. Suda, T., J. Suda and M. Ogawa. 1983. Disparate differentiation in mouse hemopoietic cultures derived from paired progenitors. Proc. Natl. Acad. Sci. USA 81:2520-2524.

20. Goding, J. 1976. The chromic chloride method of coupling antigens to erythrocytes: Definition of some important parameters. J. Immunol. Method. 10:61-66.

21. Linch, D.C., L.M. Nadler, E.A. Luther and J.M. Lipton. 1984. Discordant expression of human Ia-like antigens on hematopoietic progenitor cells. J. Immunol. 2324-2329.

22. Falkenburg, J.H.F., J. Jensen, N. van der Vaart-Duinkerken, W.F.J. Veenhof, J. Blotkamp, H.M. Goselink, J. Parlevliet and J.J. van Rood. 1984. Polymorphic and monomorphic HLA-DR determinants on human hematopoietic progenitor cells. Blood 63:1125-1132.

23. Pelus, L.M., S. Saletan, R.T. Silver and M.A.S. Moore. 1982. Expression of Ia-antigens on normal and chronic myelogenous leukemic human granolocyte-macrophage colony forming cells (CFU-GM) is associated with the regulation of cell proliferation by prostaglandin E. Blood. 59:284-292.

24. Falkenburg, J.H.F., N. van der Vaart-Duinkerken, W.F.J. Veenhof, H.M. Goselink, G. van Eden, J. Parlevliet and J. Jansen. 1985. Complement-dependent cytotoxicity in the analysis of antigenic determinants on human hematopoietic

progenitor cells with HLA-DR as a model. Exp. Hematol. 12:817-821.

25. Accolla, R.S. 1983. Analysis of the structural heterogeneity and polymorphism of human Ia antigens. J. Exp. Med. 159:378-393.

26. Robinson, J., C. Sieff, D. Delia, P.A.W. Edwards and M. Greaves. 1981. Expression of cell surface HLA-DR, HLA-ABC and glycophorin during erythroid differentiation. Nature 289:68-69.

HLA-TYPING OF FETAL CELLS USING INTERFERON TREATMENT IN VITRO

Catherine ROYO, Jean-Louis TOURAINE, and Hervé BETUEL
Transplantation and Immunobiology Unit, INSERM U80, Pav.P, Hôpital Edouard Herriot, 69374 Lyon Cédex 08, FRANCE

Determination of the HLA phenotype of fetal cells is important in several circumstances: in fetal liver transplantation, it permits to look for the initial development of donors cells and the establishment of chimeric state; in HLA-associated diseases, it allows prenatal diagnosis of certain conditions. The expression of HLA antigens at the surface of fetal cells, below the age of 3 or 4 months, is relatively low, as compared to adult cells. Several methods can be envisioned to detect either the HLA antigens or their genes: culture of fibroblasts from the fetus then absorption of antisera of known specificities (Singh et al. 1979, Forest et al. 1981), use of cDNA probes for HLA genes. We report herein a more rapid and less tedious method which consists in enhancing the expression of HLA antigens by incubation of fetal cells with interferon *in vitro*, then carrying out the HLA typing as usual. Several authors have previously described the capacity of α-interferon (α-IFN) to increase the density of cell-surface HLA molecules (Class I HLA antigens and β_2-microglobulin (β_2-m)) (Fellous et al. 1979, Basham et al. 1982).

MATERIALS AND METHODS

Tissue samples

Human fetuses originated from induced-abortions performed for therapeutical purposes (in accordance with recommendations issued by the Ethical Committee of the Claude Bernard University). Their gestational ages, ranging from 7 to 23 weeks, were calculated from both the date of the last menstruation period and the crown-rump length, following Streeter's indications.

Cell preparation

Cell suspensions were prepared from fetal thymus, liver and spleen. The organs were gently homogenized in RPMI-1640 medium, using a Tissue Grinder. Enrichment in mononuclear cells from liver and spleen cell suspensions was then performed by centrifugation on a Ficoll-Hypaque gradient(Boyum 1968). The cell viability, determined by the trypan blue exclusion method, was always above 90%.

Induction assay

The recombinant α_2-IFN was provided to us by Dr A. Waitz (Schering Plough, Kenilworth, N. J. and DNAX Research Institute, Palo Alto, Ca., U. S. A.).

Fetal mononuclear cells from thymus, liver and spleen were suspended in RPMI-1640 medium (10^6 cells/ml), supplemented with 10% heat-inactivated human AB serum, glutamine, penicillin and streptomycin. Cells were incubated with α-IFN, at the concentration of 30U/ml, for 24 hrs, at 37°C in an humidified atmosphere of 5% CO_2-95%air. These optimal dose and time of incubation with α-IFN had been previously determined on peripheral blood lymphocytes of adults and children, as well as on lymphoblastoid cell lines, using cytofluorometric analysis of HLA expression. Cells were then washed twice and checked for viability by the trypan blue exclusion method. It was found above 85% in every sample. Finally, cells were processed either for immunofluorescence staining or for HLA A and B typing.

Immunofluorescence staining

The anti-β_2-m murine monoclonal antibody was purchased from Becton-Dickinson (Sunnywale, Ca.). The fluorescein-isothiocyanate conjugated (FITC) goat anti-mouse immunoglobulin (Ig) serum was obtained from Coulter Immunology (Hialeh). It was used at the 1:5 dilution.

Fetal cells (10^6 cells in 50μl of phosphate buffer saline with 2% bovine serum albumin) were incubated with 5μl of monoclonal antibody for 30 min at 4°C and washed twice. Cells were then incubated with 20μl of the FITC goat anti-mouse Ig serum diluted in phosphate buffer saline solution containing 2% bovine serum albumin. Cells stained with FITC only were used as controls for fluorescence background.
After 30 min of incubation at 4°C, and three washes, the fluorescence intensity of the stained cells was determined by cytofluorometry on an Ortho H50 (Ortho Instruments, Westword, Massachussetts). The lymphoid population was gated on the basis of their scatter characteristics. Fluorescence histograms were developed by the DEC LSI.11/23 associated

computer. The percentage of positive cells and the median fluorescence intensity, defined as the channel above and below which 50% of the cell population lay, were then determined.

HLA A and B typing

It was performed by Dr H. Bétuel (Histocompatibility Laboratory, Blood Transfusion Center, Lyon, France), using the two-stage cytotoxicity method (Mittal et al. 1968) with minor modifications (Bétuel et al. 1975). Only thymocytes and spleen cells from from a 13 week-old fetus, following incubation with α-IFN —or with a control medium— were typed, at the present time.

RESULTS

Following incubation of mononuclear cells from fetal thymus, liver and spleen with α-IFN, no increased mortality and no alteration of the scatter profiles were observed. When cells were labeled with anti-β_2-m antibodies, an increase in fluorescence intensity of α-IFN-treated cells, as shown by the shift to the right of the fluorescence curve, was consistently found (Fig.1). This increased β_2-m expression was found on cells from each of the three fetal organs: thymus, liver and spleen (Tables 1,2 and 3). A weaker β_2-m expression was found on untreated thymocytes as compared to untreated splenocytes.

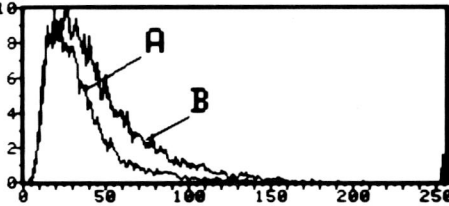

Fig.1. Cytofluorometric analysis of β_2-m expression on fetal liver cells of a 15 week-old fetus. The data are presented as histograms with cell number (Y-axis) versus linear fluorescence intensity (arbitrary units) (X-axis). Cells (10^6/ml) were incubated for 24 hrs with 30U/ml of α-IFN (curve B), and were compared to untreated cells (curve A). Cells were stained with an anti-β_2-m murine monoclonal antibody, revealed by an FITC goat anti-mouse Ig serum. The shift to the right of the curve B, as compared to the control curve A, illustrated an increased β_2-m expression on α-IFN-treated cells.

Table 1. *In vitro* effect of α-IFN on the β_2-m expression on fetal thymocytes

Gestational age (weeks)	0	IFN
7	87/15[a]	20/42[b]
14	86/22	85/46
15	97/38	96/61
16	86/25	88/52
17	85/40	90/96
20	93/64	90/102
21	94/52	98/105
23	61/40	72/96

Table 2. *In vitro* effect of α-IFN on the β_2-m expression on fetal liver cells

Gestational age (weeks)	0	IFN
7	4/13	12/31
12	17/20	29/37
13	14/20	19/82
14	10/11	21/80
15	19/11	26/41
16	26/39	35/73
21	46/54	50/120

Table 3. *In vitro* effect of α-IFN on the β_2-m expression on fetal splenocytes

Gestational age (weeks)	0	IFN
15	84/33	89/51
16	83/70	85/125
17	89/90	87/210
20	62/84	72/165
21	91/134	96/223

[a] Percentage of positive cells determined by cytofluorometry
[b] Median fluorescence intensity determined by cytofluorometry

A and B antigens of the studied fetus have been determined, on thymocytes and on splenocytes. HLA A and B typing was easier performed on α-IFN-treated fetal cells than on control fetal cells, which have a weaker expression of Class I HLA antigens. Corresponding HLA A and B reactions were found on thymocytes and splenocytes, and HLA phenotype of the fetus was: A1 A24 B12 B40.

DISCUSSION

The capacity of α-IFN to enhance H2 antigens on murine adult lymphocytes has been demonstrated by several investigators (Lindahl et al. 1974, Vignaux and Gresser, 1977, Sonnenfeld et al. 1981). Similarly, it has been found that α-IFN could increase the surface density of β_2-m and class I HLA antigens on human lymphoid cells (Fellous et al. 1979, Hokland et al. 1981). The expression of class II antigens did not appear to be enhanced by α-IFN, but it was increased at the murine macrophage surface (Steeg et al. 1982), on human fetal monocytes (Kelley et al. 1984) and on human monocyte cell lines (Koeffler et al. 1984, Virelizier et al. 1984). Hokland et al.(1984) have observed that 18-21 week-old thymocytes responded to α-IFN with an augmentation of HLA expression. Our studies have established that such a phenomenon could be seen with cells of younger fetuses, at a period when the normal HLA density is much lower and difficult to detect with conventional typing method. We have also demonstrated that not only fetal thymocytes were sensitive to this effect of α-IFN, but also fetal liver and spleen cells.

The cytofluorometric analysis of fetal liver cells suggested that both an increased expression of β_2-m-positive cells and the acquisition of some surface β_2-m by previously negative cells were responsible for this enhancement of β_2-m expression.

In association with the increased density of β_2-m, class I HLA antigens were found in higher concentrations at the surface of fetal cells incubated with α-IFN. The mechanism of this effect is likely to be comparable with that demonstrated on MOLT-4 lymphoblastoid cells, namely an augmentation of mRNA synthesis mostly restricted to class I HLA antigen production (Burrone & Milstein, 1982).

When comparing the HLA expression on cells from various organs, it was found to be lower on thymocytes than on splenocytes (Danilovs et al. 1979). Our results are similar and show that the increased concentration of HLA molecules on thymocytes is sufficient to permit HLA typing of fetal thymocytes.

This enhancement of HLA expression can be used for HLA typing of fetuses, at the age of 14 weeks and probably even earlier. Studies on 7 to 13 week-old fetuses are in progress. It will also be of crucial importance, for diagnostic purposes, to extend this investigation to other varieties of fetal cells, expecially those which can be obtained by punction without any damage to the fetus.

In conclusion, enhancement of HLA A and B expression on fetal cells enabled us to readily type fetal cadavers used for transplantation purposes. Fetal thymocytes and splenocytes can be employed for such a determination. Fetal liver cells of less than 15 weeks are more difficult to analyze in this respect. Typing of other cells of fetal origin, following *in vitro* incubation with IFN, should permit easier and more rapid diagnosis of HLA-associated diseases than did conventional methods. Alternatively, methods for "DNA typing" of the HLA region will become very useful in the same clinical context.

REFERENCES

Basham, T.Y., Bourgeade, M.F., Creasey, A.A. & Merigan, T.C. (1982) Interferon increases HLA synthesis in melanoma cells : interferon-resistant and -sensitive cell lines. Proc. Natl. Acad. Sci. USA 79, 3265.

Bétuel, H., Camoun, M., Colombani, J., Day, N.E., Ellouz, R. & De The, G. (1975) The relation between nasopharyngeal carcinoma and the HLA system among Tunisians. Int. J. Cancer, 16, 249.

Boyüm, A. (1968) Scand. J. Clin. Lab. Invest. 21 (suppl.97) 9, 109.

Burrone, O.R. & Milstein, C. (1982) Control of HLA A, B, C synthesis and expression in interferon treated cells. Embo J. 1, 345.

Danilovs, J.A., Brown, J., Terasaki, P. & Clark, W.R. (1983) HLA DR and HLA-A,B,C, typing of human fetal tissue. issue Antigens, 21, 296.

Fellous, M. , Kamoun,M., Gresser, I. & Bono, R. (1979). Enhanced expression of HLA antigens and β_2-microglobulin on interferon-treated human lymphoid cells. Eur. J. Immunol. 9, 446.

Forest, M.G., Bétuel,H., Couillin, P. & Boue, A. (1981) Prenatal Diagnosis of Congenital Adrenal Hyperplasia due to 21-Hydroxylase Deficiency by steroid analysis in the amniotic fluid of mid-pregnancy : comparison with HLA typing in 17 pregnancies at risk for CAH. Prenatal Diagnosis , 1, 190.

Hokland, M., Heron, I. & Berg, K. (1981) Increased expression of β2-microglobulin and histocompatibility antigens on human lymphoid cells by interferon. J. of interferon Research, 1, 483.

Hokland, M, Ritz, J., & Hokland, P. (1983) Interferon-Induced Changes in Expression of antigens defined by monoclonal antibodies on Malignant and non-malignant Mononuclear Hematopoietic Cells. J. of Interferon Research, 3, 199.

Kelley, V.E., Fiers, W. & Strom, T.B. (1984) Cloned human interferon γ, but not interferon α or β, induces expression of HLA-DR determinants by fetal monocytes and myeloid leukemic cell lines. J. Immunol. 132, 240.

Koeffler, H.P., Ranyard, J., Yelton, L., Billing, R. & Bohman R. (1984) interferon induces expression of the HLA-D antigens or normal and leukemic human myeloid cells.

Lindahl, P., Leary, P. & Gresser, I. (1974) Enhancement of the expression of histocompatibility antigens of mouse lymphoid cells by interferon in vitro. Eur.J.Immunol. 4, 779.

Mittal, K.K., Mickey, M.R., Singal, D.P. & Terasaki, P.I. (1968) Serotyping for homo-transplantation.XVIII; Refinement of microdroplet lymphocyte cytotoxicity test. Transplantation 6, 913.

Singh, S.P.N., Vyramuthu, N., Margoles, C & Lawler, S.D. (1979) HLA typing of human fetal fibroblasts. Transplantation 28, 262.

Sonnenfeld, G., Mervelo, D. Mc Devitt, H.O. & Merigan, T.O. (1981) Effect of type I and type II interferons on murine thymocyte surface antigen expression : induction or selection ? Cell. Immunol. 57, 427.

Steeg, P.S., Moore, R.N., Johnson, H.M. & Oppenheim, J.J. (1982) Regulation of murine macrophages Ia antigen expression by a lymphokine with immune interferon activity. J. Exp. Med. 156, 1980.

Vignaux, F. & Gresser, I. (1977) Differential effects of interferon on the expression of H-2K, H-2D and Ia antigens on mouse lymphocytes. J. Immunol. 118, 721.

Virelizier, J.L., Perez, N., Arenzana-Seisdedos, F. & Devos, R. (1984) Pure interferon gamma enhances class II antigens on human monocyte cell lines. Eur. J. Immunol. 14, 106.

REGULATION OF IN VITRO GRANULOPOIESIS BY HUMAN FETAL LIVER STROMAL CELLS

Y. Barak, Y. Karov, S. Levin, A. Barash, H, Ben-Hur and M. Lancet
Departments of Pediatric Research and Obstetrics and Gynecology, Kaplan Hospital, Rehovot-76100, Israel

Recent studies have shown that fibroblasts of the hemopoietic stroma probably play an important role in the regulation of hemopoiesis. A long-term murine bone marrow culture system developed by Dexter et al (1977), permits the proliferation of hemopoietic stem cells for several months. Hemopoiesis in this system is dependent on the presence of a marrow-derived adherent population, consisting of a variety of cell types, of which the fibroblastic cells (FC) represent a major component (Allen and Dexter, 1976). The efforts to adapt this culture system for human bone marrow culture have as yet achieved only limited success (Hocking and Golde, 1980, Toogood et al, 1980, Suda and Dexter, 1981). This is probably either due to an insufficient hemopoietic inductive capacity by the human adherent cell population, or to excessive promotion of differentiation by these cells, leading to termination of the culture (Moore et al, 1980).

Previous studies clearly demonstrated that early human fetal livers (HFL) lack mature granulocytes but contain abundant numbers of granulocyte-macrophage colony-forming cells (GM-CFC) (Barak et al 1980), suggesting that HFL stromal cells are geared specifically to promote more proliferation and less differentiation, and their use as adherent cells in human long term Dexters' culture may possibly lead to prolonged proliferation in these cultures.

In the present study we have tested this hypothesis by employing a combination of long-term liquid culture and short-term semi-solid culture systems, in order to investigate the effects of FC obtained from early human fetal livers on the growth of normal human marrow-derived GM-CFC, as compared with the in vitro granulopoietic effect of bone marrow derived FC.

MATERIALS AND METHODS

HFL cells: Five human embryos at 7-11 weeks of fetal age were obtained by therapeutic vaginal abortions performed for reasons not involving disease of the fetus, using the manual dilatation and curetage method. The livers were removed aseptically and converted into single cell suspensions by gentle manipulation of small blocks of liver through a fine mesh. In order to obtain FC from other fetal sources, pieces of skin from the same embryos were processed into single cell suspensions by the same method.

Liquid culture for FC: A modification of the technique described by Greenberg et al (1981) was used. 5.10^6 HFL cells, fetal skin (FS) cells or normal adult marrow cells (BM) obtained by aspiration from the posterior superior iliac crest were placed in 50 ml tissue culture flasks (Nunc, Denmark) containing 10 ml Modified McCoys 5A medium (Bio-lab, Israel) with 20% fetal-calf serum (Gibco, Grand Island, N.Y.). The cells were incubated in a $37°C$, 10% CO_2 humidified environment. Following 48 h of incubation, the supernatant and non-adherent cells were removed, fresh medium added, and the cultures reincubated for an additional 7 days. The flasks were examined repeatedly for the presence of adherent fibroblastic colonies. Upon reaching proximately 75% confluency, cells were detached and passaged several times by treatment with 0.25% trypsin in phosphate-buffered saline until "pure" populations of FC were obtained. These FC were maintained in culture for 13 weeks.

Stimulation of granulopoiesis The ability of FC derived from the HFL, FS and BM liquid cultures to stimulate granulopoiesis was determined using a short term, semi-solid, double-layer culture technique. From the 3rd to the 13th weeks of liquid cultures, FC were removed weekly from the flasks with trypsin, resuspended in supplemented McCoys 5A medium and reseeded into 30 mm culture dishes (Nunc, Denmark) at several concentrations, from $0,5x10^4$ to $50x10^4$ cells per dish. Following overnight incubation, the medium above the FC was removed and the dishes refilled with 1 ml of 0,3% agar-medium, $2x10^5$ fresh normal human bone marrow cells supplemented with or without 0,1 ml of human placental-conditioned medium (HPCM), prepared according to the method of Burgess et al (1977), which served as a source of granulocyte-macrophage colony stimulating factor (GM-CSF). Colonies were counted following 7 days of incubation at $37°C$ in a fully humidified atmosphere with 10% CO_2. Control cultures consisted of bone marrow cells in agar-medium-HPCM in plates without FC.

Conditioned medium studies To determine the granulopoietic effect of medium conditioned by the HFL, FS and BM adherent cells in the liquid cultures, the medium in the flasks was collected weekly and frozen until just prior to use. The granulopoietic effect of the FC conditioned medium (CM) collected at 1,2,4,8 weeks of culture was assayed in agar cultures according to a modification of the method of Pike and Robinson (1970). Suspension of 2×10^5 normal human bone marrow cells in modified McCoys 5A medium with 20% fetal calf serum and 0,3% agar were plated in 30 mm culture dishes, with or without 10% HPCM and 10% CM from the various sources. Discrete colonies were scored after 7 days of incubation at $37^\circ C$ in a fully humidified atmosphere with 10% CO_2.

RESULTS

Fetal livers Details on human fetal liver studied are summarized in table 1. The livers obtained ranged in weight from 90 to 340 mg and contained from 6 to 120×10^6 cells/liver.

TABLE 1. Details on Human Fetal Livers Studied

No.	Fetal Age (wks)	Weight (g)	Length (C-R)[1] (mm)	Cell Yield ($\times 10^6$)
1	7	2,2	20	12
2	12	3,4	41	120
3	11	2,7	30	25
4	7	1,0	26	18
5	7	0,9	15	6

1) Crown-Rump

Granulopoietic effects of fibroblastic cells Granulocyte-macrophage colonies derived from normal marrow GM-CFC grown on top of HFL FC underlayers are shown in Fig 1. The results of the effect of FC from HFL, FS and BM in cultures supplemented with HPCM on GM-CFC production by normal human marrow targets, are presented in Fig 2 and table 2. Without HPCM, FC from all three sources stimulated only 0-7 colonies per 2.10^5 BM cells seeded. When cultures were supplemented with HPCM, the results obtained with FC derived from different fetuses and BM aspirates were not significantly different throughout the 10 weeks of study and are therefore grouped together. The number of GM-CFC observed in cultures containing 0,5x, 1x and 2×10^4 FC/plate derived from FS or BM did not differ significantly from the number of GM-CFC obtained with HPCM alone.The ability of HFL derived FC to stimulate GM-CFC production under the same conditions was significantly increased (P<0.0005). With all 3 FC sources at 5×10^4 FC/plate, mild granulopoietic inhibition was apparent (with HFL-FC - 0.1>P>0.5) (Fig 3).

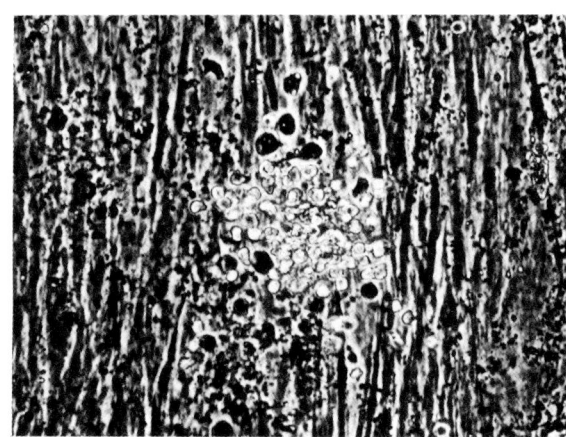

Fig. 1. Granulocyte-macrophage colony grown on top of underlayers composed of human fetal liver FC after 4 weeks of liquid culture. x160

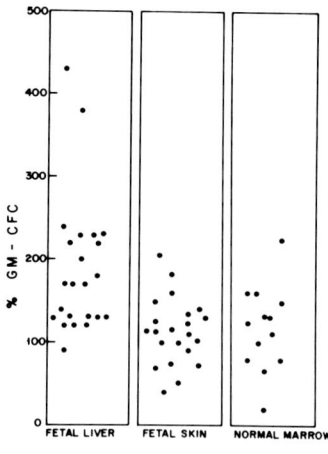

Fig. 2. In vitro granulopoietic effects of fibroblastic cells at $0,5-2\times10^4$ cells/plate from various sources upon normal bone marrow targets, stimulated also by human placental conditioned medium (HPCM), expressed as % of GM-CFC produced by HPCM alone (100%).

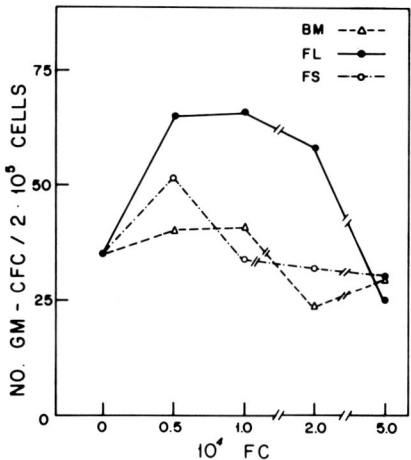

Fig. 3. The effect of fetal liver (FL), fetal skin (FS) and bone marrow (BM) FC concentrations on GM-CFC production by normal BM targets.

TABLE 2. Stimulation of Normal Bone Marrow GM-CFC by FC.

Source of FC	No. of Experiments	GM-CFC/2×10^5 Cells [4]	p [2] Value
HPCM [1] only (No FC)	11	34,4 ± 10,1	-
Fetal livers+HPCM (0.5-2$\times 10^4$ cells/plate)	9	62,8 ± 10,1	<0.0005
Fetal livers+HPCM (5$\times 10^4$ cells/plate)	6	24,9 ± 17	<0.1, >0.05
Fetal skins+HPCM	10	37,1 ± 18	N.S [3]
Normal marrows+HPCM	7	36,3 ± 17,7	N.S

1) Human placental conditioned medium
2) Calculated by Student's t test
3) Not significant
4) Mean ± SD

Granulopoietic effect of FC-conditioned medium: Supernatant obtained from the HFL, FS and BM liquid cultures at 1,2,4 and 8 weeks of culture added alone to normal marrow cultures had no effect on GM-CFC production by the marrow targets. In cultures containing both HPCM and conditioned medium, the numbers of GM-CFC observed were significantly increased when HFL derived CM was supplemented (<0.005), and not significantly changed when FS or BM derived CM preparations were used (table 3).

TABLE 3. Effect of CM[1] from FC Cultures on GM-CFC Production

GM-CFC/2.10^5 cells (mean + SD) in cultures supplemented by CM conditioned by FC from:

Wks in culture	None (HPCM)[2]	Fetal liver	Fetal skin	Bone Marrow
1	42,6+15,3	60,3+19,6	47 + 9,9	44,3+15,5
2	32,7+23	64,6+17,9	41,1+ 2,1	42,3+15,5
4	42,6+15,3	52,6+ 8,14	43,3+ 2,9	36,3+ 2,1
8	42,6+15,3	69 + 7,93	54,3+ 9,4	43 + 7
P value[3]	-	<0.005	NS[4]	NS

1) Conditioned medium
2) Human placental conditioned medium
3) Calculated by Student's t test
4) Not significant

DISCUSSION

The present study was concerned with the in vitro granulopoietic capacities of human fetal liver stromal cells, while detailed analysis of their morphologic, cytochemical and ultrastructural characteristics will be reported elswhere (Barak et al, in preparation). The study has shown that unlike FC from bone marrows of normal subjects, those derived from human fetal liver significantly enhanced HPCM-stimulated target marrow GM-CFC. This effect clearly depended on the concentration of FC seeded. While FC at $0,5x - 20x10^4$ cells/plate stimulated enhanced growth of marrow targets GM-CFC, actual inhibitory effects of FC were observed if large numbers of FC ($50x10^4$ cells/plate) were present. This granulopoietic enhancing capacity was found to be unique for the fetal liver, as fetal FC from other sources studied did not exhibit this augmentation effect. Greenberg et al (1981), employing a similar system, have studied the effect of adherent bone marrow FC from normal humans. When using target marrows containing few spontaneous colonies, increased numbers of GM-CFC were stimulated by the FC. Actual inhibition was produced by these FC if target marrows contained large numbers of spontaneous GM-CFC. In another study by Blackburn and Goldman (1980) it was reported that human FC enhanced the growth of co-cultured GM-CFC and BFU-E. In the mouse, Zipori (1981) reported short-range inhibition of colony formation by marrow adherent cells, and proposed a model in which this inhibitor and GM-CSF together regulate GM-CFC growth. The discrepancy between our and the previous results concerning stimulation and inhibition of marrow GM-CFC by human marrow-derived FC may be related to different culture conditions. We have shown, however, that in identical culture conditions, HFL-derived FC differed significantly from human BM-derived FC, by their capacity to enhance significantly the growth of normal marrow targets. HFL FC did not produce GM-CSF in this system. Their enhancing capacity has been shown to be dependent on exogenous GM-CSF, and most probably mediated by contact, short range interactions, suggesting an in vitro granulopoietic microenvironmental effect.

The results of our studies demonstrated that conditioned medium derived from HFL liquid stromal cell cultures significantly increased colony production by HPCM-stimulated normal marrow GM-CFC, in contrast to negative results obtained with BM or FS-derived conditioned medium (table 3). This HFL-derived granulopoietic stimulating factor lacked GM-CSF characteristics, as it was totally dependent on an exogenous supply of GM-CSF. Other reports have indicated either no production of GM-CSF by adherent cells in mouse long-term cultures (Dexter et al, 1980), low levels of GM-CSF (Shadduck et al, 1983, Zipori, 1982) or inhibition of GM-CFC growth by human BM-derived FC-conditioned media (Greenberg et al, 1981, Castro-malaspina et al, 1980).

The results of the present study, demonstrating a unique in vitro cellular and humoral hemopoietic effect of early human fetal liver stromal cells, do not in themselves establish a physiologic role for these cells in the regulation of in vivo fetal hemopoiesis. It is interest., however, that in several reports of HFL-grafted aplastic anemia patients, permanent or transient reconstitution of the patients own stem cells occured, suggesting hemopoietic "helper" effect

of some populations within the HFL cellular suspension.
(Lucarelli, 1978, Kelman, 1973, Kansal et al, 1979). Further
studies on the morphology and biology of HFL stromal cells
as well as studies on the nature of the interactions between
HFL stromal cells and hemopoietic cells in Dexter's long-
term culture system are clearly indicated.

REFERENCES

Allen TD, Dexter TM (1976). Cellular interactions during in
vitro granulopoiesis. Differentiation 6:191.
Barak Y, Karov Y, Levin S, Soroker N, Barash A, Lancet M,
Nir E (1980). Granulocyte macrophage colonies in cultures of
human fetal liver cells: Morphologic and ultrastructural
analysis of proliferation and differentiation. Exp Hematol.
8:837.
Blackburn MJ, Goldman JM (1980). Increased survival of
haemopoietic progenitor cells in vitro induced by marrow
stromal cells. Exp. Hematol. 8 (Suppl 7):79.
Burgess AW, Wilson WMA, Metcalf D (1977). Stimulation by
human placental conditioned medium of hemopoietic colony
formation by human marrow cells. Blood 49:573.
Castro-malaspina-H,Gay RE, Resnick G, Kapoor N, Meyers P,
Chiarieri D, McKenzie S, Broxmeyer HE, Moore MAS (1980).
Characterization of human fibroblast colony forming cells
(CFU-F) and their progeny. Blood 56:289.
Dexter TM, Allen TD, Lajtha LG (1977). Conditions controlling
the proliferation of haemopoietic stem-cells in vitro. J.
Cell. Physiol. 91:335.
Dexter TM, Spooncer E, Toxsoz D, Lajtha LG (1980). The role
of cells and their products in the regulation of in vitro
stem cell proliferation and granulocyte development. J.
Supramol.Struct. 13:513.
Greenberg BR, Wilson FD, Woo L (1981). Granulopoietic effects
of human bone marrow fibroblastic cells and abnormalities in
the "granulopoietic microenvironement". Blood 58:557.
Hocking WG, Golde DW (1980). Long term human bone marrow
cultures. Blood 56:118.
Kansal V, Sood SK, Batra AK, Adhar G, Malviya AK, Kucheria K,
Balakrishnan K (1979). Fetal liver transplantation in
aplastic anemia. Acta Haemat. 62:128.
Kelman E (1973). Recovery from chronic idiopathic bone marrow
aplasia of a young mother after intravenous injection of
unprocessed cells from the liver of her embryo. Scand. J.
Haemat. 10:305.

Lucarelli G (1978). Fetal liver transplantation in severe aplastic anemia. Haematologica 63:93.
Moore MAS, Broxmeyer HE, Sheridan APC, Meyers DA, Jacobsen N, Winchester RJ (1980). Continuous human bone marrow culture: Ia antigen characterization of probable pluripotential stem cells. Blood 55:682.
Pike BL, Robinson WA (1970). Human bone marrow colony growth in agar gel. J. Cell Physiol. 76:77.
Shadduck RK, Waheed A, Greenberger JS, Dexter TM (1983). Production of colony stimulating factor in longterm bone marrow cultures. J. Cell Physiol. 114:88.
Suda T, Dexter TM (1981). Effect of Hydrocortisone on long term human bone marrow cultures. Brit. J. Haemat. 48:661.
Toogood IRG, Dexter TM, Allen TD, Suda T, Lajtha LG (1980). The development of a liquid culture system for the growth of human bone marrow. Leuk. Res. 4:449.
Zipori D (1981). Cell interactions in the bone marrow microenvironement: role of endogeneous colony stimulating activity. J. Supramol. Struct. 17:347.
Zipori D (1982). Properties of bone marrow stromal cell and derived liver from SJL/J mice. Exp. Hematol. 10:10.

MORPHOLOGICAL PATTERN OF HEMATOPOIESIS IN HUMAN FETAL LIVER

S. Sharma, M. Bhargava and V. Kochupillai

All-India Institute of Medical Sciences,
New Delhi - 110 029, India

Fetal liver cell suspensions were prepared from 60 abortuses of 8-32 weeks gestation. Their slides stained with Jenner and Giemsa stains were studied under light microscope. Erythropoietic cells were the most numerous (median, M-94%; range 60.5-98.5%); intermediate and late normoblasts outnumbered early and pronormoblasts ($p < 0.001$). Myeloid precursors were less than 5% in 49 abortuses and more than 5% in 11 abortuses. Lymphoid cells were signficantly less up to the gestation period of 15 weeks than beyond ($p < 0.05$). No megakaryocytes could be identified in 41 abortuses; in the remaining they constituted 0.5-1% of the total cells.

Numerical preponderance of erythroid cells over myeloid, lymphoid and megakaryocytic cells may be because of decreased demand for the latter three types due to the protected germ free environment of the embryo.

INTRODUCTION

Pattern of hematopoiesis is different in the fetal liver than in the adults bone marrow; the former being predominantly myeloid. Thus the erythroid to myeloid cell population ratio is 25 in the fetal liver and 0.33 in the adult bone marrow (Calvo 1980, Shadduck 1980, Cappeline 1984, Kubanek 1980, Gale 1980).

MATERIAL AND METHODS

Sixty abortuses (50 following hysterotomy, 6 after prostaglandin injection and 4 spontaneous abortions) were collected in normal saline from the obstetrics department of the All-India Institue of Medical Sciences. Fetal age estimated from last date of menstruation and crown to rump length (Hamilton 1957) ranged between 8 and 32 weeks; 2 between 8-11, 17 between 12-15, 33 between 16-19 and 8 between 20-32 weeks.

Fetal liver was dissected under sterile conditions and its cell suspension prepared according to the details described earlier (Kochupillai 1985). A drop of the cell suspension was taken on a glass slide, a thin smear prepared and fixed in methanol for 2 minutes and then stained with Jenner and Giemsa stains. Cell morphology was studied under light microscope. Two hundred cells were counted from each slide for counting the individual population of various hematopoietic cells.

RESULTS (Table 1)

Throughout 8-32 weeks of gestation period, erythropoiesis predominated among erythroid precursors, pronormoblasts and early normoblasts numbered clearly less than intermediate and late normoblasts ($p < 0.001$). Up to 15 weeks of gestation intermediate normoblasts and numbered more than other erythroid precursors ($p < 0.01$), however, from 20-32 weeks of gestation late normoblasts were most prominant ($p < 0.01$). In the early gestation period, primitive cells (hemocytoblasts) varied between 0-4%; such cells were non-existent beyond 19 weeks of gestation.

Myeloid precursors varied between 0-34%; they were less than 5% in 49 and more than 5% in 11 abortuses. Difference in the number of myeloid precursors did not vary signficantly between various gestation periods.

Lymphoid cells varied between 0-12% (M-1.5%). They were 2% or less in 42 and more than 2% in 18 abortuses. Up to 15 weeks of gestation, lymphoid cells varied between 0-2.5% (M-1.5%); beyond 15 weeks, there was increase in lymphoid cells to 0-12 (M-2%). This difference was statistically significant ($p < 0.05$). Megakaryocytes were

TABLE:I MORPHOLOGICAL PATTERN OF HEMATOPOIESIS IN HUMAN FETAL LIVER

Gestation period in week	No.of Abortuses	Total Erythroid precursors	Erythroid Precursors % Median(M) and (Range)				Erythroid precursors in mitosis	Myeloid precursors % M and (range)	Lymphoid cells % M and (range)	Megakaryocytes % M and (range)	Hemocytoblasts % M and (range)
			Pronormoblasts	Early normoblasts	Intermediate normoblasts	Late normoblasts					
8-11	2	88-97	11-7.5	9-13	29.5-45	31-31.5	3.5-4	0.5-8	0.5-2	0	2-2
12-15	17	M-94.5 (91-98)	M-11 (5-20.5)	M-15 (8-26)	M-39.5 (25-50)	M-28.5 (11-42.5)	M-2 (0-6)	M-2 (0.5-6.5)	M-1.5 (0-2.5)	M-0 (0-1)	M-1 (0-4)
16-19	33	M-94 (60.5-98.5)	M-11 (1.5-23)	M-13.5 (4-29)	M-33 (5.5-55)	M-31 (9-70.5)	M-2 (0-6.5)	M-3 (0-34.5)	M-1.5 (0-4.5)	M-0 (0-1)	M-0.5 (0-2)
20-32	8	M-92 (72-96)	M-7.75 (4-15)	M-12.75 (3-15.5)	M-27.75 (12-38)	M-42.75 (25.5-57)	M-1.25 (0-6)	M-3.25 (1-16)	M-3.5 (1-12)	M-0.25 (0-1)	0
Total 8-32	60	M-94 (60.5-98.5)	M-10.25 (1.5-23)	M-13.25 (3-29)	M-33.25 (5.5-55)	M-31.25 (9-70.5)	M-2 (0-6.5)	M-3 (0-34.5)	M-1.5 (0-12)	M-0 (0-1)	M-0.5 (0-4)

not seen in 41 abortuses; in the remaining 19 they varied between 0.5-1% of the total cells.

DISCUSSION

The present study confirms the preponderance of erythropoiesis and paucity of myelopoiesis, lymphopoiesis and megakaryopoiesis during intrauterine development (Calvo 1980, Shadduck 1980, Cappeline 1984, Kubanek 1980, Gale 1980). Paucity of the latter 3 cell lines may be due to the decreased demand of such cells during intrauterine life on account of protected, germ free environment (Kubanek 1980). Of the erythroid precursors intermediate and late normoblasts predominate but as the fetal age advances, late normoblasts become the most prominant. Unlike myeloid precursors there is a tendency for the lymphoid cells to increase numerically as the fetal age advances; difference in number of these cells calculated before and after 15 weeks of gestation was statistically significant ($p < 0.05$).

Paucity of lymphopoiesis during intrauterine life has practical implications and is consistent with observations made in animal and human studies that fetal liver cells have minimal or no potential for the occurence of graft-versus-host disease (Kochupillai 1985, Uphoff 1958, Lucarelli 1980).

Morphological patterns of hematopoiesis in human fetal liver did not vary significantly with hysterotomy, prostaglandin induced or spontaneous abortion.

ACKNOWLEDGEMENT

We extend our sincere thanks to Professor N.K. Bhide, Head of the Department of Pharmacology, All-India Institute of Medical Sciences, for his help in the preparation of this manuscript.

Financed by Department of Science and Technology, Government of India.

REFERENCES

Calvo W and Carbonell E (1980). The development of liver granulopoiesis in the human fetus. In Fetal Liver Transplantation. Current Concepts and Future Directions. Lucarelli G, Fliedner TM and Gale RP (eds). Excerpta Medica, p. 14.

Cappelline BD, Petter CG and Wood WG (1984). Long term hemopoiesis in human fetal liver cell cultures. Br J Haemat; 57:61.

Gale RP (1980). Concepts of fetal liver transplantation in man. In Fetal Liver Transplantation. Current Concepts and Future Directions. Lucarelli G, Fliedner TM and Gale RP (eds). Excerpta Medica, p. 247.

Hamilton WB, Body JJ and Monhan HW (1957). Human embryology. Cambridge, Hefton and Son, p. 104.

Kochupillai V, Sharma S, Francis S, Mehra NK, Nanu A, Kalra V, Manon PSN and Bhargava M (1985). Bone marrow reconstitution following human fetal liver infusion (FLI) in sixteen severe aplastic anemia patients. In Fetal Liver Transplantation. Gale RP (ed). Alan R. Liss, N.Y.

Kubanek, Bern Hard, Heit, Wolfgang and Rich I (1980). Fetal erythropoiesis. In Fetal Liver Transplantation. Current Concepts and Future Directions. Lucarelli G, Fliedner TM and Gale RP (eds). Excerpta Medica, p. 71.

Lucarelli G, Izzi T, Porcellini A, Delfine C, Polchi P, Moretti L, Manna A and Grilli G (1980). Fetal liver transplantation in aplastic anemia and acute leukemia. In Fetal Liver Transplantation. Current Concepts and Future Directions. Lucarelli G, Fliedner TM and Gale RP (eds). Excerpta Medica, p. 284.

Shadduck RK, Pigoli G, Waheed A and Boegal F (1980). Characterization of hemopoietic progenitor cells in fetal liver. In Fetal Liver Transplantation. Current Concepts and Future Directions. Lucarelli G, Fliedner TM and Gale RP (eds). Excerpta Medica, p. 29.

Uphoff DE (1958). Preclusion of secondary phase of irradiation syndrome by inoculation of fetal hematopoietic tissue following lethal body X-irradiation. J Antl Cancer Inst; 20:625.

SECTION III
FETAL LIVER TRANSPLANTATION–ANIMAL MODELS

HEMOPOIESIS AND IMMUNE FUNCTIONS IN DOGS FOLLOWING FETAL LIVER TRANSPLANTATION

Otto Prümmer, Wenceslao Calvo, Christine Werner, Felix Carbonell, and Theodor M. Fliedner

Department of Clinical Physiology and Occupational Medicine, University of Ulm, D-7900 Ulm, FRG

ABSTRACT Ten beagles were exposed to total body X-irradiation (3x6 Gy) and rescued with cryopreserved fetal liver cells from DLA-identical siblings obtained around the 52nd day of gestation. Grafts contained $0.2-1.6 \times 10^8$ mononuclear cells/kg and $0.9-19.8 \times 10^4$ granulocyte-macrophage progenitor cells/kg. Hemopoiesis and immune functions were followed for up to one year after fetal liver transplantation (FLT). There was a prompt engraftment in all recipients. Bone marrow metaphases were always of donor origin, whereas some host lymphocytes circulated for 2-3 months. Blood granulocytes and monocytes rose to pre-treatment levels within 2-3 weeks of FLT and platelets and erythrocytes were normal within 3-4 and 5-6 weeks, respectively. The relative incidence of bone marrow CFU-GM was normal by day 14 and the absolute numbers of circulating CFU-GM remained elevated for one year after day 14. Blood lymphocytes reached control numbers between days 35 and 101 with a faster B cell than T cell recovery. Their response to mitogen stimulation was normal by day 75, while the mixed lymphocyte reaction tended to be reduced for one year. Serum levels of IgM (day 35) and IgG (day 49) recovered earlier than IgA levels (day 270). Thus, cryopreserved canine fetal liver cells can restore hemopoiesis and immunocompetence with considerable rapidity in histocompatible, adult siblings pre-treated with total body irradiation, and, since they lack mature T cells, may be used to analyze effector mechanisms that mediate rejection of T cell-depleted allografts under less favourable conditions.

INTRODUCTION

Transplantation of fetal liver cells (FLC) may correct radiation-induced bone marrow aplasia in small rodents, even under circumstances, where graft donors and recipients differ strongly in their major histocompatibility antigens (Uphoff 1958; Löwenberg 1975; O'Reilly 1983). Presumably owing to the lack of mature T lymphocytes, FLC grafts, as opposed to bone marrow cells, do not elicit severe, acute graft-versus-host disease (GVHD) under these conditions (Löwenberg 1975). Attempts to reduplicate these encouraging experiences in larger, outbred mammals and in man have been largely unsuccessful, most often because of the failure of the histoincompatible fetal stem cells to engraft durably (Thomas et al. 1963; Van Putten et al. 1983; O'Reilly et al. 1983). Similarly, depletion of T cells from allogeneic bone marrow increases the probability of graft rejection in clinical bone marrow transplantation (Trigg et al. 1984).

Canine FLC are able to initiate hemopoiesis in histocompatible, related recipients which have previously been subjected to high-dose cytoreductive treatment (Prümmer et al. 1983a; Stitzel et al. 1983). Increasing the genetic disparity between donor and recipient or reducing the severity of immunosuppression leads to graft rejection, unless fetal thymocytes are added to the FLC transplants (Saltzstein et al. 1974; Champlin et al. 1982; Prümmer, unpublished observations). Fetal liver cell transplantation (FLT) in dogs, therefore, constitutes a convenient and sensitive model for studying on a preclinical level of effector mechanisms active in hemopoietic allograft rejection and may aid in designing more effective conditioning regimens. Moreover, it may provide insight into the conditions of tolerance development. This communication reviews our experiences with the grafting of ideally matched, cryopreserved FLC from histocompatible sibling donors; the results may provide a framework for the reconstitution processes to be expected after FLT in dogs. Part of these results has been described in detail elsewhere (Prümmer et al. 1985; Prümmer, Werner et al.)

MATERIALS AND METHODS

Animals

Ten beagles of either sex, aged 7-11 months and weighing between 10.2 and 15.5 kg were given FLC transplants from littermates or non-littermate siblings that were identical for dog leukocyte antigens (DLA). Recipients were vaccinated against parvovirus, distemper, hepatitis, leptospirosis, and rabies and had been dewormed prior to entering the study.

Procurement, Storage and Transfer of Fetal Liver Cells

Parents of FLC donors and recipients were unrelated but homozygous and identical for DLA-A, -B, and -D. Sire and dam were date-mated for 24 hours and fetuses were obtained by total or partial hysterectomy 52 days later in the middle of the third trimester of the gestation period, which is 60-63 days in beagles. Partial hysterectomy involved the removal of one uterine horn to provide FLC donors; the prospective graft recipients were left in situ and allowed to continue to term and to be born normally. Details of the procedure have been described (Prümmer et al. 1985).

Fetal livers were removed aseptically from the donors, cut in pieces, and were gently disrupted in glass tissue grinders. All preparatory steps were carried out on ice in Hanks' balanced salt solution without Ca^{2+} and Mg^{2+} (HBSS). Quickly sedimenting clumps were removed and supernatant cells were washed in HBSS and suspended in Earl's minimal essential medium (S-MEM) containing 20% of horse serum. From aliquots the yield of mononuclear hemopoietic cells (MNC) and of granulocyte-macrophage progenitor cells (CFU-GM) was determined according to established procedures (Nothdurft et al. 1984). Cells were frozen in S-MEM containing 10% horse serum and 10% dimethylsulphoxide (DMSO) in plastic bags using a standard program (Fliedner et al. 1977) and were stored under liquid nitrogen for 7-11 months. After thawing, FLC were washed once in S-MEM containing deoxyribonuclease to dissociate aggregates. The recovery after cryopreservation of MNC was poor ranging between 5% and 16% (median 9%), whereas CFU-GM recoveries were 62-182 % (median 85%), when assessed immediately after washing (dogs 86-115)(Table 1). Storage of thawed FLC for about one hour at room temperature

TABLE 1. Data on dogs given 3 x 6 Gy TBI and grafts of cryopreserved fetal liver cells from DLA-identical siblings

Recipients			Grafts			GVHD	Survival
Dog no.	Sex / Age (mo)	No. of livers	MNC/kg ($\times 10^{-8}$)	CFU-GM/kg ($\times 10^{-4}$)			(days)
70	F / 7	3	1.6	0.9		None	74
72	F / 7	3	1.0	1.0		Skin	60
74	F / 7	2	1.3	2.0		Skin	90
86	F / 7	1	0.3	1.9		None	60
90	F / 7	1	0.2	4.1		None	57
93	M / 7	1	0.3	6.3		None	77
108	F / 11	1	0.3	5.5		None	450+
109	M / 8	1	0.6	16.2		None	520+
113	M / 8	1	0.5	18.4		None	520+
115	M / 8	1	0.4	19.8		None	520+

in the presence of 0.5-1.0 % DMSO reduced CFU-GM recoveries (median 15%) in dogs 70-74.

Recipients were exposed to three fractions of TBI from an X-ray source (6 Gy each; 0.07 Gy/min), separated by 48-hour intervals. After completion of TBI, animals were intravenously infused with the cell yield of 1-3 fetal livers (Table 1). Grafts contained $0.2-1.6 \times 10^8$ MNC/kg body weight and $0.9-19.8 \times 10^4$ CFU-GM/kg. Recipients were kept in individual cages for 3-4 weeks after FLT and subsequently returned to open kennel conditions. Details of the post-transplant care, antibiotic treatment, platelet support, and the substitution of pancreas enzymes have been described (Prümmer et al. 1985).

Laboratory Studies

For most of the parameters evaluated three control values were obtained at weekly intervals prior to TBI. Complete blood cell counts and differential counts, including enumeration of platelets and reticulocytes, were carried out for 42 days after FLT and at intervals thereafter. Serum concentrations of alanine aminotransferase (ALT) and alkaline phosphatase (AP) were assessed by standard procedures as were blood glucose levels.

The assay system for growing CFU-GM has been described (Nothdurft et al. 1984). Briefly, $\leq 1 \times 10^6$ MNC from heparinized venous blood or 1×10^5 MNC from bone marrow (iliac crest) were cultured in 0.3% agar in 35-mm petri dishes in the presence of 1.5×10^6 irradiated granulocytes and 0.3 ml post-irradiation dog serum as a source of colony-stimulating activity (CSA). After seven days of culture (37°C, 3% CO_2), aggregates of more than 40 cells were scored as colonies in 3-6 parallel cultures. Serum from FLC recipients was evaluated for CSA content by adding 0.3 ml of the serum to indicator cultures containing in agar 4×10^5 MNC from dog blood which had been obtained after dextran sulfate (DS) administration and had been further enriched for CFU-GM by Ficoll-Isopaque and albumin density gradient centrifugation. The radiosensitivity after FLT of CFU-GM from blood and bone marrow was assessed by in vitro X-irradiation as described previously (Nothdurft et al. 1983). The fraction of CFU-GM in the S-phase of the cell cycle was determined by pre-incubating the cells with cytosine-arabinoside (ARA-C, 40 µg/ml) for 30 min at 37°·C and assessing the percentage of ARA-C-induced reduction in colony numbers. Velocity sedimentation for 4 hours at unit gravity (Miller 1973) was used to characterize the size distribution of CFU-GM after FLT. The number of CFU-GM mobilizable into the circulation was assessed by injecting i.v. DS (15 mg/kg) and recording the maximal increase in CFU-GM numbers, which occured 1-3 hours later (Nothdurft et al. 1982). Details of the procedures mentioned have been described (Prümmer, Werner et al.).

T lymphocytes were detected on smears of buffy coat cells stained for α-naphthyl acetate esterase (ANAE). Lymphocytes with 1-5 distinct, brown dots were scored as T cells. B cells were enumerated by direct immunofluorescent staining of surface immunoglobulins. Lymphocytes that stained with the $F(ab')_2$-fragments of a polyclonal, rhodamine-labeled goat-anti-dog Ig antiserum (Cappel Laboratories) and which excluded latex particles were scored as B cells. Serum levels of immunoglobulins IgG, IgM, and IgA were quantitated by single radial immunodiffusion (RID-Kit dog IgG, IgM, IgA; Miles). Lymphocyte transformation (LT) assays were carried out by incubating 5×10^4 blood MNC with optimal amounts of concanavalin A (Con A, 20 µg/ml; Pharmacia) or pokeweed mitogen (PWM, 2 µl/ml; GIBCO) in Waymouth's medium plus 10 % normal dog serum. Triplicate cultures in round-bottomed microwells were labeled with ^{3}H-thymidine after 3 days of culture (37°C, 5 % CO_2) and harvested and processed for scintillation counting 18-20 hours later. In mixed lymphocyte cultures (MLC), 5×10^4 blood MNC were stimulated with 5×10^4 irradiated (20 Gy), incompatible blood MNC in microwells. Cultures were labeled on day 4 and processed as described for the LT assay. Details of the various tests have been given elsewhere (Prümmer, Raghavachar, Fliedner).

Chimerism was proved by cytogenetic analysis of spontaneous bone marrow metaphases and metaphases of blood MNC after stimulation with phytohemagglutinin (Carbonell et al. 1984).

After death, animals were subjected to complete autopsies.

The two-sided Wilcoxon U-test, or Student's t-test where indicated, were applied to determine significance levels.

RESULTS

The intravenous administration of thawed FLC was well tolerated by all recipients. Transient weakness and dyspnea resolved within half an hour of cell infusion. In each instance, the fetal stem cells engrafted readily as evidenced by foci of hemopoiesis in bone marrow smears 3-7 days after FLT and rising blood leukocyte counts subsequent to day 6. Furthermore, in seven informative transplants, spontaneous bone marrow metaphases were always of donor sex; this was true as early as ten days after treatment and repeatedly for one year thereafter.

Six of ten animals had to be sacrificed 2-3 months after transplantation owing to progressive inanition, which most likely was a consequence of radiation-induced pancreatic fibrosis and exocrine insufficiency of that organ. Blood glucose levels remained in the normal range.

Granulopoiesis and Monocytopoiesis

Granulocytes and monocytes disappeared from the blood within 3 days (monocytes) to 7 days (granulocytes) after initiation of the fractionated TBI. Both cell types started to rise in parallel 6 days after FLT; mean pre-treatment numbers were attained on days 17-18 for monocytes and on days 19-20 for granulocytes. Between days 21 and 42, there was an overshoot in blood cell counts, which was more pronounced for monocytes (169 percent of control; $p < 0.001$) than for granulocytes (123 percent of control; $p < 0.001$). Granulocyte numbers tended to increase more rapidly in those animals that were grafted with more than 10^5 CFU-GM/kg as opposed to the remaining recipients (Table 2). Mean pre-treat-

TABLE 2. Recovery of blood granulocytes after FLT

Graft	n	Granulocyte count ($\times 10^{-9}$/1)		
CFU-GM/kg ($\times 10^{-4}$)		Before FLT	> 0.5	> 1.0
2.0 (0.9- 6.3)[a]	7	6.6 ± 0.8[b]	10 (9-11)[c]	11 (11-13)
18.4 (16.2-19.8)	3	5.0 ± 0.3	9 (8- 9)	10 (9-11)

[a] Median (range); [b] Mean $\pm$ SD; [c] Days after FLT, median (range)

ment levels were attained on day 14 in the former and on day 20 in the latter group. No such difference was recorded for the monocyte recovery. Granulocyte and monocyte counts remained stable for more than a year in long-term survivors.

Erythropoiesis

Although maturing hemopoiesis in livers of fetal graft donors was predominantly erythropoietic, erythropoiesis appeared to recover later than granulopoiesis after transplantation. Reticulocytes were detected in the circulation on days 9-10 after FLT and increased to rebound values 2-3 weeks later. Erythrocyte counts and hemoglobin concentrations, which initially dropped to about 70 % of control values, recovered after day 14 and were transiently normal 5-6 weeks after transplantation. During the following months, both values fell again, presumably reflecting the poor nutritional status of the animals during this interval. After day 100, erythrocyte counts and hemoglobin concentrations recovered again in surviving animals.

Megakaryopoiesis

Platelet counts dropped below $20 \times 10^9/l$ 5-6 days after FLT, when platelet support was initiated. Animals grafted with more than 10^5 CFU-GM/kg needed fewer platelet transfusions than recipients of smaller grafts (Table 3) and had

TABLE 3.   Platelet transfusions in FLC recipients

Graft	n	Platelet transfusions	
CFU-GM/kg ($\times 10^{-4}$)		number	duration
2.0 (0.9- 6.3)[a]	7	4 (2-5)	14 (7-14)[b]
18.4 (16.2-19.8)	3	2 (-)	7 (-)

[a] Median (range)
[b] Day of last transfusion, median (range)

restored their platelet counts to normal a few days earlier than the latter group (day 24 versus days 26-28).

Granulocyte-Macrophage Progenitor Cells (CFU-GM)

The CFU-GM compartments may recover slowly or even remain defective for extended periods of time after transplantation of hemopoietic stem cells from adult donors (Barrett, Adams 1981; Raghavachar et al. 1983b). Three days after FLT, low numbers of CFU-GM were detected in bone marrow aspirates from 5 of 10 animals (Table 4). After day 10, their relative

TABLE 4. CFU-GM in blood and bone marrow of ten FLC recipients

Time	CFU-GM	
	Blood (per ml)	Bone marrow (per 10^5 MNC)
Pre-FLT	39 ± 12[a]	210 ± 13
Day 3[b]	0 ± 0	13 ± 9
Day 10	20 ± 13	158 ± 20
Day 21	177 ± 66	241 ± 22
Day 370[c]	140 ± 12	269 ± 39

[a] Mean ± SE
[b] Day after FLT
[c] Only four recipients

incidence continued to be normal for at least one year. Blood CFU-GM appeared at a low frequency per 10^6 MNC in two recipients on day 3; by day 14, the average frequency was 20 times the control value. In contrast, the absolute CFU-GM concentration per ml blood surpassed unity only after day 7 (Table 4); however, subsequent to day 14, it remained at least twice as high as prior to treatment for the following year.

The interval of the most rapid replenishment of the CFU-GM compartment coincided with a peak in the serum levels of the colony-stimulating activity 3-7 days after transplantation.

Significance of Elevated Blood CFU-GM Levels

Under steady state conditions, circulating CFU-GM differ from the bulk of marrow CFU-GM by their smaller size, a higher radiosensitivity, and a smaller proportion of cells engaged in DNA synthesis and are, therefore, considered to represent a relatively immature subpopulation of myeloid progenitor cells (Metcalf, Mac Donald 1975; Gerhartz, Fliedner 1980; Nothdurft et al. 1983). Furthermore, they are supposed to equilibrate with the pool of immature - and likewise total - CFU-GM in bone marrow. For this reason, assessing the number of circulating CFU-GM may provide a more reliable estimate of the total CFU-GM compartment size than is indicated by the relative incidence of marrow CFU-GM. Thus, elevated levels of blood CFU-GM early after FLT suggested a rapid restoration of the total body pool of these progenitors. This view was further supported by the observation that DS mobilized normal numbers of CFU-GM into the circulation as early as 46 days post-grafting (control: net increase of 168 ± 55 CFU-GM/ml; day 46: 168 ± 53 CFU-GM/ml). When tested 4-7 months after FLT, blood CFU-GM did not differ from their counterparts in normal dogs with respect to radiosensitivity (D_o:0.26 ± 0.02 Gy), sedimentation velocity (monophasic sedimentation pattern, peak 4.37 ± 0.12 mm/h), or fraction of cells in S-phase of the cell cycle (20.5 ± 2.6 %). However, these circulating progenitors were clearly distinct from the recipient's bone marrow CFU-GM (D_o: 0.60 ± 0.04 Gy; biphasic sedimentation pattern, peak 5.06 ± 0.20 mm/h; S-phase fraction 19.7 ± 1.9%). Thus, increased leakage of CFU-GM from the bone marrow or from sites of extramedullary hemopoiesis into the circulation appeared to play no major role in the enhancement of blood CFU-GM numbers during this interval. It cannot be excluded that these mechanisms were partially active for the first 1-2 months after grafting (Prümmer, Werner et al.). Since additional factors such as hypercellularity of the marrow, altered cloning efficiencies, or prolonged transit times in the blood of CFU-GM were presumably of little importance, the most likely explanation for the sustained increase in circulating CFU-GM numbers is an absolute and relative expansion of the pool of migratory CFU-GM in the bone marrow.

Lymphocytes

Lymphocyte numbers in the blood had dropped to low or undetectable levels 4-8 days after initiation of TBI. Between days 6 and 38 after FLT, a steady increase was noted; then lymphocyte numbers leveled off at about 50 % of control. Between days 75 and 101, mean pre-treatment values (3422 ± 208/µl) were reached and were maintained thereafter. The pace of the lymphocyte reconstitution was associated with the size of the liver cell inoculum. Three animals transfused with more than 10^5 CFU-GM/kg had normal lymphocyte counts within 5 weeks of FLT, while it took more than 3 months in the remaining recipients rescued with smaller numbers of CFU-GM.

The regeneration of circulating T cells proceeded with similar kinetics as noted for total lymphocytes; a transient subnormal plateau 6-11 weeks post-grafting was followed by normal values (2028 ± 150/µl) after day 101.

While substantial numbers of T cells could be detected in the circulation within two weeks of FLT, B cells were almost absent on day 14. Thereafter, they rose more rapidly than T cells and reached control values (406 ± 42/µl) within 5 weeks after treatment. Up to day 270, their mean concentration remained slightly above control levels.

Serum Immunoglobulins

The serum levels of the major immunoglobulin classes were depressed for 3-4 weeks after FLT. Owing to various half-lives of the different isotype classes and also to influence by previous platelet transfusions, different nadir values were recorded. The IgG concentrations were lowest 4 weeks after FLT (76 % of control). Mean pre-treatment values (8.9 ± 2.3 g/l) were attained 3 weeks later. The nadir for the IgM concentrations was recorded on day 21 (37 % of control) and control values (1.17 ± 0.29 g/l) were reached two weeks later. After day 101, IgM values were again slightly reduced. Serum IgA levels dropped almost at the same rate as noted for IgM with a nadir (37 % of control) on day 21. In contrast to IgM and IgG concentrations, however, IgA levels remained low for extended periods of time and it was not until day 270 that the lower normal range was approached. Thus, IgM levels recovered earlier than IgG values, which in turn rose prior to IgA, a sequence that compares favourably with the maturation of the B cell system in the course of mammalian ontogeny.

In Vitro Blastogenesis

The functional integrity after FLT of circulating MNC was assessed by mitogenic and alloantigen stimulation in vitro. Cryopreserved cells were used throughout and recipient MNC obtained before and after transplantation were tested simultaneously. The proliferative responses after stimulation with Con A tended to be reduced up to seven weeks post-FLT and were well in the normal range thereafter. Clear-cut reductions up to day 49 were noted when PWM was used as a stimulant; again, blastogenesis was normal at later time points. In contrast to the LT responses, blood MNC after FLT reacted poorly to alloantigen activation; MLC responses were severely impaired for seven weeks after grafting (34-40 % of control) and approached the lower normal range only between days 270 and 370.

Chimerism of Circulating Lymphocytes

Bone marrow metaphases, as detected by a direct method, were exclusively of donor origin throughout the observation period. In contrast, substantial numbers of host type metaphases were found 5 weeks after FLT, when blood MNC were stimulated for four days with phytohemagglutinin (Table 5). Thus,

TABLE 5. Origin of PHA-responsive blood MNC after FLT

Days post-transplant	No. of animals	Percent host metaphases	
		Median	Range
35	6	35	4 - 80
55 - 81	5	4	0 - 48
192	3	0	-
340 - 370	3	0	-

some radioresistant host cells survived the fractionated TBI of 3x6 Gy and retained at least part of their functional potential. As time elapsed, the proportion of these host type cells decreased and they had completely disappeared from the circulation when analyses were carried out 6-12 months after transplantation.

Graft-Versus-Host Disease

In two of the ten FLC recipients, macroscopic skin alterations were noted which were compatible with a moderate form of GVHD. Dog 72 showed a faint rash in both ears and at the bridge of the nose after day 20, which evolved into mild hyperkeratosis at later stages. Foci of karyorrhexis were apparent within basal layer cells of the epidermis in tissue samples taken from lips and nose after death. Histological evaluation revealed no pronounced mononuclear cell infiltrates. Dog 74 had hyperkeratotic plaques on the chest and abdomen with central necroses and granulocytic infiltrates at about day 70. Neither the liver nor the intestinal tract from any of the recipients subjected to autopsy revealed clear-cut signs of GVHD. Increases in the serum levels of the AP and ALT after day 21 were comparable to enzyme changes noted after autologous stem cell transplantation in our dog model and did not aid in discerning GVHD from late effects of irradiation (Prümmer et al. 1985).

DISCUSSION

The experiments described in this communication clearly indicate that cryopreserved, canine FLC obtained in the middle of the third gestational trimester are able to seed the aplastic marrow of an adult, DLA-identical sibling which has previously been exposed to high-dose TBI. Moreover, FLC gave rise to both myeloid and lymphoid progeny and restored hemopoiesis and immune functions.

Cryopreservation of FLC was carried out under routine conditions (Fliedner et al. 1977; Prümmer et al. 1985). The loss of about 90 % of mononuclear, hemopoietic cells was largely due to the damage of late stages of erythropoiesis (Prümmer et al. 1985). In contrast, the recovery of CFU-GM was fairly good and comparable with recovery rates after cryopreservation of CFU-GM from adult bone marrow, provided there was no undue delay between thawing and injection of the grafts.

The intravenous administration of FLC was followed by a prompt engraftment of the fetal stem cells, which was indicated by the emergence of CFU-GM in bone marrow and blood and by rapidly rising blood leukocyte counts. Moreover, marrow hemopoiesis was consistently of donor type at ten days after grafting and for at least one year thereafter. This was concluded from the analysis of spontaneously dividing bone marrow cells. The technique applied did not allow us to distinguish whether non-cycling hemopoietic cells of host origin remained in the marrow or not (Lawler et al. 1984).

The restoration of granulopoiesis and monocytopoiesis proceeded fairly rapidly after FLT and there was a simultaneous rise in circulating numbers of both cell types. Normal blood counts were attained 2-3 weeks after FLT. In contrast, after identical pre-treatment of canine recipients it took about ten weeks until blood granulocyte numbers rose to control levels, when autologous stem cells (equivalent to about 1×10^5 CFU-GM/kg) from adult blood or bone marrow were transfused (Raghavachar et al. 1983a). In some animals, the emergence of mature blood cells was preceded by the appearance of the respective progenitor cells (CFU-GM) in marrow and blood and serum levels of the colony-stimulating activity were maximal when granulocyte and monocyte numbers were lowest and CFU-GM reduplicated at a maximal rate. Dissimilar to some observations in man (Barrett, Adams 1981; Arnold et al. 1982) and dogs (Raghavachar et al. 1983b) after transplantation of hemopoietic stem cells from adult or juvenile donors, CFU-GM frequencies in bone marrow continued to be normal after day 14 following the transfer of FLC. An intriguing finding was the high number of circulating CFU-GM. Biophysical properties of these cells and the number additionally mobilizable from extravascular sites by DS suggested that enhanced levels of circulating CFU-GM reflected an expansion of the total pool of these migratory progenitors throughout the body - at least more than four months after transplantation. At earlier stages, extramedullary hemopoiesis or leaky bone marrow-blood barriers might have facilitated the immigration of CFU-GM into the circulation (Prümmer, Werner et al.). Since no comparable levels of blood progenitors were noted after autologous stem cell transplantation (Raghavachar et al.1983b), the cited mechanisms cannot completely explain the prompt recovery of circulating CFU-GM after FLT. Owing to their biophysical features, migrating CFU-GM appear to represent a relatively immature subpopulation of myeloid progenitor cells (Metcalf, Mac Donald 1975; Gerhartz, Fliedner 1980). Thus, all features described argue in favour of a rapid and efficient restoration of granulopoiesis after FLT, which was reflected both at the level of mature blood cells and of their respective progenitors.

Similar to granulopoiesis, megakaryocytopoiesis was rapidly restored after FLT when compared to the kinetics after transfer of autologous, adult stem cells (Raghavachar et al. 1983a). However, normalization of platelet counts took 1-2 weeks longer as compared to the recovery of granulocytes and monocytes.

Of all hemopoietic lineages followed, erythropoiesis was the last to recover. It was not until 5-6 weeks after grafting that blood erythrocyte counts and hemoglobin concentrations rose to pre-treatment levels. This delayed reconstitution contrasts with the predominance of erythropoiesis in fetal livers of graft donors. Thus, microenvironmental conditions in adult bone marrow might favour the maturation of granulopoiesis relative to erythropoiesis, as is the case in long-term cultures of human fetal liver cells (Cappellini et al. 1984).

The reconstruction of the immune system after marrow transplantation is a slow process (Witherspoon et al. 1984). The same was true for most of the FLC recipients in our series of transplants. On the average, it took about three months for circulating lymphocyte numbers to reach control values. For comparison, in recipients of 10^5 autologous CFU-GM/kg from blood or marrow, lymphocyte counts were only 30-40 % of control on day 101 (Prümmer, Raghavachar, Fliedner). The restoration of circulating lymphocyte pools was in line with autopsy findings in animals sacrificed 2-3 months postgrafting. Lymph node cellularity and the frequency of germinal centers were well within normal limits, as was the number of plasma cells (Calvo, unpublished observation). However, on gross inspection no thymuses were discernible in these animals, though they were present in age-matched controls. Only histological evaluation of the fatty, mediastinal tissue revealed tiny remnants of the organ with some lymphatic repopulation but largely irregular structure (Bödey et al. 1984). Since T cells recovered at about the same rate as total lymphocytes, the question arose whether there was kind of extrathymic T cell maturation. Normal blastogenic responses more than 7 weeks post-FLT of lymphocytes stimulated with Con A or PWM in vitro might support this view; FLC throughout gestation do not respond to mitogenic activation in vitro (Prümmer et al. 1983b). The slow recovery of the mixed lymphocyte reaction is in line with MLC reactivities of blood lymphocytes after bone marrow transplantation (Abb et al. 1978).

The rapid increase in circulating B cell numbers was paralleled by an early rise in serum concentrations of IgM and IgG. B cells or their precursors present among FLC (Prümmer et al. 1983b) might account for this sequence of events. The relative role played by radioresistant B lineage cells of host type (Witherspoon et al. 1984) is unclear. So are the factors operative in the delayed recovery of serum IgA levels, which may also be observed after bone marrow transplantation (Witherspoon et al. 1984; Prümmer, Raghavachar, Fliedner).

When following the immunoreconstitution after FLT one has to recognize the presence among blood MNC of radioresistant host cells, which have retained at least some of their functional properties. Although there remains some doubt as to the nature of these cells, they constitute candidates for effector cells that mediate rejection of hemopoietic allografts.

The pace of the recovery after FLT of granulocytes, platelets, and lymphocytes was associated with the number of CFU-GM transfused. Thus, the CFU-GM content in FLC grafts of similar origin and pre-treatment may be taken as an indicator of the restorative potential or the content of pluripotent hemopoietic stem cells of the respective grafts. In addition, since reconstitution processes proceeded at a similar pace in the present experiments as after transplantation of comparable numbers of fresh fetal liver CFU-GM (Stitzel et al. 1983), one may conclude that the pluripotent stem cells after cryopreservation were recovered to the same extent as CFU-GM.

Two of ten dogs exhibited skin alterations compatible with moderate acute and protracted GVHD, respectively. The significance of these findings has been discussed (Prümmer et al. 1985). It remains questionable whether the intermittent plateau phase in the recovery of lymphocytes and the secondary depression of red blood cell counts and hemoglobin concentrations reflected the presence of subclinical GVHD that escaped both macroscopic and histological detection. Alternatively, malnutrition as a consequence of pancreatic fibrosis might have influenced both lymphocyte and erythrocyte reconstitution (Deeg et al. 1981; Floersheim 1979; Prümmer et al. 1985).

In summary, the present studies demonstrate that a single fetal liver from the middle of the third gestational trimester contains enough stem cells to restore both hemopoiesis and immune functions in a histocompatible adult sibling. The high repopulating potential of these FLC is retained after cryopreservation and compares favourably with the quality of murine FLC (Schofield 1970; Yunis et al. 1976). Moreover, FLC share some properties with adult bone marrow grafts depleted of T cells: they are exquisitely prone to graft rejection mechanisms under matched and mismatched histocompatibility conditions and they may be transplanted without eliciting severe GVHD. Thus, the transplantation of canine FLC may serve as a preclinical model for the analysis of both graft rejection and tolerance induction after the transfer of hemopoietic stem cell grafts lacking mature T lymphocytes.

ACKNOWLEDGEMENTS

We are indebted to all members of the Department of Clinical Physiology and Occupational Medicine, University of Ulm, who provided technical and secretarial help. Part of the antibiotics used were the generous gift of Beecham-Wülfing, Neuss; Boehringer Mannheim; Byk-Essex, Munich; and of Grünenthal, Stolberg. Supported by the Deutsche Forschungsgemeinschaft, SFB 112, and the Radiation Protection Programme of the Commission of the European Communities, Contract No. BIO-C 345-80-D, Contribution No. BIO 2182.

REFERENCES

Abb J, Kolb HJ, Grosse-Wilde H, Rieder I, Thierfelder S (1978). Cell-mediated immunity in canine marrow graft recipients given cyclophosphamide. Exp Hematol 6:58.

Andreani M, Agostinelli F, Manna M, Gaudenzi G, Proietti A, Grianti C, Lucarelli G (1983). Fetal liver transplantation in the mini-pig. In Gale RP (ed): "Recent Advances in Bone Marrow Transplantation," New York: Alan R Liss, p 849.

Arnold R, Heit W, Heimpel H, Frickhofen N, Schmeiser T, Kubanek B (1982). The reconstitution of haemopoietic precursors after bone marrow transplantation. Exp Hematol 10, Suppl 10:79.

Barrett AJ, Adams J (1981). A proliferative defect of human bone marrow after transplantation. Br J Haematol 49:159.

Bödey B, Calvo W, Prümmer O, Carbonell F, Fliedner TM (1984). Regeneration of thymus after total body irradiation in dogs rescued by transfusion of fetal liver cells. Exp Hematol 12:451.

Cappellini MD, Potter CG, Wood WG (1984). Long-term haemopoiesis in human fetal liver cell cultures. Br J Haematol 57:61.

Carbonell F, Calvo W, Fliedner TM, Nothdurft W, Ross WM (1984). Cytogenetic studies in dogs after total body irradiation and allogeneic transfusion with cryopreserved blood mononuclear cells: observations in long-term chimeras. Int J Cell Cloning 2:81.

Champlin RE, Stitzel KA, Gale RP (1982). Fetal liver cell transplantation (FLCT) in dogs. Exp Hematol 10, Suppl 11:31.

Deeg HJ, Storb R, Weiden PL, Schumacher D, Shulman H, Graham T, Thomas ED (1981). High-dose total-body irradiation and autologous marrow reconstitution in dogs: dose-rate-related acute toxicity and fractionation-dependent long-term survival. Rad Res 88:385.

Fliedner TM, Körbling M, Calvo W, Bruch C, Herbst E, Fache I, Rüber E (1977). Cryopreservation of blood mononuclear leukocytes and stem cells suspended in a large fluid volume: a preclinical model for a blood stem cell bank. Blut 35:195.

Floersheim GL (1979). Immunosuppressive effects of miscellaneous agents. In Turk JL, Parker D (eds): "Drugs and Immune Responsiveness," London: Macmillan Press, p 1.

Gerhartz HH, Fliedner TM (1980). Velocity sedimentation and cell cycle characteristics of granulopoietic progenitor cells (CFUc) in canine blood and bone marrow: influence of mobilization and CFUc depletion. Exp Hematol 8:209.

Lawler S, Baker MC, Harris H, Morgenstern GR (1984). Cytogenetic studies on recipients of allogeneic bone marrow using the sex chromosomes as markers of cellular origin. Br J Haematol 56:431.

Löwenberg B (1975). "Fetal Liver Transplantation," Rijswijk: Publication of the Radiobiological Institute TNO.

Metcalf D, Mac Donald HR (1975). Heterogeneity of in vitro colony- and cluster-forming cells in the mouse marrow: segregation by velocity sedimentation. J Cell Physiol 85:643.

Miller RG (1973). Separation of cells by velocity sedimentation. In Pain RH, Smith BJ (eds): "New Techniques in Biophysics and Cell Biology, Vol 1," London: John Wiley & Sons, p 87.

Nothdurft W, Steinbach KH, Ross WM, Fliedner TM (1982). Quantitative aspects of the granulocyte progenitor cell (CFUc) mobilization from extravascular sites in dogs using dextran sulphate (DS). Cell Tissue Kinet 15: 331.

Nothdurft W, Steinbach KH, Fliedner TM (1983). In vitro studies on the sensitivity of canine granulopoietic progenitor cells (GM-CFC) to ionizing radiation: differences between steady state GM-CFC from blood and bone marrow. Int J Radiat Biol 43:133.

Nothdurft W, Braasch E, Calvo W, Prümmer O, Carbonell F, Grilli G, Fliedner TM (1984). Ontogeny of the granuloyte/macrophage progenitor cell (GM-CFC) pools in the beagle. J Embryol exp Morph 80:87.

O'Reilly RJ, Pollack MS, Kapoor N, Kirkpatrick D, Dupont B (1983). Fetal liver transplantation in man and animals. In Gale RP (ed): "Recent Advances in Bone Marrow Transplantation," New York: Alan R. Liss, p 799.

Prümmer O, Raghavachar A, Calvo W, Carbonell F, Fliedner TM (1983a). Restoration of hemopoiesis by cryopreserved fetal liver cells in a canine model. In Gale RP (ed): "Recent Advances in Bone Marrow Transplantation," New York: Alan R. Liss, p 857.

Prümmer O, Calvo W, Fliedner TM, Nothdurft W (1983b). Immunological characterization of canine fetal liver cells. In Gale RP (ed): "Recent Advances in Bone Marrow Transplantation," New York: Alan R. Liss, p 841.

Prümmer O, Raghavachar A, Werner C, Calvo W, Carbonell F, Steinbach I, Fliedner TM (1985). Fetal liver transplantation in the dog. I. Restoration of hemopoiesis with cryopreserved fetal liver cells from DLA-identical siblings. Transplantation, in press.

Prümmer O, Werner C, Raghavachar A, Nothdurft W, Calvo W, Steinbach KH, Fliedner TM. Fetal liver transplantation in the dog. II. Repopulation of the granulocyte-macrophage progenitor cell compartment by fetal liver cells from DLA-identical siblings. Submitted for publication.

Prümmer O, Raghavachar A, Fliedner TM. Recovery of immune functions after total body irradiation and transplantation of autologous stem cells from peripheral blood or bone marrow. Submitted for publication.

Raghavachar A, Prümmer O, Fliedner TM, Calvo W, Steinbach IBE (1983a). Stem cells from peripheral blood and bone marrow: a comparative evaluation of the hemopoietic potential in the dog. Int J Cell Cloning 1:191.

Raghavachar A, Prümmer O, Fliedner TM, Steinbach KH (1983b). Progenitor cell (CFUc) reconstitution after autologous stem cell transplantation in lethally irradiated dogs: decreased CFUc populations in blood and bone marrow correlate with the fraction mobilizable by dextran sulphate. Exp Hematol 11:996.

Saltzstein EC, Bortin MM, Rimm AA, Hussey JL (1974). Long lived canine allogeneic radiation chimera produced with combined fetal liver and thymus cells. Transplantation 18:461.

Schofield R (1970). A comparative study of the repopulating potential of grafts from various haemopoietic sources: CFU repopulation. Cell Tissue Kinet 3:119.

Stitzel KA, Champlin R, Gale RP (1983). Fetal liver transplantation in dogs: a possible alternative source of hematopoietic cells for transplantation. In Gale RP (ed): "Recent Advances in Bone Marrow Transplantation," New York: Alan R. Liss, p 831.

Thomas ED, Collins JA, Kasakura S, Ferrebee JW (1963). Lethally irradiated dogs given infusions of fetal and adult hematopoietic tissue. Transplantation 1:514.

Trigg ME, Bozdech MJ, Sondel PM, Billing R, Finlay JL, Peterson AD, Stuiber M, Hong R (1984). Depletion of T-cells from mismatched allogeneic bone marrow: results of transplantation in 23 patients with malignancy or aplastic anemia. Exp Hematol 12: 412.

Uphoff DE (1958). Preclusion of secondary phase of irradiation syndrome by inoculation of fetal hematopoietic tissue following lethal total-body X-irradiation. J Natl Cancer Inst 20:625.

Van Putten LM, Van Bekkum DW, De Vries MJ (1968). Transplantation of foetal haemopoietic cells in irradiated rhesus monkeys. In: "Radiation and the Control of the Immune Response," Vienna: International Atomic Energy Agency, p 41.

Witherspoon RP, Lum LG, Storb R (1984). Immunologic reconstitution after human marrow grafting. Sem Hematol 21:2.

Yunis EJ, Fernandes G, Smith J, Good RA (1976). Long survival and immunologic reconstitution following transplantation with syngeneic or allogeneic fetal liver and neonatal spleen cells. Transplant Proc 8:521.

FETAL LIVER CELL TRANSPLANTATION IN DOGS: RESULTS WITH DLA-COMPATIBLE AND INCOMPATIBLE GRAFTS

Richard Champlin, M.D., Gary Cain, D.V.M. Katherine A. Stitzel, D.V.M., Robert Peter Gale, M.D., Ph.D. UCLA School of Medicine, Los Angeles, California 90024 and Laboratory for Energy Related Helath Research, University of California-Davis, Davis, California 95616

ABSTRACT

We evaluated the ability of fetal liver hematopoietic cells to reconstitute hematopoiesis and immunity in lethally irradiated dogs. Nineteen consecutive dogs received transplants of fetal liver cells from donors identical or mismatched for DLA antigens. Six animals received 16 Gy fractionated total body irradiation (TBI) followed by transplantation of DLA-identical fetal liver. Three other dogs received transplants of fetal liver that was homozyous for a DLA haplotype shared by the recipient. No post-transplant immunosuppressive treatment was administered. All nine dogs had rapid and sustained restoration of hematopoiesis and none developed graft-versus-host disease. T and B-lymphocyte function recovered slowly over several months in all animals with sustained engraftment and they remained free of infection in open kennel conditions. These data indicate that a single DLA-identical fetal liver can reconstitute hematopoiesis in lethally irradiated dogs. This conditioning regimen was inadequate for transplantation of DLA-mismatched fetal liver cells; 6 of 6 dogs failed to engraft. We evaluated whether more intensive conditioning with 18 Gy fractionated TBI or 16 Gy TBI followed by post transplant treatment with methotrexate was feasible in 4 dogs. These regimens produced severe mucositis and gastrointestinal toxicity; 2 recipients of DLA-matched fetal liver transplants survived but 2 dogs receiving DLA-haploidentical fetal liver had engraftment but died of toxicity. Further studies are required to develop an effective, yet tolerable conditioning regimen in this setting. Fetal liver transplantation may ultimately be useful as a source of hematopoietic cells for transplantation in human patients if an effective conditioning regimen can be developed to allow engraftment of histoincompatible transplants.

Transplantation of hematopoietic cells derived from bone marrow is an effective treatment for selected hematologic, neoplastic and immunologic diseases (Champlin 1984; O'Reilly 1983; Thomas et al 1975). Several major problems may complicate the use of allogeneic bone marrow transplatation including graft rejection and the development of graft-versus-host disease (GVHD). The pathophysiology of GVHD is incompletely understood but most data indicate it is mediated by T lymphocytes present in the graft which react against recipient (host) tissues (Grebe and Streilen 1976; Korngold and Sprent 1982; Mitsuyasu et al 1985). Because of these problems of graft rejection and GVHD, bone marrow transplantation is currently reserved for patients with an HLA-identical sibling donor.

There is considerable interest in identifying alternative sources of hematopoietic stem cells with a decreased capacity to induce GVHD. The fetal liver is a prominent site of hematopoiesis during mid-gestation and contains abundant numbers of hematopoietic stem cells. Unlike the bone marrow, fetal liver contains few if any immunocompetent lymphocytes (Champlin 1980). Transplantation of fetal liver cells can restore hematopoiesis and immune function in lethally irradiated rodents. The ensuing GVHD is absent or mild and is typically delayed compared to that associated with transplantation of bone marrow cells. Long term survival has been achieved following fetal liver transplants between donor-recipient pairs completely mismatched for major histocompatibility complex (MHC) antigens (Uphoff 1958; Lowenberg 1975).

In contrast to these favorable results in rodents, fetal liver transplants have been largely unsuccessful in outbred animals and man (Lowenberg 1975; Thomas 1963; Perryman 1980; Van Putten 1978; Lowenberg 1977; O'Reilly 1978; Gale 1980). Failure of engraftment or incomplete hematologic and immune reconstitution have been major problems. The basis for these failures is unknown and it is unclear if they result from insufficient numbers of hematopoietic and lymphoid stem cells or qualitative differences between fetal liver or bone marrow derived stem cells. To study this problem, we developed a model of fetal liver cell transplantation in dogs (Stitzel et al 1983). We report studies which indicate successful hematologic and immune reconstitution after transplantation of cells from a single fetal liver in DLA-identical recipients. In contrast to these favorable results, graft failure was a major problem in recipients of DLA-nonidentical transplants. These data suggest that fetal liver transplantation may potentially be successful in human candidates for bone marrow transplantation who lack an HLA-identical donor provided that an effective immunosuppressive conditioning regimen for HLA-nonidentical transplants can be developed.

METHODS

One to 9 year old beagles, 10-13 kg in weight, were selected from a colony of dogs at the Laboratory for Energy Related Health Research. Dogs that were genotypically homozygous or heterozygous for DLA antigens were identified and bred to produce fetuses of specified DLA profiles (see Figure). Fetal liver cells from these fetuses were transplanted into lethally irradiated recipients that were identical or mismatched for one or more DLA-haplotypes.

Recipient dogs were prepared for transplantation with one to three fractions of total body irradiation (TBI) from a Co^{60} source at a dose rate of 3 cGy/min. Fetal liver tissue was obtained by hysterotomy at 53-55 days gestation. Fetuses were exsanguinated from the brachial artery and the liver removed surgically. A single cell suspension of hematopoietic cells was prepared by disrupting the tissue with surgical forceps irrigating the liver in RPMI-1640 tissue culture media. The resulting cell suspension was passed through cotton gauze to remove debris and assessed for viability by trypan-blue dye-exclusion. Nucleated hematopoietic cells and CFU-GM were enumerated (Wilson 1978). The fetal liver cell suspension was infused intravenously into a recipient dog of the opposite sex within 24 hours of the last dose of radiation (day 0). Dogs received either no immunosuppressive treatment, or methotrexate post-transplant. Methotrexate was given at a dose of 0.25 mg/kg on days 1,3,6 and 11.

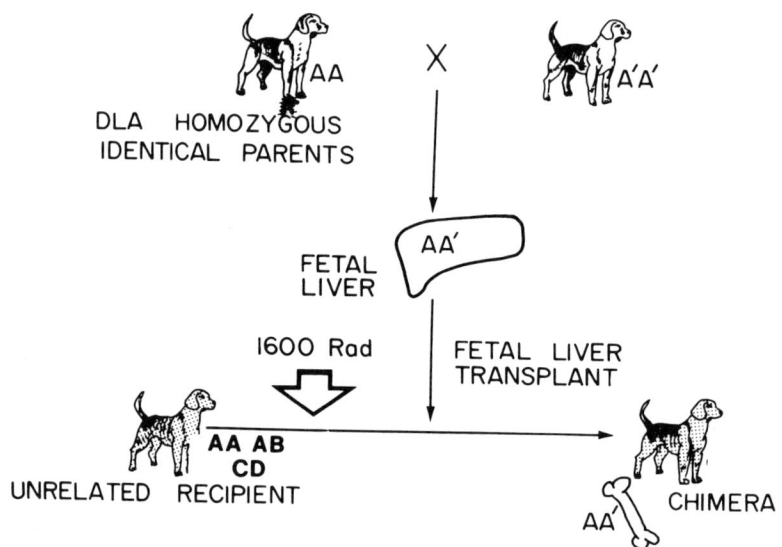

Figure: Scheme of study design. DLA-homozygous and identical beagles were bred giving rise to a litter of a uniform DLA type. The fetal liver was transplanted into DLA-identical or -nonidentical recipients who were prepared with total body irradiation.

Engraftment was confirmed by serial cytogenetic analyses of recipient bone marrow cells (Taylor 1975) and by DLA-antigen typing of peripheral blood mononuclear cells (Vriesendorp 1977). All dogs received oral and parenteral antibiotics. The animals were followed by daily physical examinations, serial blood counts, bone marrow biopsies, and biochemistry studies. Immune reconstitution was assessed by peripheral blood lymphocyte counts, proliferative response to phytohemagglutinin, reactivity in mixed lymphocyte culture and quantitative serum immunoglobulins (Stitzel 1983). Biopsies of lymphoid tissue was performed in selected animals. The animals were returned to open outdoor kennels 3 months post-transplant.

RESULTS

Nineteen dogs received fetal liver transplants. DLA histocompatibility, conditioning regimen, number of fetal livers, cell dose and CFU-GM transplanted are indicated in the table. A single fetal liver was utilized if it contained $\geq 10^8$ nucleated hematopoietic cells; otherwise cells from 2 or more fetal livers were transplanted. Engraftment was documented in each indicated case by the presence of exclusively donor karyotypes in the bone marrow of sex-mismatched recipients as well as presence of cells with donor DLA-antigens.

Six dogs received pretransplant conditioning with 16 Gy total body irradiation given as two 8 Gy fractions on day -3 and -1 followed by a transplant of DLA-identical fetal liver cells. All six had prompt engraftment with recovery of granulocytes to $> 0.5 \times 10^9/\ell$ by day +11 and platelets to $> 20 \times 10^9/\ell$ by day +15. Peripheral blood lymphocytes recovered more slowly and with considerable variability requiring 30 to 80 days to exceed $1.0 \times 10^9/$. All six dogs survived > 6 months with sustained engraftment, full recovery of peripheral blood counts and evidence of immune reconstitution. One animal subsequently developed adrenal insufficiency and two, pancreatic exocrine insufficiency. Another dog developed myasthenia gravis documented by anti-neuromuscular junction antibodies and a positive response to edrophonium (Cain 1985).

Three dogs received the same 16 Gy conditioning radiation scheme followed by transplants of DLA-haploidentical fetal liver cells. In these dogs the fetal livers were homozygous (AA) and matched for one DLA-haplotype of the recipient (AB). This donor-recipient combination would tend to allow engraftment but favor development of graft-versus-host disease. All 3 had prompt engraftment; GVHD did not occur. Two of the 3 dogs survived > 6 months. The remaining dog died on day +139 of fibrosing alveolitis.

Four dogs received the same 16 Gy TBI conditioning regimen followed by transplants of DLA haploidentical fetal liver cells. In this instance the fetal liver cells were heterzygous (AB) and matched for one DLA haplotype of the recipient (AA or AC). This combination would favor graft-rejection. Each animal had initial recovery of hematopoiesis followed by abrupt loss of the graft with pancytopenia and an acellular marrow within 2 weeks of transplantation. These findings are most consistant with graft-rejection. Graft failure also occurred in 2 similarly prepared dogs who received completely DLA-mismatched fetal liver cells.

In an attempt to develop a more effective preparative regimen 4 dogs received intensive immunosuppressive conditioning with 16 Gy TBI plus methotrexate (0.25 mg IV d 1,3,6,11) or 18 Gy TBI in 3 fractions without methotrexate. These regimens produced unacceptable mucositis and gastrointestinal toxicity as shown in Table 1. Two DLA-identical recipients survived; two DLA-haploidentical recipients engrafted but died of toxicity. Although these regimens allowed initial engraftment in DLA-haploidentical recipients the early deaths in these animals preclude critical analysis.

DISCUSSION

These data indicate that cells from a single DLA-matched or partially mismatched fetal liver can reconstitute hematopoiesis and immunity in lethally irradiated dogs. Hematologic recovery was rapid, similar to that observed following bone marrow transplantation. Immunologic recovery occurred at a slower rate but was sufficient to allow prolonged survival without infections in open kennel conditions. Graft-versus-host disease did not occur even in animals receiving DLA-haploidentical fetal liver cells; transplants of bone marrow cells in this setting predictably results in severe, fatal GVHD. One dog developed myasthenia gravis suggesting that abnormal regulation of immunity may develop. This may be more common in dogs receiving fetal liver than in bone marrow transplant recipients. No other animals had evidence of rheumatologic or autoimmune related diseases. Adrenal insufficiency, pancreatic exocrine insufficiency and fibrosising alveloitis also occured in these animals, probably secondary to the effects of high-dose radiation.

Engraftment was consistently achieved in dogs

Fetal Liver Transplantation in Dogs

DLA Match	N	Radiation Gy x Fractions	No. Fetal Livers	Cell Dose/kg x 10⁸	CFU-C/kg x 10⁴	Engraftment	GVH	Survival No. (m)
Identical	6	8 x 2	1(4)*,2,4	0.9-32.4	1.1-5.8	+	-	5(8+ to 36+) 10m myasthenia gravis
AA → AA	1	6 x 3	2	4.0	ND	+	-	12+
	1	8 x 2 + MTX	3	3.1	ND	+	-	12+
Haplo-identical AA → AA	3	8 x 2	1	1-1.6	0.3-6.6	+	-	2(8+, 36+) 4m fibrosing alveolitis
AB → AA	4	8 x 2	1	0.6-2.6	0.2-6.7	-	NE	< .5
	1	6 x 3 or	2	0.6	0.2	?+	NE	< 1 died GI toxicity
	1	8 x 2 +MTX	2	2	2.25			
Mismatch AB → CD	2	8 x 2	2	0.9-1.2	1.6-15	-	NE	< .5

*( ) = number of dogs transplanted

receiving 16 Gy of total body irradiation in two 8 Gy fractions followed by DLA-identical cells from a single fetal liver or with fetal liver cells that were homozygous for a DLA-haplotype present in the recipient. This conditioning regimen was inadequate, however, to ensure sustained engraftment when the fetal liver contained DLA-antigens not shared by the recipient. When more intensive immunosuppressive conditioning was utilized 16 Gy TBI plus post-transplant methotrexate or 18 Gy TBI without methotrexate, engraftment occured in 2 dogs but both animals died of severe gastrointestinal toxicity.

These data indicate that a single fetal liver contains sufficient stem cells to restore hematopoiesis and immunity in lethally irradiated dogs. Severe graft-versus-host disease did not occur, even in dogs receiving DLA-nonidentical grafts. Failure of engraftment is a major problem with DLA-nonidentical fetal liver transplants. This may be overcome by more effective immunossuppressive conditioning. Further studies are required to develop an effective conditioning regimen with acceptable toxicity.

These results are relevent to the preliminary studies of fetal liver transplants in man where HLA-nonidentical fetal liver cells are typically transplanted and where failure of engraftment has been a major problem. Most patients received immunosuppression with high-dose cyclophosphamide and 10 Gy total body irradiation. This is unlikely to be sufficient to allow engraftment in otherwise immunocompetent transplant recipients. Our data in dogs suggest that more intensive immunosuppressive conditioning is probably required to allow sustained engraftment. Further studies are required to develop effective yet tolerable conditioning regimens for major histocompatibility complex mismatched fetal liver transplants in both dogs and man.

This work was supported in part by Grants CA 23175 and AM 30296 from the National Cancer Institute and Grant DE-AM03-76SF00472 from the U.S. Department of Energy

References

Cain GC, Cardimet GN, Cuddon PC, Gale RP, Champlin RE.

Myasthenia gravis and polymyositis in a dog following fetal hematopoietic cell transplantation. Transplantation 1985, (in press).
Champlin RE, Gale RP. The role of bone marrow transplantation in the treatment of hematologic malignancies and solid tumors: a critical review of syngeneic, autologous and allogeneic transplants. Cancer Treat Rep 1984; 68:145-161.
Champlin RE, Gale RP. Hematopoiesis and immune reactivity of human fetal liver cells. In Lucarelli G, Fliedner TM, Gale RP (eds). Fetal LIver Transplantation, Amsterdam, Excerpta Medica 1980; pp 117-125.
Gale RP. Fetal Liver Transplantation in man. In: Fetal Liver Transplantation: Current concepts and future directions (Eds. G. Lucarelli, T. Fliedner, R.P. Gale). Elsevier, Amsterdam, 1980. pp. 268-76.
Grebe SC, Streilen JW. Graft-versus-host reactions: a review. Adv Immunol 1976; 22:119-221.
Korngold R, Sprent J. Features of T cells causing H-2 restricted lethal graft-versus-host disease across minor histocompatibility barriers. J Exp Med 1982; 155:182.
Lowenberg B. Fetal liver cell transplantation role and nature of the fetal haematopoietic stem cell. Publication of the Radiobiological Institute of the Organization for Health Research TNO, Rijswijk (Z.H.), The Netherlands, 1975.
Lowenberg B, Vossen JMJJ, Dooren LJ. Transplantation of fetal liver cells in the treatment of severe combined immunodeficiency disease. Blut 1977; 34:181-195.
Mitsuyasu RT, Champlin RE, Ho WG, et al. Prospective randomized controlled trial of ex-vivo treatment of donor bone marrow with monoclonal anti-T cell antibody and complement for prevention of graft-versus-host disease: a preliminary report. Transplant Proc 1985; 17:482-485.
O'Reilly R. Allogeneic bone marrow transplantation: current status and future directions. Blood 1983; 62:941-954.
O'Reilly RJ, Pahwa R, Dupont B, Good RA. Severe combined immunodeficiency: transplantation approaches for patients lacking an HLA genotypically identical sibling. Transplant Proc 1978; 10:187-199.
Perryman LE. Use of fetal liver for immunoreconstitution in horses with SCID. IN Lucarelli G, Fliedner TM, Gale RP (eds). Fetal Liver Transplantation Amsterdam, Excerpta Medica 1980; pp 183-197.
Stitzel KA, Champlin RE, Gale RP. Fetal liver

transplantation: a possible alternative to bone marrow as a source of hematopoietic cells for transplantation. In Gale RP (ed). Recent Advances in Bone Marrow Transplantation. Alan R. Liss, Inc, New York 1983; pp 29-38.

Taylor N, Shifrine M, Wolf HG, Trommershausen-Smith A. Canine karyotypes from an original tumor, its metastasis, and tumor cells in tissue culture. Transplant Proc 1975; 7:485-493.

Thomas ED, Storb R, Clift RA, et al. Bone marrow transplantation. N Engl J Med 1975; 292:832-843, 895-902.

Thomas ED, Collins JA, Kasakura S. Lethally irradiated dogs given infusions of fetal and adult hematopoietic tissue. Transplant 1963; 1:514-520.

Uphoff DE. The preclusion of secondary phase of irradiation syndrome by innoculation of fetal hematopoietic tissue following total body irradiation. J Nat Cancer Inst 1958; 20:625.

Van Putten LM, Van Bekkum D, DeVries J. Transplantation of foetal hematopoietic cells in irradiated Rhesus monkeys. In Radiation and Control of the Immune Response, Vienna: International Atomic Energy Commission, 1978.

Vriesendorp HM, Gross-Wilde H, Dorf ME. The Major Histocompatibility Complex in Man and Animals, Berlin: Springer Verlag, 1977.

Wilson FD. Quantitative response of bone marrow colony forming units (CFU-C and PFU-C) in weaning beagles exposed to acute whole body gamma irradiation. Radiat Res 1978; 74:289-297.

FETAL LIVER TRANSPLANTATION IN THE MINI-PIG

Andreani M, De Biagi M, Centis F, Manna M,
Agostinelli F, Filippetti A, Gaudenzi G*, Muretto P§,
Grianti C§, Sotti G**, Rigon A**, Lucarelli G.

Divisione di Ematologia, § Servizio di Anatomia
Patologica, USL-3, Pesaro. ** Servizio di Radio-
logia, USL-21, Padova. * Veterinary Sourgeon, Pesaro.
Italy.

SUMMARY

After the characterisation of the hematological and
immunological status of the mini-pig fetus at different gestational ages of development was performed, two different
groups of animals receiving 800 rads of TBI given by a radioactive cobalt source at a dose/rate of 5/6 rad/min or 750
rads of TBI given by a Linear Accelerator at a dose/rate of
25/26 rad/min, both in a single dose exposure, were transplanted with a pool of allogeneic fetal liver cells whose
age ranged between 55 and 75 days of gestation.

In the first group 1 animal out of 6 is alive and well
30 months post-transplant. In the second group one of the
nine transplanted animals survived 78 days. Engraftment was
proved by the presence of the donor chromosome in the proliferating bone marrow cells in one animal.

INTRODUCTION

Totipotent stem cells present in the fetal liver are
able to restore hemopoiesis in supralethally irradiated recipients. Pioneer experimental observations in the rodent

(Andreani 1982; Bortin 1976; Lowenberg 1976) are now supported by many data reported in the literature on fetal liver transplantation in large animals (Perryman 1980; Prümmer 1983; Stitzel 1983). In our Department we initiated a study on fetal liver transplantation in the mini-pig (Andreani 1983). After evaluation of the immunological and hematological characteristics of the fetuses at different ages of development (Delfini 1980) we investigated the possibility of obtaining a bone marrow reconstitution in supralethally irradiated mini-pigs after infusion of allogeneic fetal liver cells.

MATERIALS AND METHODS

Animal

4 to 12 month old mini-pigs, weighing 20 to 35 Kg, were obtained from the Morini-Canosa random out-bred colony. The treated animals were housed in single cages and observed for disease at least one month before use. Blood products, hypernutrition and liquid infusion were given through an atrial catheter (Silicon catheter Vygon, France) from which blood for tests was withdrawn. MSLA typing was not performed.

Fetal Tissue Suspensions

Fetuses were obtained by hysterectomy at various times after the beginning of the pregnancy which was considered 24 hours after mating. Fetal liver, thymus and spleen suspensions were obtained by mincing the fetal tissues and passing the cells through decreasing needles in RPMI for a final single cell suspension. 55 to 75 day old fetal liver cells were used for the transplant.

Mitogen Test

Mini-pig peripheral blood lymphocytes (PBL) or fetal liver, thymus and spleen cells were cultured at a concentration of 10^5 cells per 200 μl in RPMI 1640 medium (GIBCO) supplemented with 5% FBS (GIBCO), glutamine (0.3 mg/ml), non essential aminoacids (0.1 mM - GIBCO) sodium pyruvate (1 mM), penicillin (100 units/ml) streptomycin (100 mg/ml) and gentamycin (40 μg/ml) that will be referred to as Complete Medium (CM). Cultures were maintained at 37°C in 5% CO_2 for 48 hours, at which time H-thymidine, 1 μCi in 50 μl medium, was added at each culture well. 18 hours after addition of 3H-thymidine incorporation was observed by means of liquid scintillation counting.

Immunoglobulin Positive Cells

A polyvalent isothiocyanate conjugate rabbit anti-swine IgG (Kirtegaard Perry Laboratories Inc, Gaithersberg, Maryland) diluted 1/4 was used to detect the percentage of B cells in the mini-pig PBL and in the different fetal tissues.

E-Rosette

The percentage of E-rosette forming cells (E-RFC) determining the number of T cells present in the PBL and fetal tissues was evaluated by mixing 2×10^6 in 200 μl RPMI (CM) with 7×10^7 sheep red blood cells. After centrifuging gently, cells were stored for 4 to 6 hours at 4°C and counted.

Chromosome Test

The mini-pig karyotype is constituted of 38 chromosomes. Proliferating bone marrow cells were blocked in the mytosis phase with Colchicine (Kolcemid). Hypotonic solution and subsequently methyl alcohol and acetic acid glacial were added to the suspension in proportion of 1 and 3 parts respectively. 10% Gimsa solution was used as colorant.

Conditioning Regimen

800 rads at a dose/rate of 5/6 rad/min from a Cobalt radioactive source or 750 rads at a dose/rate of 25/26 rad/min from a linear accelerator were used as the conditioning regimen for 2 different groups of animals treated.

Support

Platelets were obtained by bleeding a healthy donor. Whole blood was gently centrifuged at 35 g for 30 minutes, the supranatant collected and centrifuged again at 450 g for 10 minutes.

RESULTS

Table 1 summarizes the peripheral blood values of fetuses at different ages of intrauterine life.

Days (Gest.)	RBC $\times 10^6$	Hb gr/100 ml	WBC $\times 10^3$	Plat. $\times 10^3$	Retic. %	PMN %	Lymph. %	Monoc. %	EOS %	RCP %
50	2.96	9.0	4.0	380	26	0	100	–	–	50
60	4.08	9.8	2.9	483	29	15	85	–	–	38
75	4.34	10.1	2.2	423	25	22	78	–	–	30
95	4.9	9.7	4.1	410	16	19	79	2	–	10
New born	6.1	10.9	10.3	660	19	60	40	–	–	7
Adult	6.08	13.1	10.5	445	2	55	41	3	1	–

Table 1. Peripheral blood values of fetuses at different ages of intrauterine life.

A very high percentage of circulating red cell precursors is detectable in the peripheral blood at the earlier stage of development decreasing progressively with age. The percentage of reticulocytes throughout the interuterine life of the mini-pig is also high. Platelet levels are found in the normal range at 50 days of fetal life while red blood cells reach adult level after 95 days of gestation.

The fetal liver is the major sight of hemopoiesis from 25 to 95 days of gestation. During this period the bone marrow is almost completely depleted of hemopoietic activity. From day 95 active hemopoiesis is observed in the bone marrow which presents the normal aspect of hemopoietic adult organ at the time of birth while only a few foci of erythropoiesis are still present in the liver.

The response to the mitogens such as Con-A, PHA, PWM of fetal liver, thymus and spleen suspensions has been evaluated and reported as stimulation index in table 2.

Gestational age (days)	Organ	Con.A	PHA	PWM
30-39	Liver	0.4	0.7	0.4
40-49	Liver	0.7	1	0.7
50-59	Liver	1.5	1.6	1.7
	Thymus	15.1	5.1	5.3
	Spleen	2.3	1.9	2.1
60-69	Liver	1.6	1.2	1
	Thymus	12.5	36.7	8.5
	Spleen	1.1	1.2	1.2
70-79	Liver	0.9	1.7	1.3
	Thymus	12.9	18.4	20.9
	Spleen	1.3	3.5	1.2
95-110	Liver	1.6	1.5	0.9
	Thymus	55.3	42.2	25
	Spleen	20.4	58.6	28.5
New born	Liver	3	1.7	1.3
	Thymus	35.3	125.5	21.7
	Spleen	19.1	141.6	31.6

Table 2. Response to Mitogens

No response to lectins was detected in the liver suspension while a high cell proliferation was observed in the spleen suspension in the period of development and in the thymus from 40 days of gestation onwards. The presence of T and B lymphocytes was also investigated performing the E sheep rosette test and by using an antiswine immunofluorescent antibody. Table 3 reports the results obtained. E rosette forming cells were not detected in the liver suspensions while a high percentage of T cells is always present in the thymus and appears in the spleen at the time of birth.

Positive cells for an immunofuorescent antiswine antibody are present only in the spleen suspension and in a very low concentration throughout the different gestational periods studied.

Gestational age (days)	Thymus E-RFC	Thymus SIFl	Spleen E-RFC	Spleen SIFl	Liver E-RFC	Liver SIFl
30 - 39	N.D.	N.D.	N.D.	N.D.	0	0
40 - 49	N.D.	N.D.	N.D.	N.D.	0	0
50 - 59	56	0	0	2	0	0
60 - 69	57	0	1	1	1	0
70 - 79	59	0	3	3	2	0
95 - 110	53	0	11	3	6	0
New born	68.5	0	23	5	7	0

Table 3. E Rosette forming cells (E-RFC) and surface immunoglobulin fluorescent (SIFl) percentage.

Two groups of animals were transplanted using two different conditioning regimens. The first consisting of 800 rads given by a Cobalt 60 source at a dose rate of 5/6 rad/min., the second consisting of 750 rads given at 25/26 rad/min. from a Linear Accelerator (L.A.). Both these conditioning regimens resulted as being supralethal since all the non-transplanted controls died with bone marrow aplasia, within 15 days from TBI (Fig. 1, 3).

One animal out of six in the first group, transplanted with a pool of 75 days old fetal liver cells at a dose of 4×10^8/Kg is alive 30 months after transplant with a complete bone marrow reconstitution (Fig. 1).
The pattern of peripheral blood reconstitution of this surviving recipient is reported in fig. 2.
Graft in this amimal was not proved with sex chromosome makers.

Of the remaining 5 animals one died at days +65 after transplant for an alveolar pneumonia with fully reconstituted hemopoietic bone marrow.

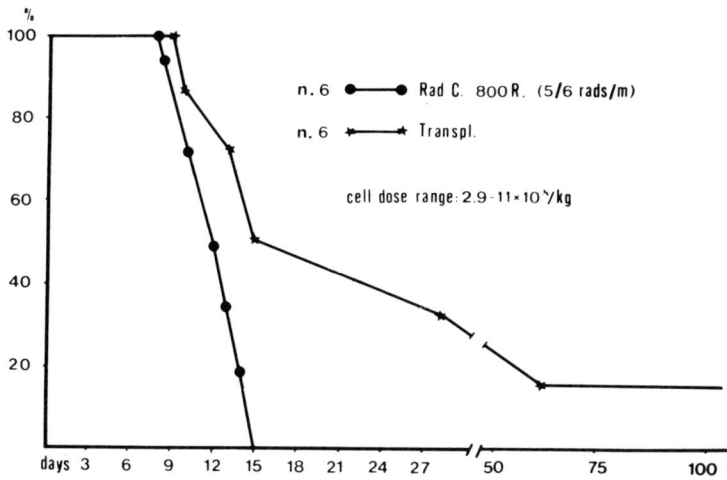

Fig. 1 – Percent of survival of irradiated controls (800 R – 5/6 rad/min.) and recipients of FLT.

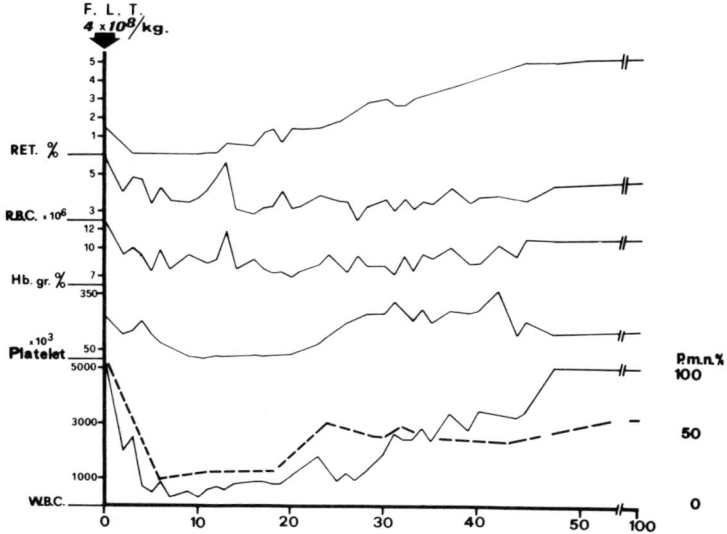

Fig. 2 – Recipient no. 1, pattern of peripheral blood reconstitution after FLT.

The rest of the animals died early during the post irradiation aplastic phase due to hemorrhage and infections. Autoptic bone marrow sections showed initial hemopoietic activity in all cases.

None of the transplanted animals conditioned with 750 rads and transplanted with a pool of fetal liver cells of 55 to 69 days of gestational age survived longer than 78 days from the transplant (Fig. 3).

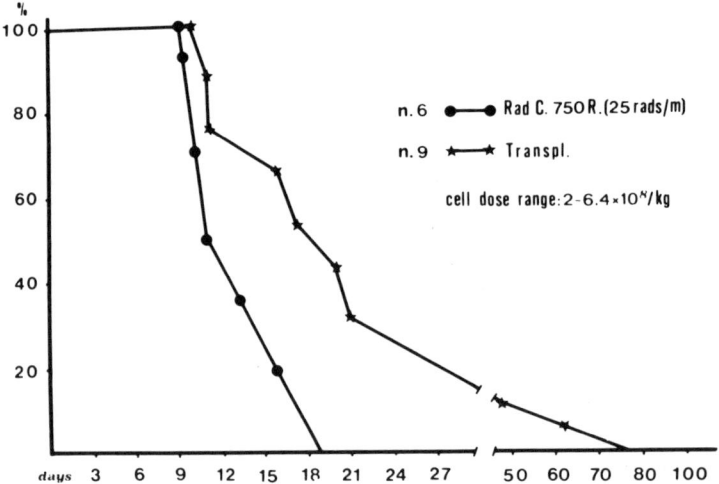

Fig. 3 - Percent of survival of irradiated controls (750 R - 25/26 rads/min.) and recipients of FLT.

Two animals died at day +15 and +16 respectively from the transplant with no signs of engraftment. Four animals died between days 15 and 21 due to infections and hemorrhage.

The histology of the bone marrow of these animals showed initial signs of hemopoietic activity at the autopsy.

Animal no. 2 and no. 5 received pools of 55 and 61 days old fetal liver cells at a dose of 5.1×10^8 cells/Kg and 2.9×10^8 cells/Kg respectively. They both had good bone marrow reconstitution after the transplant as shown by the biopsy performed at day +15 and +30. Fig. 4 and 5 show how peripheral blood counts of these two animals reached normal values early after the transplant.

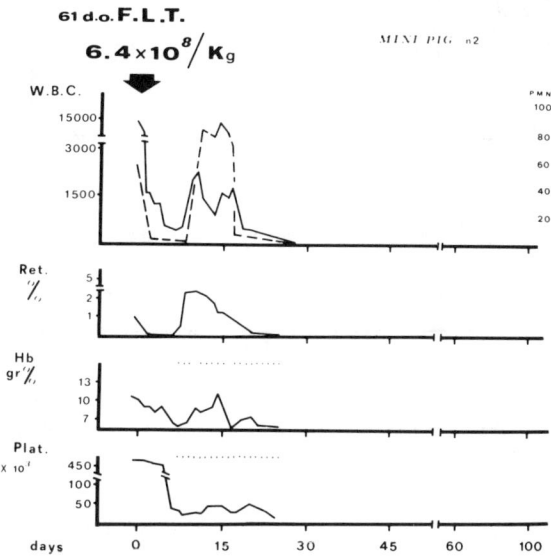

Fig. 4 - Recipient no. 2, pattern of peripheral blood reconstitution after FLT.

At time of death, due to hemorrhage for animal no. 2 and alveolar pneumonia for animal no. 5, the bone marrow of these mini-pigs resulted completely aplastic. Allogeneic engraftment, although transient, was not proved in both these animals.

Peripheral blood lymphocytes of animal no. 5 were responsive to the mitogens such as Con-A, PHA and PWM as tested at day +30. At that time the percent of E-rosette forming cells and the immunofluorescent anti-swine immunoglobin positive cells were 55 and 8 respectively (Fig. 5).

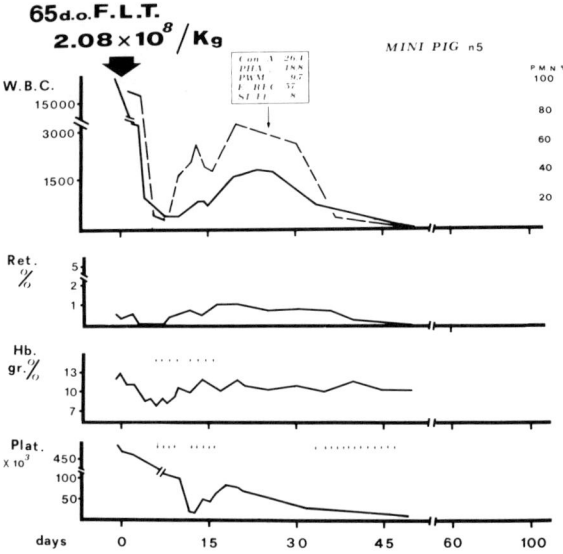

Fig. 5 - Recipient no. 5, pattern of peripheral blood reconstitution after FLT.

Animal no. 6 received 2.9×10^8 cells/Kg from a pool of 69 days old fetal livers.

This animal had complete bone marrow reconstitution following fetal liver transplantation. His peripheral blood counts reached normal values at day +18 (Fig.6). The peripheral blood lymphocytes responded to the mitogens and formed E sheep rosettes while the percent of positive cells for an immuno-fluorescent anti-swine immunoglobin was found to be 4%.
At day +15 and +40 after transplant allogenic engraftment was proved by the changing of the sex chromosome in the bone marrow proliferating cells. Unfortunatly this animal died at day +78 while in good clinical conditions with no signs of GVHD for massive bleeding due to the rupture of the jugular catheter.

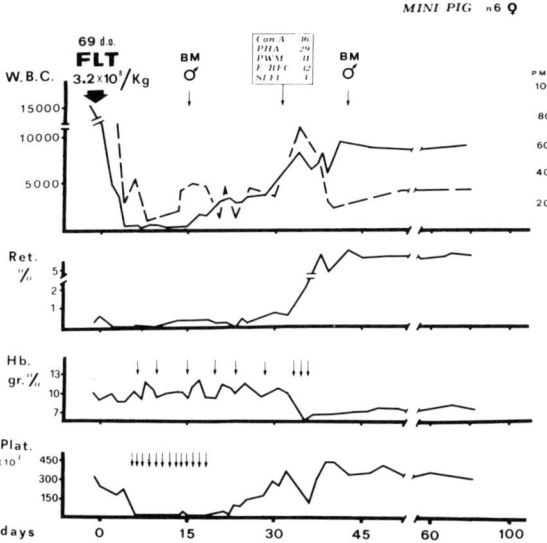

Fig. 6 - Recipient no. 6, pattern of peripheral blood reconstitution after FLT.

CONCLUSIONS

Autologous hemopoietic reconstitution after graft has been observed in all the transplanted animals. If this represents lack of pre-transplant immunosuppresion or a rescue of residual stem cell stimulated by the transient fetal liver graft, remains an open question that requires further studies.

REFERENCES

Andreani M., Agostinelli F., Manna M., Gaudenzi G., Proietti
A., Grianti C., Lucarelli G. (1983).
Fetal Liver Transplantation in the mini-pig.
In Recent Advances in Bone Marrow Transplantation
pages 849-856. 1983 Alan R. Liss, Inc., New York, N.Y.

Andreani M., Agostinelli F., Stramigioli S., Manna M.,
Donati M., Moretti L., Polchi P., Proietti A., Lucarelli G.,
Di Pietrantony F. (1982).
Transplantation of cryopreserved fetal liver cells in
lethally irradiated rats.
Haematologica, 67: 5.

Bortin M.M., Rimm A.A., Rose W.C., Truitt P.L., Saltzstein
F.C.(1976).
Transplantation of hemopoietic and lymphoid cells in mice.
Transplantation 21: 4.

Delfini C., Izzi T., Porcellini A., Lucarelli G.(1980).
Immunologic features of human fetal liver, spleen and
thymus at various gestational ages.
In fetal liver transplantation, Current concepts and future
directions.
Excerpta Medica, Amsterdam.

Lowenberg B., Dicke K.A., van Bekkum D.W., Dooren L.J. (1976).
Quantitative aspects of fetal liver cell transplantation.
Transplantation Proc., 8: 4.

Pennington L.R., Lunney J.K., Sachs D.M..(1981).
Transplantation in miniature swine.
Transplantation, 31: 1.

Perryman L.E.(1980).
Use of fetal tissue for immunoreconstitution in horses with
severe combined immunodeficiency.
In Fetal Liver transplantation, Current concepts and future

directions. Excerpta Medica, Amsterdam.

Prümmer O., Raghavachnar A., Calvo W., Carbonell F., Fliedner T.M., (1983).
Restoration of hemopoiesis by criopreserved fetal liver cells in a canine model.
In Recent Advances in Bone Marrow Transplantation, pages 857-863. 1983 Alan R. Liss, Inc.,New York, N.Y.

Stitzel K.A., Champlin R., Gale R.P. (1983).
Fetal Liver cell transplantation in dogs: a possible alternative source of hemopoietic cells for transplantation.
In Recent Advances in Bone Marrow Transplantation, pages 831-840. 1983 Alan R. Liss, Inc., New York, N.Y.

Supported by C.N.R. Roma, Italy.

FETAL HEMOPOIETIC-CELL TRANSPLANTATION IN SHEEP: AN APPROACH TO THE CELLULAR CONTROL OF HEMOGLOBIN SWITCHING

Christopher BUNCH, W.G. WOOD, and Susan J. KELLY

Nuffield Department of Clinical Medicine
and the MRC Molecular Haematology Unit,
University of Oxford, John Radcliffe Hospital,
Headington, Oxford, OX3 9DU, U.K.

Introduction

In all vertebrates there are developmental changes in the pattern of hemoglobin synthesis; in most species the earliest (embryonic) hemoglobins are replaced by the definitive (adult) hemoglobin early in fetal development in parallel with the shift from yolk-sac to hepatic hemopoiesis. In man, primates and ruminants on the other hand, production of embryonic hemoglobins gives way to that of a specific **fetal** hemoglobin (Hb F, $\alpha_2\gamma_2$), which is replaced by **adult** hemoglobin (Hb A, $\alpha_2\beta_2$), towards the end of gestation. Underlying all these developmental events are changes, or **switches** in expression of different globin-chain genes. For example, in man the γ-chain genes are fully-expressed from about 6 weeks to about 32 weeks gestation, after which Hb F synthesis declines to very low levels; β-chain gene expression begins at a low level at 8 weeks and increases sharply from 32 weeks gestation, so that Hb A is the major hemoglobin produced by the time of birth (Wood and Weatherall 1983).

An important consequence of these changes is that inherited disorders affecting the β globin gene — such as sickle-cell disease and β thalassemia — do not become clinically apparent until shortly after birth. These common disorders represent a major health problem world-wide, and it is thus of some interest that both conditions run a much milder clinical course in patients who

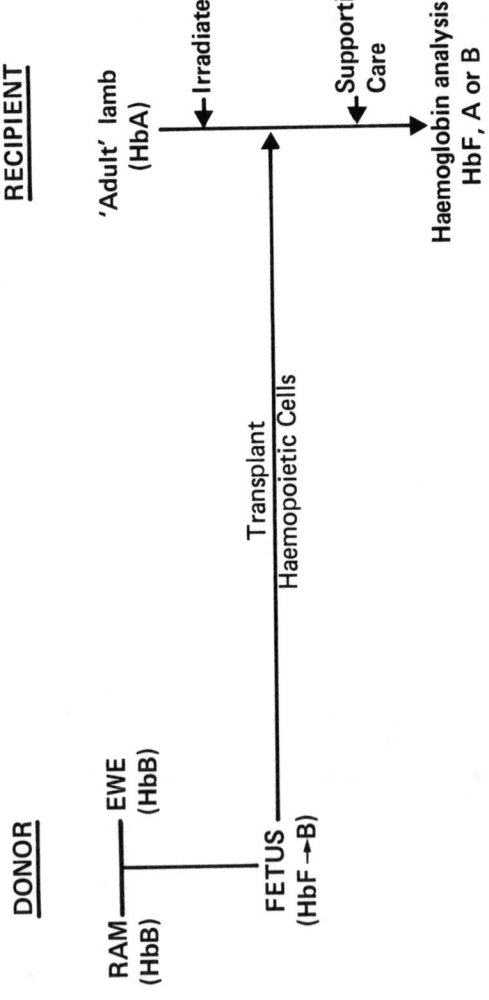

Figure 1. Fetal ⟶ Adult Haemopoietic Cell Grafts. General Experimental Design.

have also inherited an ability to produce increased amounts of fetal hemoglobin throughout adult life (Wood et al 1976; Perrine et al 1978). This suggests that less fortunate patients might benefit if the fetal-to-adult switch could be manipulated in some way to increase fetal hemoglobin production throughout post-natal life.

Whilst our understanding of some of the molecular changes that accompany gene expression, such as DNase sensitivity and cytosine methylation, has increased in recent years (Bird 1984), the cellular mechanisms involved in the control of these developmental switches remains largely unknown. Some years ago the discovery that the small amounts of fetal hemoglobin produced during adult life were confined to only a few erythrocytes led to the suggestion that different populations or clones of hemopoietic progenitors might be responsible for directing fetal and adult hemoglobin production (Weatherall et al 1976). However, very little support for this concept has been forthcoming and the overwhelming balance of evidence (reviewed by Wood 1985) now suggests a common lineage for all erythroid cells. More important questions relate to how the timing of the switch is determined: for example, are there changes in the environment towards the end of gestation which influence the type of hemoglobin produced, or is there a transient environmental signal which triggers a switch in gene expression within the hemopoietic cells? Alternatively, is the pattern of gene expression wholly-controlled by the hemopoietic cells themselves, perhaps by some time-clock mechanism?

In an attempt to answer some of these questions, we have transplanted fetal hemopoietic cells into adult animals in order to examine the effect of the adult hemopoietic environment on the pattern of hemoglobin production (Bunch et al 1981; Wood and Bunch 1983; Wood et al 1985). Our experiences related here may be of relevance to fetal-liver transplantation in general as well as to the control of hemoglobin switching.

Experimental Approach (Figure 1)

The lack of a distinct fetal hemoglobin in the majority of animal species commonly used for transplantation research has been a disadvantage. Following earlier work which established the time course of the fetal-to-adult hemoglobin switch in sheep (Wood et al 1976), we and others have attempted fetal-liver and marrow transplantation in this species (Zanjani et al 1979; Bunch et al

1981). Sheep have one particular advantage for these experiments in having a polymorphism at the β-chain locus with two common alleles, β^A and β^B (Figure 2). By selecting donors and recipients which are homozygous for β^B and β^A respectively, it is possible to unambiguously determine the origin of any adult hemoglobin synthesized after transplantation.

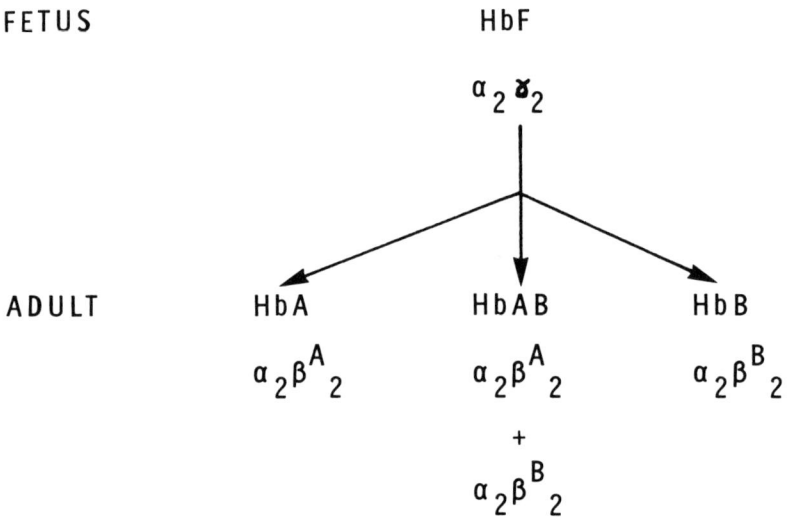

Figure 2. Sheep Hemoglobins

Donor fetuses of 70-110 days gestation (term = 145 days) were obtained by cesarian section from 1-2 year-old ewes of various breeds which had been mated at known times with Dorset rams. All rams and ewes were homozygous for Hb B. Haemopoietic-cell suspensions were prepared from fetal livers by gentle scraping with a scalpel into calcium-free Hanks BSS, and depleted of hepatocytes by centrifugation after addition of calcium (Schwartz et al 1976). Cell yields ranged from 0.2 to 2.63×10^{10}, and were proportional to gestational age. Marrow suspensions were prepared from the long bones of fetuses of 90 days or more gestation (Bunch et al 1981); yields ranged from 0.1 to 30.0×10^8 cells. Marrow development in younger fetuses was insufficient for useful harvest. In 11 instances the graft was augmented by 0.08 to 3.4×10^9 thymus-cells, prepared as a single-cell suspension by mincing with scissors and passage through progressively finer needles.

Recipients were fully-weaned and wormed 2 – 12 month wethers or ewe-lambs, weighing 15 – 40 kg. A variety of different breeds were used for these experiments; in only 7 instances were recipient lambs and donor ewes (but not rams) from the same flock, and no attempts were made to ensure histocompatibility. In our initial experiments we did not attempt to select on the basis of hemoglobin type, but the value of this marker became evident in control experiments when some residual hemoglobin synthesis could be detected for up to 12 – 14 days in irradiated animals that were not transplanted (Bunch et al 1981). Accordingly, the subsequent 31 recipients were selected to be homozygous for Hb A. All recipients had fully completed the switch to adult hemoglobin production. 32 lambs had Hickman or Raaf silicon-rubber right-atrial catheters inserted prior to transplantation to aid supportive care.

Conditioning. Recipients were conditioned with ^{60}Co total-body irradiation (TBI) as follows: 29 unsedated lambs were mounted in a sling and exposed to 4 uncollimated sources as previously described (Bunch et al 1981). A single dose of 10 or 12 Gy, or 12 or 14 Gy in two fractions 18 hr apart, was given at a rate of 6.5 – 10 cGy/min (Table 1). The midline absorbed dose for each animal was estimated on the basis of its size and previous measurements in air using an ionization chamber.

Conditioning Regime	Number of Lambs			Survival (d)	
	tx	eval	graft	median	range
1 x 10 Gy TBI	9	5	0	15	0 – 23
1 x 12 Gy TBI	9	6	3	14	4 – 23
" + MTX	4	2	0	9	3 – 15
2 x 0.6 Gy TBI	5	4	1	18	13 – 22
2 x 0.7 Gy TBI	2	1	0	–	11, 24
3 x 0.6 Gy TBI	11	5	3	12	2 – 41

Table 1. Effect of Conditioning Regime on Engraftment.
tx = number transplanted, eval = number surviving>14 d
graft = successful engraftment (see text)

11 lambs received 18 Gy in three fractions 48 hr apart at 4-5 cGy/min from a collimated cobalt radiotherapy machine (Mobaltron). These lambs were sedated with pentobarbitone and placed in a ventilated perspex box padded with water-equivalent material and were irradiated in both prone and lateral positions. Dosimetry in this group was performed using thermo-luminescent dosimeter chips; actual doses were with one exception within 7% of intended dose. Finally, 4 lambs given a single dose of 12 Gy received in addition intermittent i.v. methotrexate (MTX) after transplantation (Storb et al 1970) in an attempt to improve the rate of engraftment.

Supportive care with parenteral fluid and irradiated platelets was given as required. Platelet concentrates were prepared by standard differential centrifugation techniques from 400-800 ml CPD-anticoagulated whole blood obtained from unrelated ewes (often the mother of the fetal donor). All recipients surviving more than 12 days were given at least one platelet transfusion; one was often sufficient when engraftment was successful. Ampicillin (1 g) and gentamicin (80 mg) were given intravenously twice-daily during periods of neutropenia, and it has been our recent practice to give in addition amphotericin 1-20 mg daily as an 8-hour infusion. Animals receiving single doses of TBI were starved before and after radiation, otherwise free access to food and water was allowed. Several animals received additional nutritional support with 500-1000 ml 20% dextrose daily.

Evaluation. Engraftment was assessed by regular peripheral blood counts, marrow examination, and hemoglobin and/or chromosomal analysis when appropriate. Marrow was aspirated at intervals after transplantation and incubated with [^{3}H]leucine; globin chains were separated by cellulose chromatography as previously described (Clegg et al 1966; Bunch et al 1981). Although some persistent β^A chain synthesis (of recipient origin) was seen in some of these experiments, γ and β^B chain synthesis were both presumed to be of donor origin, as reactivation of recipient fetal hemoglobin synthesis was not seen in a previous series of control experiments (Bunch et al 1981).

Results

Engraftment. Successful engraftment, as judged by return of peripheral blood counts and marrow cellularity toward normal, occurred in only 7 of 40 attempted transplants (Table 1).

Engraftment was confirmed in each instance by hemoglobin analysis, and by chromosomal analysis when donor and recipient were of opposite sex. In the majority of unsuccessful transplants, marrow samples on day 7 or 10 post-transplant showed several foci of hemopoiesis; these foci may have resulted from transient engraftment of committed progenitors, as they were usually either all myeloid or all erythroid rather than mixed. In some instances there was an associated slight but transient rise in peripheral-blood granulocytes. Failure of engraftment was in most cases associated with severe marrow aplasia; partial recovery of autologous marrow function was observed in one recipient conditioned with 10 Gy.

Although the numbers involved are small, the dose and schedule of radiation appeared to influence the rate of engraftment, which was most successful after 18 Gy given in three fractions (Table 1), and after a single fraction of 12 Gy, although the latter regime was associated with severe gastrointestinal toxicity. No effect of donor gestational age (and thus the number of cells transplanted) on engraftment was observed (Table 2). Because of the low rate of engraftment, the graft was augmented in 12 instances by a suspension of fetal thymus cells. These were given to 5/9 animals conditioned with 10 Gy, and 7/11 conditioned with 18 Gy. No grafts were seen in the former group, but 3/4 in the 18 Gy group who were given thymocytes and who survived >14 days grafted successfully (Table 3). Further experiments are required to define the effect of thymus supplements on engraftment using different conditioning regimens.

Gestational Age	Cells Transplanted		Number of Lambs		
	liver x 10^{10}	marrow x 10^8	tx	eval	graft
<90 d	0.94 (0.45 – 1.5)	—	14	7	3
>90 d	1.42 (0.2 – 2.63)	8.68 (0.1 – 30.0)	26	15	3

Table 2. Effect of Donor Gestational Age on Engraftment

Toxicity and Complications. The major non-hemopoietic toxicity was to the gastrointestinal tract. Presumably because of the anatomical arrangement of the ruminant digestive system, recipients did not vomit during or after irradiation. Extreme anorexia was the rule, however, and very few animals resumed a normal pattern of feeding after transplantation. Marked weight-loss occurred in all animals not fed parenterally. Even when engraftment was successful, recipients failed to thrive, and this undoubtedly contributed to their disappointing long-term survival. Ruminant digestive physiology is complex and relies heavily on bacterial decomposition of cellulose; this process may have been adversely affected by broad-spectrum antibiotics as well as by radiation. Diarrhoea occurred in all animals within 48 hr of irradiation and lasted 1-2 weeks. This was attributed to the radiation, but again broad-spectrum antibiotics may have contributed. It did not recur to any significant extent in successfully-engrafted animals, and no manifestations of graft-versus-host-disease were observed. Gastrointestinal toxicity appeared to be less after 18 Gy given in three fractions 48 hr apart, although severe diarrhoea was common following the second fraction. This may have been responsible for the early death of some of these animals, but with aggressive fluid replacement has been less of a problem.

Conditioning Regime	Number of Lambs		
	tx	eval	graft
10 Gy + Thy	5	0	–
10 Gy – Thy	4	4	0
18 Gy + Thy	7	4	3
18 Gy – Thy	4	1	0

Table 3. Effect of Addition of Thymic Cell Suspension to Graft

Major small-bowel necrosis producing obstruction and/or perforation was found at autopsy in 10/20 animals given 12 Gy TBI, but not following other doses. This was not necessarily an acute effect, and was found in animals dying 4-24 days after transplant. The necrosis affected particularly the abomasal area and in some instances was associated with a haemorrhagic pancreatitis. Evidence for chronic pancreatitis was not seen in our longer-term survivors. This has been a problem in dogs given 18 Gy in a similar regime, but generally only after 6 weeks post-transplantation (Deeg et al 1981).

All irradiated animals shed their fleece; return of wool growth occurred after 14 days in animals given 10 Gy, but was not seen in

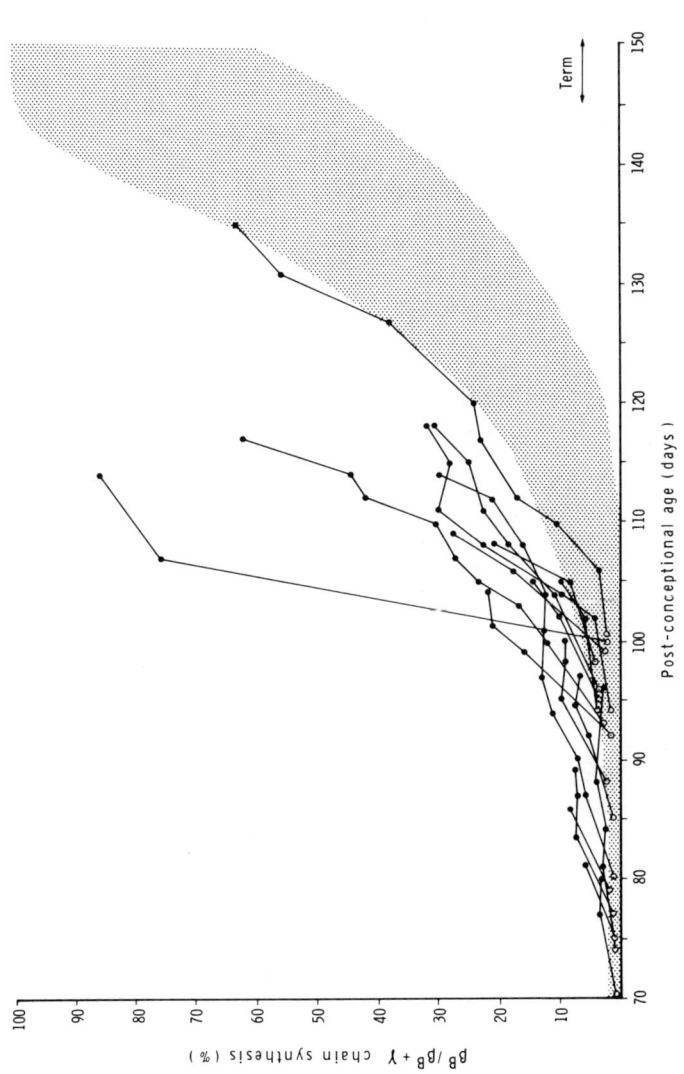

Figure 3. Combined globin synthesis data from 18 transplants comparing the relationship of increased β chain synthesis to gestational age with the normal pattern in utero (shaded).

other groups, even in those surviving 4-6 weeks.

Documented infection was fatal in 13 animals, and infection was presumed to be a major if secondary factor in the death of the remainder. A variety of organisms were isolated from blood cultures, and 7 animals developed multiple fungal or candidal abscesses in the liver, prompting our now routine use of amphotericin. One successfully-engrafted animal died of bacterial meningitis despite an adequate marrow response, whilst another developed severe, protracted but localized orf.

Hemoglobin Synthesis. In all animals which survived the first week after transplant, marrow incubation at 7 days showed predominantly fetal hemoglobin synthesis. At a variable time thereafter, a progressive rise in adult hemoglobin synthesis of donor origin was observed. Hemoglobin production could also be detected (but at a low level) in some animals who did not otherwise engraft successfully, and the cumulative results of 18 transplants in which satisfactory serial data was obtained are shown in Figure 3. This demonstrates that (with the exception of one, unexplained, experiment) the timing of the increase in adult hemoglobin synthesis is related to the gestational age of the donor cells. When compared with observations in a large number of intact fetuses (Wood et al 1976; Bunch and Wood, unpublished), this increase occurred on average about 20 days earlier than expected.

Discussion

The most direct approach to unravelling the control mechanisms involved in the timing of fetal→adult hemoglobin switching is to study the effect of transplantation of fetal hemopoietic cells into an adult hemopoietic environment. When fetal cells of 100 days gestation were first successfully transplanted into an adult sheep (Zanjani et al 1979), they produced predominantly adult hemoglobin, suggesting an immediate environmental effect. In two later experiments using 94-96 day fetuses (Bunch et al 1981), recipient lambs survived 24-26 days during which time the engrafted cells produced predominantly fetal hemoglobin, although a gradual increase in β-chain production by donor cells was noted subsequently. These reports appear to exclude a control mechanism involving a transient environmental trigger, as this should have been by-passed by the experiment unless it were active at least 30 days before the onset of switching. However, further studies were clearly necessary to resolve the conflicting evidence in favor of a more general environmental effect on one hand, and an internal program on the other. Accordingly, we have performed a series of transplants using progressively younger fetal donors; we expected that if switching is controlled by an internal program then the transplanted cells would switch in their own time, whilst if they are susceptible to environmental differences then switching should occur rapidly, irrespective of gestational age.

The results described above show that switching was delayed when cells of around 70 days gestation were used, but occurred almost immediately after transplantation in 100-day cells (Figure 3). This strongly favors the existence of an internal program or time-clock, but some environmental effect cannot be completely excluded as the timing of the switch in the transplanted cells occurred overall about 20 days earlier than expected from previous studies of normal, intact fetuses. It is possible that the grafts included cells from the fetal hemopoietic microenvironment which were able to exert a continuing influence on the transplanted hemopoietic cells in their new environment. Marrow stromal cells of donor origin have been detected following human marrow transplantation (Keating et al 1982), but we have found that the karyotype of stromal cells recovered from long-term marrow cultures obtained from recipient lambs at various times after transplantation shows a predominantly **recipient** pattern, suggesting that donor hemopoietic cells were producing largely fetal hemoglobin whilst differentiating amongst predominantly **adult** environmental cells (Wood et al 1985).

Mechanisms for the control of switching involving environmental factors or an internal program are not necessarily mutually-exclusive. It is possible, for example, that an internal program could simply regulate the expression at around 100 days gestation of a receptor for an environmental factor which is itself responsible for initiating the switch, but which is not normally present until after 120 days. An alternative explanation for the observed acceleration of the switch after transplantation suggests a means by which an internal program could operate. Recipient lambs were heavily irradiated — primarily to prevent graft rejection — and the relatively small numbers of cells transplanted would thus be under considerable pressure to increase their numbers by cell division in order to repopulate the empty marrow. Switching could therefore be controlled by a 'clock' within each stem-cell which counts the number of divisions it undergoes. This possibility could be tested by experiments which artificially increase the rate of stem-cell division in intact fetuses, and it is of interest that control of gene expression by numbers of cell divisions has been demonstrated in other developmental systems (Satoh 1984).

Several other papers in this volume attest to the potential value of fetal liver as a source of hemopoietic cells for transplantation in clinical situations where bone-marrow transplantation has been successfully employed, but when a suitable marrow donor is not available. Permanent, complete hemopoietic reconstitution is at present uncommon following fetal liver transplantation (FLT), but temporary engraftment has occurred in several instances, and occasional recovery of autologous marrow function has been described by several groups. Although it is likely that autologous recovery reflects inadequacy of the conditioning regimen, a non-specific stimulatory effect of FLT itself cannot be wholly excluded. Partial autologous recovery following 10 Gy was noted in only one of our recipients, but the true incidence may have been higher as animals without a successful graft generally succumbed quickly to the effects of marrow failure.

Although the importance of histocompatibility in BMT is widely accepted, matching for MHC determinants was not feasible in our experiments, partly because of our wish to use the hemoglobin polymorphism as a transplantation marker, and partly because understanding of the sheep MHC has lagged behind that of other species commonly used for transplantation research (Cullen et al 1982). The lack of histocompatibility between donor and recipient and the limited numbers of cells available for transplantation closely parallels the clinical situation, and was probably the major reason for the low rate of engraftment. We have attempted to improve this by alterations in the conditioning regime, but simply increasing the dose of radiation, with or without the addition of methotrexate, was associated with an unacceptable increase in gastrointestinal toxicity. In common with other groups' experiences with dogs given DLA-nonidentical, unrelated marrow (Deeg et al 1982), or DLA-identical, cryopreserved sibling fetal liver cells (Prümmer et al 1983), we have had some success with a total radiation dose of 18 Gy given in three fractions, 48 hr apart. Nevertheless, even when engraftment has been successful animals have failed to thrive and we have so far been unable to achieve long-term survival. Our difficulties in this respect may have been complicated by the nature of the ruminant digestive system, but it is noteworthy that a high proportion of dogs given similar conditioning have developed a wasting disorder associated with pancreatic fibrosis some months after otherwise successful transplantation (Deeg et al 1981).

There is thus good reason to be circumspect about the use of high-dose fractionated TBI, and studies of less toxic conditioning agents are urgently required. It has been suggested that fetal hemopoietic stem cells are more sensitive to allogeneic inhibition than adult cells (Gale 1980); this has prompted us to examine the effect of adding fetal thymocytes to the graft (Saltzstein et al 1974), in the hope of counteracting such inhibition, but the numbers so far studied do not justify comment (Table 3). Alternative approaches could include the use of cyclosporine, or pre-conditioning with cyclophosphamide, which has been shown to reduce the gastrointestinal toxicity of TBI in mice (Millar and Hudspith 1976) and of high-dose melphelan in sheep (Millar et al 1978).

Acknowlegements

We are indebted to the many people who have helped with this project. In particular we would like to thank H Elvidge, C Hanson, S Ayres and S Howes for invaluable technical assistance, MJ Corp, Dr DW Barnes and Dr Y Gunn of the Medical Research Council for help with irradiation, and Mr G Breckon for performing chromosomal analyses.

References

Bird AP (1984). DNA methylation - how important in gene control? Nature **307**:503.
Bunch C, Wood WG, Weatherall DJ, Robinson JS, Corp MJ (1981). Haemoglobin synthesis by fetal erythroid cells in an adult environment. Br J Haematol **49**:325.
Clegg JB, Naughton MA, Weatherall DJ (1966). Abnormal human hemoglobins. Separation and characterization of the α and β chains by chromatography, and the determination of two new variants, Hb Chesapeake and HbJ (Bankok). J Mol Biol **19**:91.
Cullen PR, Bunch C, Brownlie J, Morris PJ (1982). Sheep lymphocyte antigens: a preliminary study. Anim Blood Grps Biochem Genet **13**:149.
Deeg HJ, Storb R, Weiden PL, Schumacher D, Shulman H, Graham T, Thomas ED (1981). High-dose total-body irradiation and autologous marrow reconstitution in dogs: dose-rate-related acute toxicity and fractionation-dependent long-term survival. Radiat Res **88**:385.

Deeg HJ, Storb R, Shulman HM, Weiden PL, Graham TC, Thomas ED (1982). Engraftment of DLA-nonidentical unrelated canine marrow after high-dose fractionated total body irradiation. Transplantation 33:443.

Gale RP (1980). Concepts of fetal liver transplantation in man. In Lucarelli G, Fliedner TM, Gale RP: "Fetal Liver Transplantation," Amsterdam: Excerpta Medica, p 247.

Keating A, Singer JW, Killen PD, Striker GE, Salo AC, Sanders J, Thomas ED, Thorning D, Fialkow PJ (1982). Donor origin of the in vitro haematopoeitic microenvironment after marrow transplantation in man. Nature 298:280.

Millar JL, Hudspith BN (1976). Sparing effect of cyclophosphamide (NSC-26271) pretreatment on animals lethally treated with γ-irradiation. Cancer Treat Rep 60:409.

Millar JL, Phelps TA, Carter RL, McElwain TJ (1978). Cyclophosphamide pretreatment reduces the toxic effect of high dose melphelan on intestinal epithelium in sheep. Eur J Cancer 14:1283.

Perrine RP, Pembrey ME, John P, Perrine S, Shoup F (1978). Natural history of sickle cell anemia in Saudi arabs. A study of 270 subjects. Ann Intern Med 88:1.

Prümmer O, Raghavachar A, Calvo W, Carbonell F, Fliedner TM (1983). Restoration of hemopoiesis by cryopreserved fetal liver cells in a canine model. In Gale RP: "Recent Advances in Bone Marrow Transplantation," New York: A.R. Liss, p 857.

Saltzstein EC, Bortin MM, Rimm AA (1974). Long lived canine allogeneic radiation chimera produced with combined fetal liver and thymus cells. Transplantation 18:461.

Satoh N (1984). Cell division cycles as the basis for timing mechanisms in early embryonic development of animals. In Edmunds LN: "Cell Cycle Clocks," New York: Marcel Dekker, p 527.

Schwartz AL, Schwartz R, Schwartz HC (1976). Effect of hypoxia on erythroblasts from avian fetal liver: adenosine triphosphate levels nad hemoglobin synthesis. Pediatr Res 10:796.

Storb R, Epstein RB, Graham TC, Thomas ED (1970). Methotrexate regimens for control of graft-versus-host disease in dogs with allogeneic marrow grafts. Transplantation 9:240.

Weatherall DJ, Clegg JB, Wood WG (1976). A model for the persistence or reactivation of fetal haemoglobin production. Lancet 2:660.

Wood WG (1984). The cellular basis of haemoglobin switching. In Peschle C, Rizzoli C: "New Trends in Experimental Hematology," Rome: Ares Sereno Symposia, p 60.

Wood WG, Bunch C (1983). Fetal-to-adult hemopoietic cell transplantation: Is hemoglobin synthesis gestational age-dependent? In Stamatoyannopoulos G, Nienhuis AW: "Globin Gene Expression and Hematopoietic Differentiation," New York: A.R. Liss, p 511.

Wood WG, Bunch C, Kelly SJ, Gunn Y, Breckon G (1985). Control of haemoglobin switching by a developmental clock? Nature in **press**.

Wood WG, Pearce K, Clegg JB, Weatherall DJ, Robinson JS, Thorburn GD, Dawes GS (1976). Switch from foetal to adult haemoglobin synthesis in normal and hypophysectomised sheep. Nature 264:799.

Wood WG, Weatherall DJ (1983). Developmental genetics of the human haemoglobins. Biochem J 215:1.

Zanjani ED, McGlave PB, Bhakthavathsalan A, Stamatoyannopolous G (1979). Sheep fetal haemopoietic cells produce adult haemoglobin when transplanted in the adult animal. Nature 280:495.

SECTION IV
FETAL LIVER TRANSPLANTATION–MAN

FETAL LIVER TRANSPLANT IN APLASTIC ANEMIA AND ACUTE LEUKEMIA

T. Izzi, P. Polchi, M. Galimberti, C. Delfini,
L. Moretti, A. Porcellini, A. Manna, G. Sparaventi,
C. Giardini, E. Angelucci, P. Politi, G. Lucarelli

Division of Hematology, Pesaro Hospital, Italy.

Recent reports on fetal liver lymphohematopoiesis have clearly shown the increasing interest of a great number of authors in the ontogenesis of fetal liver hemopoiesis, both in animals and in man (Klein, 1983; Rabinowich, 1983; Prummer, 1983; Mandel, 1982; Zucali, 1982). The results of many studies of fetal liver transplant in animals suggested attempting this treatment in man (O'Reilly, 1983; Stitzel, 1983; Prummer, 1983). In patients affected with SCID, SAA and AL, the hemopoietic fetal liver cells from a mismatched donor can give sustained engraftment and offer a possible cure in the absence of an HLA-identical marrow donor (Kelemen, 1979; Lucarelli, 1979; Kansal, 1979; O'Reilly, 1983; Touraine, 1984).

In our Institute, besides the studies on the biology of the fetal hemopoiesis (Delfini, 1980; Porcellini, 1980; Porcellini, 1983). and fetal liver transplant in animals and in man (Lucarelli, 1980; Andreani, 1982; Andreani, 1983; Lucarelli, 1981), a clinical trial of fetal liver transplant (FLT) was begun in 1978 in a group of 18 patients (5 severe aplastic anemia, 13 acute leukemias in relapse or remission) adopting the same preparatory regimen as in the bone marrow transplant (BMT) program (Lucarelli, 1982; Lucarelli, 1983).

MATERIALS AND METHODS

Patients

   Acquired Severe Aplastic Anemia. Five patients with ASAA (age range 4-11) 1 male, 4 females, were prepared with Cyclophosphamide (Cy) 200 mg/Kg from November 1981 to February 1984 (Table 1,2). All the patients followed the protocol adopted for bone marrow transplant (BMT) patients whether for the protected environment, support therapy or the treatment of infections (Izzi, 1984). All blood products were irradiated before infusion as for BMT patients. However, no prophylaxis of Graft-versus-Host Disease (GHVD) or Pneumocystis was adopted.

N°FLT	F.AGE (Wks) F/C*	C.Susp. N°x10^9	F.Sex (M/MM)§	F.Eryth. Isoenzymes (M/MM)	Recovery after thawing (%)
10	12,10(F)	2.1/2.3	MM	MM	50,75
11	20,17,10(F) 21,20(C)	2.7/4.5/0.4 4.9/3.4	MM	–	138,182
16	21,24(C)	9.2/7.0	MM	–	92,100
17	20,21(C) 18(F)	3.7/6.3 2.2	M	N.E.	76,116
18	13,15(F) 25(C)	1.1/1.8 3.7	MM	MM	45

*F = fresh; C = cryopreserved; §M = match; MM = mismatched; N.E. = not evaluable.

Table 1. Fetal Liver Suspension-nucleated Cell Data in Severe Aplastic Anemia Patients.

Markers of Engraftment

Criteria of engraftment were the sexual chromosomes, erythrocytic isoenzymes, erythrocytic antigens, γ chain hemoglobin synthesis, HLA typing and hemopoietic recovery in the absence of other markers (table 1,2) (Lucarelli, 1983).

N°FLT	AGE SEX	FLT (Date)	C.DOSE x 10^8/Kg	ENGRAFT. MARKERS (Hem.Rec.)	SURVIVAL OUTCOME (Days)
10	10/F	19/11/81	0.75	CR	Alive, >1100
11	8/F	3/4/82	1.65	–	+120, Systemic mycosis
16	4/F	9/5/83	12.7	–	+27, Septic shock
17	10/F	9/9/83	2.2	–	+42, Septic shock
18	10/M	25/2/84	1.4	–	+29, Cerebral Hemorrhage

All patients were prepared with Cy 200 mg/Kg*

Table 2. FLT in Severe Aplastic Anemia Patients* - Clinical Data.

Acute Leukemias (Acute Lymphoid Leukemia (ALL) & Acute Myeloid Leukemia (AML)). Thirteen patients with acute leukemia (AL) (age range 2-11 yrs), all males, were prepared with Cy 120 mg/Kg and total body irradiation (TBI) 1000 rads in a single dose from September 1978 to July 1984 (Izzi, 1984). The patients followed the same protocol as Acquired Severe Aplastic Anemia (ASAA) patients for the post transplant period, the same markers were used for engraftment. Of 8 relapsed patients, 6 were ALL in 3rd or further relapse and 2 were AML in 3rd relapse (Tables 3,4). One patient had a different regimen : Vincristine (VCR) + L-Asparaginase (L-Asp) before TBI (Lucarelli, 1983). In the 5 complete remission (CR) patients, 4 were ALL in 2nd remission and 1 AML in 1st CR (Tables 5,6).

Fetal Liver Suspension. After processing fetal livers of 12-25 weeks, as previously published (Lucarelli, 1980; Lucarelli, 1982) the cell suspension, either fresh or cryopreserved (Moretti, 1979; Polchi, 1979) was infused into the patients through a blood filter (100 µ) in a time of 1-2 hours. No reactions were observed during the infusion of fresh or cryopreserved suspensions.

Cryopreserved suspensions were thawed for half an hour in a water bath at 37°C and immediately infused as for cryopreserved autologous marrow (Izzi, 1983).

N°FLT	F.AGE (Wks)	C.SUSP. N°x10^9 (F/C)	F.SEX *(M/MM)	F.ERYTHRO. ISOENZYMES (M/MM)	RECOVERY AFTER THAWING (%)
1.	12	8.3(F)	M	–	–
2.	20	5.7(C)	MM	MM	100
3.	14	5.9/4.6(F)	M	–	–
4.	14	8.4/6.0(F)	M	–	–
5.	16	2.0(F)	M	MM	–
6.	22,12	4.0/3.1(F)	MM	MM	–
7.	19,19,16	6.3/4.0/2.1(F)	M	MM	–
8.	15,20	1.8/2.1(C)	M	MM	88/90

*F = fresh; C = Cryopreserved; M = matched; MM = mismatched.

Table 3. Fetal Liver Suspension-Nucleated Cell Data in Relapsed Leukemia Patients.

N° FLT	AGE SEX	DISEASE STATUS	FLT DATE	C.DOSE x 10^8/Kg	Engraft. Markers (Hem.Rec.)	Survival Outcome (Days)
1.	9/M	ALL/4	28/9/78	0.3	–	+20, Resist.
2.	11/M	AML/3	6/5/80	2.5	K+/EI+/CR	+153,IP in CR
3.	8/M	ALL/5	4/8/80	3.6	–	+14, Sep.Shock
4.	6/M	AML/3	17/9/80	7.2	–	+20,Sep.Shock
5.	7/M	ALL/3	7/8/80	1.0	EI+/CR/γ	+30,IP in CR
6.	8/M	ALL/4	22/1/81	3.0	PR	+75,Relapse
7.	5/M	ALL/4	23/4/81	5.0	PR	+67,Sep.Shock
8.	3/M	ALL/2	15/5/81	1/2	PR	+54,Relapse

* Markers = Sexual Chromosome (K); Erythrocytic isoenzymes (EI); Hemopoietic recovery = (PR), complete (CR); γ = γ chain synthesis. All patients were prepared with Cy 120 mg/Kg and TBI 1000 rads.

Table 4. FLT in Relapsed Acute Leukemia Patients*- Clinical Data.

N°FLT	F.AGE (Wks)	C.SUSP. N°x10^8 (F/C)	F.SEX (M/MM)	F.ERYTHRO. ISOENZYMES (M/MM)	RECOVERY AFTER THAWING (%)
9	20/10	5.0/3.8(F)	M	M	88
	21	2.9(C)			
12	16	3.2(F)	MM	MM	–
14	24/20	5.1/2.3(C)	MM	MM	104,104
	19/16	5.0/2.1(F)			
15	20§	8.3(C)	M	MM	123
19	17	3.5(C)	MM	–	105

§ Twin fetal livers; F = Fresh; C = Cryopreserved; M = matched; MM = mismatched.

Table 5. Fetal Liver Suspension - Nucleated Cell Data in Complete Remission Leukemia Patients.

N°FLT	AGE SEX	DISEASE STATUS	F.DATE	C.DOSE x 10^8/Kg	ENGRAFT. MARKERS* (Hem.Rec.)	SURVIVAL OUTCOME (Days)
9	5/M	ALL/2	16/7/81	3.1	CR/EI–	+365, Relapse
12	4/M	AML/1	24/6/82	2.1	K+/EI+/CR/γ	Alive, >810
14	4/M	ALL/2	29/11/82	9.9	K+/EI–/PR/γ	+106, Relapse
15	2/M	ALL/2	21/12/82	6.3	EI–/CR/γ	+29, VOD, Relapse
19	4/M	ALL/2	26/7/84	2.9	N.E.	Alive, >60

* Markers = Sexual Chromosome, Erythrocytic Isoenzymes, EI– = After Transfusion & Transitory; EI+ = Permanent Modification; Hemopoietic Recovery, CR = Complete, PR = Partial; γ=γ Chain Synthesis.
§ All patients were prepared with Cy 120 mg/Kg and TBI 1000 rads.

Table 6. Fetal Liver Transplant in Complete Remission Leukemic Patients§ - Clinical Data.

Statistical Methods

There was no randomization between the groups of patients. Differences between percentages were evaluated by χ^2 test. There were no statistically significant results ($p = 0.8$) (Rimm, 1980).

RESULTS

1. Severe Aplastic Anemia

In 5 patients, 17 fetal liver suspensions were used; the ages varied between 10-25 weeks; 8 suspensions were fresh, 9 were cryopreserved. The cell dose was in the range of between 0.75 and 12.7 x 10^8/Kg. The number of fetuses per patient varied between 2 to 5 (Table 1). Recovery after thawing was in the range of 45 to 182%. We discussed the fact that the effect of freezing and thawing could separate cells from the islands of hepatic tissues.

Markers of engraftment were present in 4 patients (fetal sex chromosome) but it was impossible to find fetal markers in the recipient post FLT (Table 2). One patient (N°1) is alive and well after FLT from November 1981. The other four patients died without signs of engraftment (1 for cerebral hemorrhage, 1 for systemic mycosis and 2 for septic shock). No GVHD was observed. Four patients were isolated in Laminar - Air Flow rooms (LAF) 29-42 days) and one in a reverse protected room (28 days). No interstitial pneumonia was observed.

2. Relapsed Acute Leukemia

The number of fetuses per patient varied between 1 and 3. The ages of the fetuses were between 12 and 22 weeks. The cell number of fetal liver suspensions was in the range of 1.8 and 8.4 x 10^9. 11 suspensions were fresh and 3 cryopreserved. Markers of engraftment were present in 2 patients for sexual chromosomes and in 5 patients for fetal erythrocytic isoenzymes. Recovery after thawing was between 88% and 100% (Table 3). The cell dose was between 0.3 and 7.2 x 10^8/Kg (Table 4).

In two patients(N°s 2,5),we obtained CR and three patients a partial remission. The other three patients died less than one month post transplant and were not considered to be assessable.

Markers of engraftment were present in two patients (N°s 2,5). In N°2, the presence of the XYY karyotype in 20% marrow metaphases, of the double Y bodies in peripheral blood, the appearance of new HLA antigens and the red cell isoenzyme phenotypes of donor origin together with a complete hemopoietic recovery demonstrated the success of the fetal transplant (Lucarelli, 1982), though interstitial pneumonia caused the death of the patient at 5 months post transplant in complete remission.

In patient N°5, complete hemopoietic recovery was considered of donor origin because of the appearance of the fetal γ chain synthesis in the bone marrow cells together with the demonstration of fetal hemoglobin with the peroxidase anti peroxidase method applied to bone marrow sections treated with anti-fetal hemoglobin antibodies (Delfini, 1983).

3. Complete Remission Acute Leukemias

From July 1981 to July 1984 we transplanted 5 patients with AL in CR. The number of fetuses per patient was between 1 and 4. The ages of the fetuses varied from 10 to 24 weeks. The cell number of fetal liver suspensions was between 2.1 and 8.3×10^9. 5 suspensions were fresh and 5 cryopreserved. Markers of engraftment were present in 3 patients for fetal sex and in 3 patients for fetal erythrocytic isoenzymes. Recovery after thawing was between 88% and 123% (Table 5). The cell dose varied between 2.1 and 9.9×10^9/Kg (Table 6). Markers of engraftment were present in two out of five patients. The patient G.N., ALL in 2nd CR, although not showing any markers of engraftment, had a complete hemopoietic recovery but died one year post-transplant due to relapse.

The patient N°2, AML in 1st CR, presented a permanent take which lasted 6 months and is alive and well three years post-transplant with an autologous recovery without any further treatment after the transplant.

The patient N°3, ALL in 2nd CR, had a partial recovery and the presence of a female karyotype, however, relapse caused his death. Patient N°4, ALL in 2nd CR, had a prompt complete recovery and terminated isolation on day 14 post-transplant but died of a fast relapse with clinical VOD. At day 20, bone marrow incubation with ^{3}H leucine showed a pattern of hemoglobin synthesis of fetal type. The last patient, N°5, ALL in 2nd CR, is alive and well with an autologous hemopoietic recovery.

DISCUSSION

1. Severe Aplastic Anemia (SAA)

In end stage patients, without HLA identical donors and refractory to immunosuppression therapy, SAA remains a fatal disease (Champlin, 1983).

In our group of 5 patients, fetal liver transplant after immunosuppression with Cy, as in BMT, could only obtain one complete hemopoietic recovery lasting about three years. The lack of engraftment in the other four patients even after high cell doses may suggest that Cy is insufficient to engraft fetal liver cells in all SAA refractory patients. New regimens could be attempted in these end stage patients, for example Cy and TLI as adopted in BMT (Ramsay, 1980). No difference can be observed in results comparing fresh or cryopreserved FL cell suspensions.

2. Relapsed Acute Leukemias

In end stage patients in the absence of an HLA identical donor, FLT produced two complete remissions out of 8 patients, but interstitial pneumonia after TBI in a single dose caused death in both patients. In these patients fractionated TBI and earlier candidature if there are poor prognostic signs, may be suggested in further clinical trials in BMT as adopted in current BMT programs (Clift, 1982; Thomas, 1983).

3. Complete Remission Acute Leukemias

In complete remission patients, results as in patient N°2, alive 30 months following FLT in CR, may suggest that even if transient, hemopoietic liver cells can offer the possibility of achieving CR and cure to many patients. In the three patients who died in relapse, the possibility of adopting fractionated TBI and early candidature could be proposed as in BMT programs (Gale, 1983; Thomas, 1982).

CONCLUSION

In ASAA patients the preparatory regimen (Cy = 200 mg/Kg) used in our FLT trial was insufficient to give an allogeneic hemopoietic recovery (Champlin, 1983). In AL patients, all of pediatric age, the tumor response after Cy and TBI seems to follow the same pattern as well as in BMT patients (Thomas, 1983; Gale, 1983; Thomas, 1982). Thus fetal liver cells, although capable of grafting, do not present anti leukemic effects. Hemopoietic reconstitution after FLT, even though transient, can allow the patient to overcome the period of profound aplasia following the supralethal ablative regimen. Fetal liver cell suspensions may also influence autologous recovery although the promoting factors are not yet known.

In deciding a clinical trial in transplanting leukemic pediatric patients without an HLA identical sibling, FLT should be proposed as an alternative to other experimental treatments.

REFERENCES

Andreani M, Agostinelli F, Stramigioli S, Manna M, Donati M, Moretti L, Polchi P, Proietti A, Lucarelli G, Di Pietrantony F (1982) Transplantation of cryopreserved fetal liver cells in lethally irradiated rats. Haematologica 67:5.
Andreani M, Agostinelli F, Manna M, Guadenzi G, Proietti A, Grianti C, Lucarelli G (1983) Fetal liver transplantation in the mini-pig. In Gale RP (ed): "Recent Advances in Bone Transplantation" New York: Alan R. Liss, p 849.

Champlin R, Ho W, Winston DJ, Bayever E, Feig SA, Gale RP (1983). Treatment of severe aplastic anemia, a comparison of antithymocyte globulin versus allogeneic bone marrow transplantation. In Gale RP (ed): Recent Advances in Bone Marrow Transplantation", New York: Alan R. Liss, p 29.

Clift RA, Thomas ED, Buckner CD, Sanders J, Stewart PS, Sullivan KM, McGuffin R, Hersman J, Sale GE, Storb R (1982). Allogeneic marrow transplantation using fractionated total body irradiation in patients with acute lymphoblastic leukemia in relapse. Leukemia Res 6:401.

Gale RP, Champlin RE (1983). Bone marrow transplantation in leukemia. In Gale RP (ed): "Recent Advances in Bone Marrow Transplantation," New York: Alan R. Liss, p 71.

Delfini C, Izzi T, Porcellini A, Lucarelli G (1980). Immunologic features of human fetal liver, spleen and thymus at various gestational ages. In Gale RP, Fliedner TM, Lucarelli G (eds): "Fetal Liver Transplantation," Holland: Excerpta Medica, Elsevier, p 126.

Delfini C, Saglio S, Mazza U, Muretto P, Filippetti A, Lucarelli G (1983). Fetal haemoglobin synthesis following fetal liver transplantation in man. Brit J Haematol 55:609.

Izzi T, Polchi P, Galimberti M, Delfini C, Moretti L, Manna A, Porcellini A, Lucarelli G, Di Pietrantony F (1984). Allogeneic bone marrow transplant in acute leukemias and chronic myeloid leukemia. Preliminary results from the BMT Center of Pesaro. Haematologica 69:2.

Izzi T, Moretti L, Polchi P, Galimberti M, Delfini C, Porcellini A, Lucarelli G (1983). Autologous bone marrow transplantation in relapsed acute leukemias and chronic myeloid leukemia in blast crisis. Haematologica 68:3.

Kansal V, Sood SK, Batra AK, Adhar G, Malviya AK, Kucheris K, Kalakrishnan K (1979). Fetal liver transplantation in aplastic anemia. Acta Haematol (Basel) 62:128.

Kelemen E (1975). Recovery from chronic idiopathic bone marrow aplasia of a young mother after intravenous injection of unprocessed cell from the liver (and yolk sac) of her 22 mm CR-length embryo. Scand J Haematol 10:305.

Klein AK, Dyck JA, Stitzel KA, Shimizu J, Fox LA, Taylor N (1983). Characterization of canine fetal lymphohematopoiesis: studies of CFU-GM, CFU-L and CFU-F. Exp Hematol 11:263.

Lucarelli G, Izzi T, Porcellini A, Delfini C (1979). Infusion of fetal liver cells in aplastic anemia. In Heimpel H, Gordon-Smith EC, Heit W, Kubanek (eds) "Aplastic Anemia, Pathophysiology and Approaches to therapy," Berlin, Heidelberg: Springer Verlag.

Lucarelli G, Andreani M, Agostinelli F, Manna M, Moretti L, Polchi P (1981). Transplantation of fetal liver of different ages in the rat. Blut 42:337.

Lucarelli G, Izzi T, Porcellini A, Delfini C, Polchi P, Moretti L, Manna A, Grilli G (1980). Fetal liver transplantation in aplastic anemia and acute leukemia. In Gale RP, Fliedner TM, Lucarelli G (eds): "Fetal Liver Transplantation", Holland: Excerpta Medica, Elsevier, p 284.

Lucarelli G, Izzi T, Porcellini A, Delfini C, Galimberti M, Moretti L, Polchi P, Agostinelli F, Andreani M, Manna M, Dallapiccola B (1982). Fetal liver transplantation in 2 patients with acute leukemia after total body irradiation. Scand J Haematol 28:65.

Lucarelli G, Izzi T, Porcellini A, Delfini C, Galimberti M, Polchi P, Moretti L, Manna A, Sparaventi G (1983). Fetal liver transplantation in aplastic anemia and acute leukemia. In Gale RP (ed): "Recent Advances in Bone Marrow Transplantation," New York: Alan R. Liss, p 865.

Mandel TE, Jack I, Tait BD (1982). HLA-DR typing of fetal human spleen and liver lymphoblastoid cells transformed by Epstein-Barr virus. Transplantation 34:50.

Moretti L, Polchi P, Fontebuoni A, Stramigioli S, Andreani M, Agostinelli F, Izzi T, Lucarelli G (1979). Criopreservazione di cellule staminali di midollo osseo di ratto. La Trasfusione del Sangue Vol.XXIV:4.

O'Reilly RJ, Pollack MS, Kapoor N, Kirkpatrick D, Dupont B (1983). Fetal liver transplantation in man and animals. In Gale RP (ed): "Recent Advances in Bone Marrow Transplantation," New York: Alan R. Liss, p 799.

Polchi P, Moretti L, Fontebuoni A, Stramigioli S, Andreani M, Agostinelli F, Izzi T, Lucarelli G (1979). Criopreservazione di cellule staminali emopoietiche di fegato fetale di ratto. La Trasfusione del Sangue Vol.XXIV:4.

Porcellini A, Manna A, Izzi T, Delfini C, Lucarelli G (1980). In vitro culture of granulocytic colonies from liver, spleen and bone marrow of human fetuses. In Gale RP, Fliedner TM, Lucarelli G (eds): "Fetal Liver Transplantation," Holland: Excerpta Medica, Elsevier, p 45.

Porcellini A, Manna A, Manna M, Talevi N, Delfini C, Moretti L, Rizzoli V (1983). Ontogeny of granulocyte-macrophage progenitor cells in the human fetus. Int J Cell Cloning 1:92.

Prümmer O, Calvo W, Fliedner TM, Nothdurft W (1983). Immunological characterization of canine fetal liver cells. In Gale RP (ed): "Recent Advances in Bone Marrow Transplantation", New York: Alan R. Liss, p 841.

Prümmer O, Raghavachar A, Calvo W, Carbonell F, Fliedner TM (1983). Restoration of hemopoiesis by cryopreserved fetal liver cells in a canine model. In Gale RP (ed): "Recent Advances in Bone Marrow Transplantation," New York: Alan R. Liss, p 857.

Rabinowich H, Umiel T, Globerson A (1983). T cell progenitors in the mouse fetal liver. Transplantation 33:40.

Ramsey NKC, Kim T, Nesbit ME, Krivit W, Coccia PF, Levitt SH, Woods WG, Kersey JH (1980). Total lymphoid irradiation and cyclophosphamide as preparation for bone marrow transplantation in severe aplastic anemia. Blood 55:344.

Rimm AA, Hartz AJ, Kalbfleisch JM, Anderson AJ, Hoffman RG (1980). "Basic biostatistics in medicine and epidemiology". New York: Appelton-Century Crofts, p 237.

Stitzel KA, Champlin R, Gale RP (1983). Fetal liver transplantation in dogs: a possible alternative source of hematopoietic cells for transplantation. In Gale RP (ed): "Recent Advances in Bone Marrow Transplantation," New York: Alan R, Liss, p 831.

Touraine JL, Roncarolo MG, Souillet G, Betend H, Philippe N, François R, Touraine F (1984). Fetal liver transplantation, medical, immunological and ethical aspects. Exp Hematol 12 (Suppl 15): 93.

Thomas ED, Appelbaum FR, Buckner CD, Clift RA, Deeg JH, Fefer A, Sanders JE, Singer J, Stewart P, Sullivan KM, Storb R, Witherspoon RP (1983). Marrow transplantation for acute non-lymphocytic leukemia. In Gale RP (ed):"Recent Advances in Bone Marrow Transplantation," New York: Alan R. Liss, p 61.

Thomas ED (1982). The role of marrow transplantation in the eradication of malignant disease. Cancer 41:1963.

Zucali JR (1982). Self renewal and differentiation capacity of bone marrow and fetal liver stem cells. Brit J Haematol 52:295.

BONE MARROW RECONSTITUTION FOLLOWING HUMAN FETAL LIVER
INFUSION (FLI) IN SIXTEEN SEVERE APLASTIC ANEMIA PATIENTS

V. Kochupillai, S. Sharma, S. Francis, N.K. Mehra
A. Nanu, V. Kalra, P.S.N. Menon, M. Bhargava

All India Institute of Medical Sciences
New Delhi-110 029, India

Sixteen patients of severe aplastic anemia received intravenously (0.25 to 11.1)x10^8 hematopoietic cells prepared from the livers of 10-32 week old fetuses. Two patients who died within 5 days of infusion are excluded. Seven of the 14 evaluable patients responded favorably. Erythropoiesis improved within 12-30 days, followed by myelopoiesis (27-60 days) and megakaryopoiesis (1-12 months). Two of these 7 patients died of infections after 3 and 7 months. The remaining 5 are alive for 9-95 months and 3 of them have secured complete bone marrow reconstitution. Four of the 7 non-responders died within 4 months, while the remaining 3 were lost to subsequent followup. Patients of age 30 or more had significantly longer survival than the younger group ($p < 0.05$). No patient developed apparent graft Vs host disease. FLI appears a convenient and safe alternative to bone marrow transplantation, particularly for an older individual and when HLA matched donor is not available.

INTRODUCTION

In severe aplastic anemia, bone marrow transplantation is the current treatment of choice. However, difficulty to secure histocompatible donor relatives and high incidence of graft-versus-host disease (GVHD) (Camitta 1982; Gordon-Smith 1983; Gale 1981) have stimulated search of other sources of hemopoietic stem cells. Liver serves as a hematopoietic organ during intrauterine life. Uphoff suggested that fetal liver hemopoietic cells being immuno-

Financed by Department of Science and Technology, Government of India.

logically immature might not produce GVHD and she successfully grafted them in irradiated mice (Uphoff 1958). Clinical studies on fetal liver infusion (FLI) in severe aplastic anemia are comparatively few and indicate limited success (Kansal 1979; Kansal 1981; Kochupillai 1984; Scott 1961; Kelemen 1973; O'Reilly 1977; Lucarelli 1980). We report here further experience of FLI in 16 aplastic anemia patients with improvement including complete bone marrow recovery in 3.

PATIENTS AND METHODS

Twelve of the 16 patients were graded as severe aplastic anemia according to the criteria stated earlier (Kochupillai 1984). Two more patients were included because of progressive deterioration on the available therapy; the remaining 2 had pure red cell aplasia. Detailed history and physical examination preceded hemogram and histopathological examination of iliac crest bone marrow biopsy obtained with Jamshedi bone marrow aspiration biopsy needle. Preliminary results (Kansal 1979; Kansal 1981) on one patient were encouraging and further data on him are included here.

FETAL LIVER INFUSION (FLI)

Twenty four abortuses (estimated age 10-32 weeks) (Hamilton 1957) were obtained from the Department of Obstetrics. They were available following hysterotomy-15, prostaglandin injection-8 and spontaneous abortion-1. Fetal liver was dissected in sterile conditions at room temperature in a laminar flow hood. Liver was minced and mashed over sterile metallic wire mesh (100 mesh/sq.cm). RPMI 1640 culture medium (each ml fortified with 100 ug streptomycin and 100 IU crystalline penicillin) was then gently poured over the wire mesh to collect the cell suspension below in a sterile container. The suspension was allowed to stand for 15 minutes to discard sediment and the supernatant was centrifuged at 400 G x 15 minutes. Pallet with predominantly hematopoietic cells was resuspended in 2-3 ml of RPMI 1640. If Jenner and Geimsa staining indicated more than 10% of hepatocytes, the procedure of dilution, standing and centrifuging was repeated. Suspensions showing hematopoietic cells as clumps, were repeatedly passed through 21-24 gauge needles, to obtain single cell suspension. Neubaur chamber was used for counting cells. The percentage of viable cells checked by Trypan blue dye exclusion test ranged between 60-98% (median (M)-95%). Although in our laboratory, cells remained viable for 21 days, they were always used in less than 10 days, indeed most of them in less than 3 hours. On each occasion a patient received intravenously entire FLI prepared from one individual fetus. Depending upon the availability, 0.25-11.1×10^8 (M-2.05×10^8) cells were administered per patient. Decrease in blood transfusion requirement and increase in peripheral blood counts were the criteria of response. FLI was repeated if the response was poor or transient. Three to 4 weeks after FLI, 8 patients (Table II) received prednisolone 40 mgm on alternate days for 2-14 months; remaining patients did not receive prednisolone.

Where the sex of the fetus donor and the adult recipient varied, bone marrow cultures were prepared for chromosomal analysis.

HLA antigens (Terasaki 1964) were studied in all the patients before and repeatedly at 4-8 weeks interval after FLI.

Red cell antigens including AB DC with E and MN L^{ea} L^{eb} fy^a K, P were studied in all the patients before and repeatedly at 4-8 week intervals after FLI. Reagents and protocol of Ortho, USA and Hyland, USA were used.

Fetal hemoglobin (Hb), Hb_{A2} and serum iron were estimated using standard hematological techniques (Dacie 1975) before and repeatedly at 4-8 week intervals after FLI.

RESULTS

Of the 16 cases, 15 were males and 1 female, age 11-59 years (M-27 years). Fourteen patients had marked decrease of all the hematopoietic elements; case no. 9 and 15 had pure red cell aplasia. Only in case no. 7 and 12 history indicated drug intake (chloramphenicol, analgesics) as the cause; the remaining were categorized as idiopathic. Baseline clinical and hematological data before FLI are given in Table I.

Four male patients received FLI prepared from female fetuses, while the remaining 11 had it prepared from the males. The female patient received female fetus FLI (Table II). Two patients died within 5 days of FLI and are considered unevlauable (Group I). Seven patients (Group II) showed significant but variable clinical and hematological

TABLE I : INITIAL PRESENTING DATA

Case No.	Fever	Bleeding	Duration of symptoms (months)	Hemoglobin gms/dl	Reticulocytes %	Granulocytes /ul	Platelets / ul
1.	+	Nose	3	10.2	0.9	624	130,000
2.	-	Gums	0.5	3.1	1.9	253	50,000
3.	-	Gums & Skin	1	4.2	0.9	406	40,000
4.	+	Gums & Skin	5	7.0	0.1	288	30,000
5.	+	Gums & Skin	2.5	3.7	0.1	378	26,000
6.	+	Fundi, Gums & Skin	5	4.4	0.3	1020	30,000
7.	+	Gums & Skin	1	7.5	0.2	200	80,000
8.	+	Nose & Skin	3.5	3.1	0.5	1210	40,000
9.	-	-	8	2.3	0.5	4092	380,000
10.	-	Gums	8	5.2	0.1	1428	120,000
11.	+	Gums, Skin &Nose	2	6.6	0.2	90	10,000
12.	-	Gums, Skin&Nose	7	6.6	0.7	704	70,000
13.	+	Skin&Gums	1.5	3.3	2.4	476	40,000
14.	+	-	36	5.1	0.5	416	70,000
15.	-	-	12	3.0	0.1	4800	310,000
16.	-	Vagina	3	4.5	0.3	572	60,000

TABLE II : DATA OF FETAL LIVER INFUSION

Group	Case No.	Patient's Age (Yrs) and Sex	Fetal Age (weeks) and sex	No. of fetal liver cells transfused (10^9)	No. of fetal liver cells/kg body wt. (10^8)	% of fetal liver cell viability (%)	TLI/Immuno-suppression 3-4 weeks after FLI	Final Outcome and Survival Post 1st FLI (months)
1	13	14,M	32 W,M	7.2	2.0	98	Nil	0.16 died
	16	35,F	18 W,F	0.86	0.14	98	Nil	0.16 died
2	1	43,M	12 W,M (iii)	2.2	0.36	93	Pred x 3	95 alive
	2	14,M	18 V,M	1.6	0.34	99	Pred x 2	3 died
	3	45,M	16 V,M	1.9	0.31	99	Pred x 12	27 alive
	4	12,M	12 W,M	3.6	1.3	95	Pred x 14	24 alive
	9	36,M	i) 16 W,M ii) 12 W,F (iii)	1.8 0.54	0.29 0.08	98 95	Pred x 6	7 died
	10	27,M	i) 16 W,M ii) 18 W,M (iii)	3.7 5.9	0.7 1.1	92 65	Pred x 11	14 alive
	15	59,M	i) 10 W,F ii) 12 W,F (iii)	0.32 0.48	0.02 0.1	95 90	Nil	9 alive
3	5	27,M	i) 14 V,M ii) 10 V,M (iii)	1.45 1.65	0.24 0.27	92 90	Nil	2 died
	6	20,M	i) 12 W,M ii) 16 W,M iii) 16 W,M (iii)	2.55 5.7 1.7	0.43 0.95 0.29	95 92 60	Pred x 3	4 died
	7	15,M	20 W,M	7.8	1.9	99	Nil	0.7 died
	11	11,M	16 W,F	4.5	1.3	97	Nil	0.7 died
4	8	26,M	18 W,M	2.9	0.56	95	Nil	1 LFU
	12	35,M	i) 18 W,F ii) 14 W,M (iii) iii) 12 W,F (iii)	11.1 0.25 0.42	2.3 0.11 0.09	95 95 98	Pred x 4	5 LFU
	14	30,M	20 W,M	5.2	0.86	65	Nil	4 LFU

LFU :- Lost to Follow Up
Pred :- Prednisolone

Number in parentheses in column 4 indicate number of FLI received by that patient.

response between 12-70 (M-23.5) days. Four patients (Group III) died on the days - 64, 130, 22 and 20 after FLI without any response. Three (Group IV) did not respond during the 1, 5 and 4 months period, after which they stopped reporting.

Seven patients of Group II who benefitted by FLI are briefly described below.

Case No. 1

Male, 43 years, diagnosis November, 1976, first FLI December 21st, 1976, partial response, blood transfusion requirements declined, lymphoid chimerism indicated by the presence of both XX and XY complements after bone marrow culture. Second FLI May 15, 1978. Peripheral blood counts stabilized early June. No blood transfusion required. Peripheral blood counts and bone marrow, however, showed partial recovery, got 2-3 days episodes of fever at 8-10 day intervals. Third FLI on October 28, 1983. After 6 weeks Hb 11.5 gm/dl, WBC 5000/ul and platelets 210,000/ul. In August, 1984 bone marrow normal. In spite of short bouts of fever remains healthy and pursues his profession.

Case No. 2

Fourteen years, male, diagnosis July, 1981. Despite partial response to 100 mgm/day oxymetholone given for 1 year he required approximately 4 units blood transfusion per month.
FLI given on July 20, 1982. Gradual improvement over next 2 months with marked reduction in blood transfusion requirement; 3 months post FLI died in some other hospital of fever and bleeding.

Case No. 3

Male, 45 years, diagnosis February, 1982. No response to 100 mgm/day oxymetholone with 40 mgm per day prednisolone for 5 months, required about 4 units blood per month. Received FLI July 20, 1982, improvement in Hb and reticulocytes next 3 weeks. Only 2 units of blood transfused during the next 2 months and none subsequently. WBC count stabilized by May, 1983. Platelet production improved the last

and in December, 1982. Bone marrow in July, 1983 was normal and peripheral blood counts in September, 1984 are as follows: Hb 13.9 gm/dl, WBC 3,300/ul, and platelets 120,000/ul.

Case No. 4

Twelve years, male, diagnosis September, 1982. During 4 weeks required 8 units of whole blood transfusion and 4 units of platelet rich plasma infusion. FLI on October 15, 1982. Hb started improving after 3 weeks, WBC count after 8 weeks and platelet count after 4 weeks. Entire picture including bone marrow progressively improved in July, 1984. Hb 11.7 gm/dl, WBC 4250/ul and platelet count 130,000/ul. Bone marrow - normal cellularity.

Case No. 9

Thirty-six years, male, diagnosis of pure red cell aplasia in February, 1982. Received corticosteroids for 5 months, cyclophosphamide for the next 5 months and then oxymetholone for 5 months with partial temporary response followed by relapse. Required 3-4 units blood every month. FLI on August 4, 1983. Gradual improvement over 10 weeks with Hb 11.0 gm/dl, and no blood transfusions for the next 3 months. Deteriorated by December, and required 2 units blood transfusion. On January 13, 1984 received second FLI. Stopped reporting. Death elsewhere 2 months after second FLI.

Case No. 10

Male, 27 years, diagnosis April, 1983. No improvement with oxymetholone 100 mgm/day for 4 months. Required 3 units blood transfusion per month. FLI on August 12, 1983, blood transfusion requirement dropped to about one unit per month. Six months later bone marrow demonstrated paritial recovery. Blood transfusion requirement appeared to increase 3 months afterwards. Second FLI on May 14, 1984. Has required 4 units blood transfusion over 4 months after the second FLI.

Case No. 15

Fifty-nine years, male, admitted in January, 1983 with 12 months history of progressive weakness, palpitation, dyspnea and intermittent diarrhea. Bone marrow had erythroid depression and chest tomogram revealed thymoma. Thymectomy on February 9, 1983 with no improvement, 40 mgm per day prednisolone along with testosterone propionate 25 mgm twice a week for 3 months without improvement. Required 3-4 units blood transfusion per month. FLI on January 13, 1984. Required 1-2 units of blood per month after FLI. Second FLI on June 11, 1984. Needs 1-2 units blood per month.

HLA typing and red cell antigen studies carried out before and after FLI on these 7 patients demonstrated no significant changes. There was a significant rise in fetal Hb in case no. 4 after FLI from 0.0% to 9% which is now stabilized at 6.5%. Case no. 3 had milder rise of fetal Hb from 0.5% to 1.2%. After FLI serum iron lowered, though the change was not significant. Post FLI prednisolone does not seem to have clearly helped or harmed the patients, however, more evidence is required to judge its role in this therapy.

Age Factor

Patients 30 years or older had longer survival range 4-95 (M-8) months after FLI than the younger group (0.7-24 months, M-2.5-$p<0.05$).

Survival

Median survival (MS) of the 14 evaluable patients was 4.5 months (range 20 days - 95+ months). Seven patients who failed to respond to FLI had 2 months MS up to the time of their last follow up. Seven patients who responded to FLI had 14+ months MS; (up to 31st October, 1984). However, because 5 of them are still surviving, MS of this group will increase.

DISCUSSION

Two patients died within 5 days of receiving FLI. Their condition was sufficiently critical to suggest that their death was unrelated to the FLI. Data of the remaining 14 patients confirms our earlier preliminary report (Kansal 1979) that about 50% of patients with severe aplastic anemia favorably responded to FLI. Improvement after FLI is evident by decreases in blood transfusion requirements, increase in peripheral blood counts, inducement of hematopoiesis and normal cellularity of bone marrow. Comparison of MS (4.5 months) of these 14 patients with our previous 20 (MS 1 month) patients of severe aplastic anemia treated with anabolic steroids (Kochupillai 1984) demonstrates significant survival benefit for FLI group ($P<0.05$).

Fetal liver infusion in humans with aplastic anemia was first attempted by Scott et al in 1961 (Scott 1961). Of their 14 cases, however, only 2 improved with prolonged survival of more than 4 years. Remaining 10 failed to respond and 8 of them died within 6 months. Kelemen (Kelemen 1973) in 1973 infused fetal liver cells to a woman from her own 7 week old fetus; she recovered completely by 9 months. O'Reilly et al (O'Reilly 1977) reported complete recovery following FLI in a 5 year old boy suffering from posthepatitis aplastic anemia; he was preconditioned by cyclophosphamide. Lucarelli et al (Lucarelli 1980) infused fetal liver cells in 12 cases of severe aplastic anemia, 8 of whom responded in 10-55 days (M-21 days) and had MS of 302 days. These studies along with present reports clearly indicate that there exists a subset of patients of severe aplastic anemia, who respond to FLI either partially or completely.

In our previous reports on FLI (Kansal 1979; Kansal 1981) three patients showed mixed lymphoid chimerism which was temporary and within 9 months donor cells were eliminated possibly by the process of rejection. None of the 14 cases reported here manifested mixed chimerism or engraftment, as suggested by the lack of changes in HLA, red cell antigens and bone marrow chromosome patterns following FLI. Of the 12 patients treated with FLI by Lucarelli et al (Lucarelli 1980), 2 showed engraftment evidenced by the persistent modification of the pattern of red cell enzymes. On pooling the records of 43 cases of aplastic anemia treated by FLI (Kansal 1979; Kansal 1981; Kochupillai 1984; Scot 1961; Kelemen 1973; O'Reilly 1977; Lucarelli 1980) only 5 patients demonstrated initial engraftment as judged in 3 by chromosome studies in the other 2 by altered red cell enzyme pattern (Gale 1980); in only 2 of them the engraftment persisted (Lucarelli 1980).

Engraftment thus appears an unlikely mechanism of the benefit seen in most of FLI treated aplastic anemia patients. It is possible that fetal liver cells may stimulate hemopoiesis in a patient by an as yet unknown mechanism. Mismatched bone marrow infusion that fails to establish engraftment, is known to improve aplastic anemia in some patients (Nissen 1980; Speck 1980; Territo 1977). In this connection Nissen et al have postulated that transient partial chimerism which may escape detection, may have an effect in "rattling up" the immune system, and may be responsible for the recovery of autologous bone marrow which is a slow and incomplete process than bone marrow recovery by successful engraftment of the allogeneic bone marrow transplant. It is possible that similar mechanisms operate in patients who receive FLI. Such a possibility may explain the slow recovery in all of our 7 responding patients and incomplete recovery as also multiple recurrence in some of them.

Pretransplant immunosuppression to ensure quick engraftment and to prevent graft rejection is widely used in bone marrow transplantation. Immunosuppression before FLI has not been adequately studied. O'Reilly et al observed its beneficial effect in one case (O'Reilly 1977). Case no. 7 in the present study received cyclophosphamide for 3 days prior to FLI; he developed extensive pulmonary infection and hemorrhage and expired on the 22nd day of FLI. In one case of acute myeloid leukemia where prior chemotherapy caused bone marrow aplasia, FLI produced complete and quick engraftment for about 1 month which was then successfully replaced by the autologous marrow. (Kochupillai 1985). It is possible that pre-FLI immunosuppression may allow rapid, effective fetal liver engraftment.

Hematopoiesis in the fetal liver is predominantly erythroid with erythroid:myeloid ratios exceeding 25:1 (Gale 1980; Calvo 1980; Shadduck 1980; Cappellini 1984; Kubanek 1980; Sharma 1985) in contrast to adult bone marrow where myelopoiesis is more prominent than erythropoiesis (E:M ratio n-1:3). Megakaryocytes are only occasionally present in the fetal liver. Paucity of myelopoiesis and megakaryopoiesis in early fetal life could be a consequence of the germ free and mechanically protective environment which prevails during embryonic life (Kubanek 1980). Unlike the patients of successful bone marrow transplantation, those recovering after FLI show **erythropoiesis as the earliest and more dominating response** (Kubanek 1969). Thus erythropoiesis has been most marked and the earliest response followed by myelopoiesis in seven patients in this report who benefitted from FLI. Megakaryocytes were the last to respond. In this connection an interesting suggestion has been offered by Alter et al that hematopoiesis during bone marrow recovery may be associated with an "accelerated partial" recapitulation of ontogeny (Alter 1976). The fetal growth pattern of bone marrow recovery as well as rise in fetal Hb in two cases in this report following FLI support Alter's suggestion.

Present study as well as those review by Gale (Gale 1980) on fetal liver infusion indicate that the number (dose) of fetal liver cells infused bears no clear relation with recipient's response. Thus Kelemen (Kelemen 1973) reported a beneficial effect of FLI in aplastic anemia with as small a dose as 4.2×10^7 cells. Lucarelli et al (Lucarelli 1980) had similar experience. Also, in the present study, dose as small as 3.2×10^7 could partially benefit case no. 15 and the dose and response did not appear to be related.

In this work good response was seen in patients receiving FLI from fetuses aged between 10-18 weeks. Where fetal age exceeded 20 weeks, the response of their recipient appear poor. Four patients (case no. 10 (2nd FLI) 13, 6 (3rd FLI) and 14) who received FLI with cell viability of 90% or less, had poor response. More data are needed to assess the importance of fetal age and fetal cell viability in determining the outcome of FLI.

None of the patients in the present and previous studies on FLI (Kansal 1979; Kansal 1981; Kochupillai 1984; Lucarelli 1980) developed apparent graft-versus-host disease (GVHD). This was indicated by the absence of skin rash, diarrhea and significant liver abnormalities in the recipients. Animal experiments have also indicated lack of occurance of GVHD (Uphoff 1958) following FLI. This is accounted for by the fact that lymphocytes in liver throughout the fetal life are less than 2% and are functionally immature (Gale 1980; Champlin 1980; Bortin 1968). This is an important advantage of FLI over bone marrow transplantation where GVHD incidence is about 75% (Gale 1981). In this connection Lowenberg (Lowenberg 1977) has cautioned that repeated bacterial infections following FLI may be a manifestation of GVHD. Four patients in present study developed recurrent infections following FLI and two of them died. However, in these patients a possibility remains that recurrent infections are entirely due to inadequate granulocytes in the peripheral blood and not related to FLI.

It is interesting to note that in our work FLI benefitted oler age group better than the younger age group. Patients aged 30 or more responded better and had MS of 8 months as against those less than 30 who had MS of 2.5 months ($p < 0.05$). Bone marrow transplantation on the contrary is more efficacious for younger individuals (Gale 1981). FLI may thus be of particular value in a situation where bone marrow transplantation is not proimising to a patient on account of his age.

The results of the present study suggest that FLI is an important alternative to bone marrow transplantation in severe aplastic anemia. This procedure is of particular value in a country like India, where bone marrow transplantation can not be undertaken easily because of preceding immunosuppression with high requirement of support facilities. FLI is also of value when a matched donor is not available for bone marrow transplantation and when patient belongs to an older age group. Absence or lower incidence of graft-versus-host disease is also an important advantage.

The present study along with the previous studies (Kansal 1979; Kansal 1981; Kochupillai 1984; Scott 1961; Kelemen 1973; O'Reilly 1977; Lucarelli 1980) has confirmed that in certain patients FLI is capable of inducing complete bone marrow reconstitution in bone marrow failure.

Mechanism of recovery following FLI is not quite clear at present. Outcome of fetal liver cell infusion seems encouraging and deserves long term assessment.

ACKNOWLEDGEMENT

We are extremely grateful to Professor N.K. Bhide, Head of the Department Pharmacology, All India Institute of Medical Sciences, for his constructive criticism of this paper.

Alter BP, Rappaport JH, Huisman THJ, Schroeder WA, Nathan DG (1976). Fetal erythropoiesis following bone marrow transplantation. Blood 48:843.

Bortin MM, Saltstein FC. (1968). Immunologic incompetence of mouse perinatal liver hematopoietic cells against transplantation antigens. J Immunol 100:1215.

Calvo W, Carbonell F (1980). The development of liver granulopoiesis in the human fetus in fetal liver transplantation. Current concepts and future directions. In Lucarelli G, Fliedner TM, Gale RP (eds): Excerpta Medica, p 14.

Camitta BM, Storb R, Thomas ED (1982). Aplastic anemia (second of two parts); pathogenesis, diagnosis, treatment and prognosis. N Engl J Med 306:712.

Cappellini MD, Patter CG, Wood WG (1984). Long term haemopoiesis in human fetal liver cell cultures. Br J Haemat 57:61.

Champlin R, Nishanen E, Gale RP (1980). Hematopoiesis and immune reactivity of human fetal liver cells. IN Lucarelli G, Fliedner TM, Gale RP (eds). Fetal Liver Transplantation - Current Concepts and Future Directions. Excerpta Medica p 117.

Dacie JV, Lewis SM (1975). Practical hematology, 5th ed. Churchill Livingstone.

Gale RP (1980). Fetal liver transplantation in aplastic anemia. IN Lucarelli G, Fliedner TM, Gale RP (eds). Fetal LIver Transplantation - Current Concepts and Future Directions. Excerpta Medica p 268.

Gale RP (1980). Concepts of fetal liver transplantation in man. IN Lucarelli G, Fliedner TM, Gale RP (eds). Fetal Liver Transplantation - Current Concepts and Future Directions. Excerpta Medica p 247.

Gale RP, Champlin RE, Leig SA, Fitcher JH (1981). Aplastic anemia: Biology and Treatment. Ann Int Med 95:477.

Gordon-Smith EC (1983). Clinical Annotation: Management of aplastic anemia. Br J Haematol 53:185.

Hamilton WJ, Boyd JJ, MOnhan HW (1957). Human embroyology. Cambridge, Heften and Sons p 104.

Kansal V, Sood SK, Batra AK, et al. (1979) Fetal liver transplantation in aplastic anemia. Acta Hematol 62:128.

Kansal V. Fetal liver transplantation in aplastic anemia (sys lecture). J Soc Young Sci 2:8.

Kelemen E. (1973). Recovery from chronic idiopathic bone marrow aplasia of a young mother after intravenous injection of unprocessed cells from the liver (and yolk sac) of her 22 mm CR-length embryo. Scand J Haemat 10:305.

Kochupillai V (1984). Management of aplastic anemia. Ind J Hematol 3:149.

Kochupillai V, Sharma S, Sundaram KR (1984). Anabolic steroids in aplastic anemia. Ind J Med Res 80:174.

Kochupillai V, Sharma S, Francis S, et al (1985, in press). Fetal liver infusion: An adjuvant in the therapy of acute myeloid leukemia (AML). In: Fetal LIver Transplantation. Gale RP (ed). Alan R. Liss, New York.

Kubanek B, Heit W, Rich I (1980). Fetal erythropoiesis. In: Lucarelli G, Fliedner TM, Gale RP (eds). Fetal Liver Transplantation - Current Concepts and Future Directions. Excerpta Medica p. 71.

Kubanek B, Deucricca N, Porcellini A, Howard D, Stohlnan F (1969). The pattern of recovery of erythropoiesis in heavily irradiated mice receiving transplant of fetal liver. Proc Soc Exp Biol Med 131:831.

Lowenberg B, DeZeeuw HMC, Dicke KA, Van Bekkum DW (1977). Nature of the delayed graft Vs host reactivity of fetal liver transplantation in mice. J Natl Cancer Inst 58:959.

Lucarelli G, Izzi T, Porcellini A, et al (1980). Fetal liver transplantation in aplastic anemia and acute leukemia. In: Lucarelli G, Fliedner TM, Gale RP (eds). Fetal Liver Transplantation - Current Concepts and Future Directions. Excerpta Medica p 284.

Nissen C, Cornu P, Gratwohl A, Speck B (1980). Antilymphocyte globulin versus bone marrow transplantation in the treatment of severe aplastic anemia. In: Lucarelli G, Fliedner TM, Gale RP (eds). Fetal Liver Transplantation - Current Concepts and Future Directions. Excerpta Medica p 230.

O'Reilly RJ, Phawa R, Kagan W, et al (1977). Reconstitution of hematopoietic function in post-hepatic aplasia following high dose cyclophosphamide and allogeneic fetal liver transplantation. Exp Hematol 5(Suppl 2):46.

Scott RB, Matthias JQ, Constandoulakis M, et al (1961). Hypoplastic anemia treated by transfusion of fetal hemopoietic cells. Brit Med J 2:1385.

Shadduck RK, Pigoli G, Waheed A, Boegal F (1980). Characterization of hemopoietic progenitor cells in fetal liver. In: Lucarelli G, Fliedner TM, Gale RP (eds). Fetal Liver Transplantation - Current Concepts and Future Directions. Excerpta Medica p 29.

Sharma S, Bhargava M, and Kochupillai V (1985). Morphological pattern of hematopiesis in human fetal liver. In: Fetal Liver Transplantation. Gale RP (ed). Alan R. Liss, New York.

Speck B, Gratwohl A, Nissen C, et al (1980). Severe aplastic anemia: a prospective study on the value of different therapeutic approaches in 38 successive patients. Blut 41:160.

Terasaki PJ, McClelland JD (1964). Microdroplet assay of human serum cytotoxins. Nature 204:998.

Territo MC for the UCLA Bone Marrow Transplant Team (1977). Autologous bone marrow repopulation following high dose cyclosphosphamide and allogeneic marrow transplantation in aplastic anemia. Br J Haematol 36:305.

Uphoff DE (1958). Preclusion of secondary phase of irradiation syndrome, by inoculation of fetal hematopoietic tissue following lethal body x = irradiation. J Natl Cancer Inst 20:625.

FETAL LIVER INFUSION: AN ADJUVANT IN THE THERAPY OF ACUTE MYELOID LEUKEMIA (AML)

V. Kochupillai, S. Sharma, S. Francis, N.K. Mehra, A. Nanu, I.C. Verma, D. Takkar, S. Kumar, U. Gokhale
All India Institute of Medical Sciences
New Delhi-110 029, India

Twenty five acute myeloid leukemia (AML) patients received induction by daunorubicin and cytosine arabinoside and maintenance by cyclical chemotherapy. In 10 patients chemotherapy could be supplemented by fetal liver infusion (FLI) prepared from 10-24 week fetuses, in the dose of 0.07 to 34.0×10^8 liver cells. Four who had complete remission showed median survival (MS) of 21.5+ months with 3 surviving to date (2 of them showed evidence of transient engraftment by donor cells). MS in the remaining 6 patients was 1.8 months. FLI given within 48 hours after the last dose of induction therapy appeared to be more beneficial than when given later. Out of 15 patients who could not receive FLI, 2 achieved CR; one survived for 12 months and another is alive for 18 months. The remaining 13 patients had MS of 1 month. The present work suggests that FLI as an adjuvant isnot harmful and may improve remission rates and duration in AML.

INTRODUCTION

Intensive chemotherapy (3 days daunorubicin (DNR), 7 days cytosine arabinoside, Ara-C) in acute myeloid leukemia produces a high remission rate only when it is combined with equally aggressive supportive therapy (Yates 1973; Coltman 1978; Gale 1977). In the absence of such

Financed by Department of Science and Technology, Government of India.

supportive therapy, intensive chemotherapy ends up in higher mortality due to bone marrow aplasia and its main consequence which is infection (Raina 1983). Because of encouraging experience of fetal liver infusion (FLI) in severe aplastic anemia (Kansal 1981; Kansal 1981; Kochupillai 1984), we used it as an adjuvant to intensive induction and maintenance chemotherapy in acute myeloid leukemia (AML). Objectives of the present study were to ascertain if fetal liver cells (FLC) were capable of (1) improving and extending the remission status in AML and (2) engraftment in adult bone marrow.

PATIENTS AND METHODS

AML diagnosis was established on morphology of peripheral blood, bone marrow and cytochemistry. Over 32 months, from April, 1982 to November, 1984, 27 of the previously untreated AML patients were admitted to the general medical ward. Their initial presenting data are shown in Tables 1 and 2.

TABLE 1   Data at Diagnosis (Fetal Liver Group)

Case	Age	Sex	Hb gm%	WBC/ul	Platelet/ul	Subtype
1. S.S.	32	M	3.5	72,400	10,000	M_1
2. K.D.	26	F	4.0	12,000	80,000	M_5
3. V.K.	23	M	4.0	5,900	90,000	M_2
4. K.C.	32	M	9.3	11,400	70,000	M_4
5. N.K.	14	M	2.8	9,400	130,000	M_1
6. K.G.	32	M	5.8	69,000	170,000	M_1
7. M.D.	46	F	12.6	800	200,000	M_1
8. M.P.G.	53	M	4.9	52,000	90,000	M_1
9. R.R.A.	55	F	5.8	3,200	60,000	M_6
10. K.L.	31	F	4.0	35,400	100,000	M_1
11. R.P.R.	50	M	3.2	66,000	110,000	M_5
12. V.S.	25	F	8.4	16,550	150,000	M_2

TABLE 2.   Data at Diagnosis (Control Group)

Case	Age	Sex	Hb gm%	WBC/ul	Platelet/ul	Subtype
1. R.C.	18	M	5.2	72,000	40,000	M_1
2. R.L.S.	30	M	2.3	31,400	60,000	M_6
3. B.K.	14	F	5.0	114,000	40,000	M_1
4. M.A.	26	M	7.1	18,000	100,000	M_6
5. S.1.	28	M	5.4	3,600	220,000	M_4
6. M.P.	30	M	5.6	85,000	80,000	M_1
7. T.K.	39	F	4.0	1,000	20,000	M_1
8. J.G.L.	25	M	5.4	10,200	60,000	M_2
9. C.B.L.	56	F	5.9	1,950	150,000	M_1
10. S.R.	22	F	4.3	5,000	90,000	M_2
11. M.K.	16	M	6.8	176,000	70,000	M_1
12. M	18	F	3.6	30,700	90,000	M_5
13. M.K.L.	21	M	5.8	20,000	80,000	M_1
14. D.P.	49	M	12.3	1,900	150,000	M_4
15. J.G.	36	F	5.9	2,300	160,000	M_2

INDUCTION CHEMOTHERAPY

AML patients received the following intensive chemotherapy: (a) DNR in the dose of 45 mgm/m^2 intravenously (I.V.) on days 1, 2 and 3 and (b) Ara-C 100 mgm/m^2 continuous I.V. infusion from day 1 to 7. Peripheral blood counts were checked daily and Ara-C discontinued if white blood cell (WBC) count dropped to less than 1000/ul. Such a step was necessary in view of limited availability of blood components and antibiotics in our set up.

In 12 patients this chemotherapy could be supplemented by fetal liver infusion (FLI), for which a written consent was given by them. In 6 patients (case numbers 1,2,3,6,10 and 11) FLI could be administered within 48 hours of the last dose of chemotherapy; 3 (case numbers 4,5, and 8) received it after 48 hours but within one week, while the remaining 3 (case numbers 7,9 and 12) on the eighth day. Six patients refused FLI and for 9 patients it was not available.

SUPPORTIVE THERAPY

Antibiotics

Five patients who were afebrile at the start of aggressive therapy were orally administered, for pro;hylaxis, combination of trimethoprim (160 mgm) and sulphamethoxazole (800 mgm) 12 hourly and also nystatin 100,000 i.u. 6 hourly. Remaining patients who had fever at the beginning or during the 7 day therapy, received combination of gentamicin 80 mgm i.v. 8 hourly and cephalaxin or cloxacillin (500 mgm orally 6 hourly). Metromidazole (500 mgm 8 hourly) was given in 4 patients. Antibiotics were initiated after sending various body fluids for culture. Suitable changes were made in the antibiotic schedule if indicated by the bacteriology culture sensitivity. Antibiotics were continued until the patients became afebrile and the peripheral WBC counts were near-normal.

Blood Component Therapy

Patients with hemoglobin (Hb) less than 6 gms% received packed red cell transfusions. Bleeding patients with platelet counts less than 50,000/cu mm were given platelet rich plasma (Nanu 1980). Patients not repsonding to antibiotics were given buffy coat transfusion (Hughes 1981), if their white blood cell count was less than 1000/cu mm and if they were febrile. If packed red cells, platelet rich plasma or buffy coat infusion were not available fresh whole blood was transfused.

Maintenance Therapy

All patients who showed remission by criteria described earlier received cyclical maintenance chemotherapy (Raina 1983) as outpatients. During maintenance the DNR was discontinued after a maximum dose of 415 mgm/m^2. FLI was repeated when available during maintenance therapy.

Fetal Liver Infusion (FLI)

The Obstetrics Department of the hospital of this Institute could send 38 fetuses obtained during the medical termination of pregnancy by hysterotomy (26), prostaglandin injection (8) and also after spontaneous abortion (4). Fetal age determined from the last date of menstruation and from crown rump measurements (Hamilton 1957) was 10 to 24 weeks (median-M-16). Fetal liver cell suspension was prepared according to the method described earlier (Kochupillai 1985), preserved at 4°C and used within 1.5-432 hours (M-11.5). Fetal liver cell numbers that could be infused per patient varied between 0.07 to 34.0×10^8 (M-3.0×10^8). Fetal liver cell viability in the infusions varied between 55-99% (M-95%)

Studies for Evidence of Engraftment

(1) HLA A and B antigens and red cell antigens (ABO, Rh, DC with E and MNLea, Fy^a K P_1) were studied in all the cases before and one month after each FLI.

(2) Whenever there was difference in sexes of donor fetus and recipient patients, bone marrow of the latter was cultured and studied for male and female chromosomes according to the method of Tijo and Whang (Tijo 1985).

RESULTS

Of the 3 cases who received FLI on the 8th day of intensive chemotherapy only 2 survived a further 2 and 5 days. Therefore, these 2 patients are considered unevaluable. Fifteen patients who did not receive FLI are considered as the control group and are compared with the FLI group of 10 evaluable cases.

Four patients in the control group (27%) responsded, in that group 2 achieved complete remission (CR) and 2 partial remission (PR); the latter 2 survived for 3 and 4 months respectively. Eleven patients in the control group failed to respond and survived for 15 days to 2 months (mediant survival, MS-1 month). Out of 2 CR in the control group 1 relapsed and expired at 12 months. Another one relapsed at 13 months, achieved a second remission after reinduction therapy and survives at 18 months.

Five patients in the fetal liver group responded (50%) in that 4 achieved CR and one achieved PR with 3 months survival. Five who failed to respond died in 15 days to 2.5 months (MS 1.5 months). Out of 4 CR one died at 20 months during 4th relapse, the remaining 3 survive at 28, 23 and 8 months respectively. Cases 2 and 5 during induction therapy received fetal liver cells with cell viability of less than 75%. None achieved remission and both died of septicemia associated with severe hypokalemia and hyponatremia. Fetal liver cell viability varied between 90-99% in the remaining patients. Patients in CR are described below.

FLI Group

Case No. 1. Forty-eight hours after the last dose of induction chemotherapy this 32 year old male patient received FLI from a 20 week old female fetus. Over the next 19 days he required antibiotics for urine, E. coli infection, besides blood transfusions. By the 19th day, peripheral blood counts were entirely normal and bone marrow (BM) in complete remission (CR). Bone marrow culture revealed all cells with XX chromosomes; when repeated after one month, BM cultures showed all cells with XY chromosomes, indicating recovery of his own marrow cells and rejection of donor cells. The patient received cyclical maintenance therapy every three months, each course being followed by FLI. In September, 1983, 12 months from diagnosis he relapsed but achieved a second remission with Ara-C plus DNR followed by FLI. Subsequently he was maintained on cyclical therapy at monthly intervals which was often followed by FLI. Donor fetal ages varied from 12 to 24 (M-16) weeks and there were 7 male and 5 female fetuses. He has so far received a total of 5.62×10^9 fetal liver cells over 28 months. Temporary engraftment of fetal liver cells occured only after the first FLI. HLA A and B and red cell antigens have shown no significant changes. This patient is surviving at 28 months. The last bone marrow, however, indicates AML relapse.

Case No. 3. Twenty-three year old male diagnosed in January, 1983 received induction chemotherapy and after 48 hours FLI from a male fetus. This patient received cyclical maintenance therapy as case no. 1. Nine months after diagnosis he relapsed, was reinduced with Ara-C and DNR followed by FLI and achieved a second remission. Three weeks after the second remission, red cell antigen changed from Rh negative to Rh positive indicating engraftment. After 6 months, however, red cells became Rh negative indicating rejection of donor cells. Cyclical maintenance chemotherapy was then given at monthly intervals, each course being followed by FLI except on 2 occasions when FLI was not available. This patient relapsed in December, 1983 and April, 1984; remission could be achieved on both these occasions after chemotherapy which was followed by FLI. The fourth relapse in August, 1984 occured 19 months after diagnosis and despite chemotherapy and FLI resulted in death in September, 1984. Over a 20 month period this patient received a total number of 0.9×10^9 fetal liver cells on 13 occasions obtained from 9 male and 4 female fetuses.

Case No. 4. This 32 year old male patient achieved CR 4 weeks after receiving induction chemotherapy which was followed by FLI, 6 days later. This patient has been on cyclical maintenance chemotherapy at monthly intervals which could be often followed by FLI. Over a period of 22 months he has received FLI on 11 occasions from 4 male and 7 female fetuses; total 7.6×10^9 fetal liver cells. He continues to be in CR at 23 months.

Case No. 11. 50 year old male received chemotherapy followed by FLI on the 3rd day and achieved CR in 23 days. He is receiving monthly cyclical maintenance chemotherapy which was followed by FLI on two occasions. So far he has received FLI on 3 occasions from 2 male and one female fetus (total FLI cells 0.97×10^9). He continues to be in CR at 8 months.

Out of 4 patients with CR described above 3 developed Australia antigen positive hepatitis during maintenance. There was jaundice, with levels of raised bilirubin, SGOT and SGPT in serum. Hepatitis resolved within 2-3 months and Australia antigen became negative. Case No. 1 and 3 received anti-tuberculosis therapy during maintenance because of bilateral apical shadow and right mid zone infiltration respectively; the shadows disappeared on therapy.

Control Group

Case No. 4. This 26 year old male achieved CR in 6 weeks following chemotherapy. He refused to receive FLI. Maintenance therapy was given at monthly intervals in cyclical fashion. This patient relapsed in July, 1984 and was reinduced with Ara-C plus DNR. Though his bone marrow showed CR, during reinduction he developed fulminant septicemia, hypokalemia, and convulsions, and expired in August, 1984 12 months after his diagnosis.

Case No. 5. 28 year old male achieved CR in 4 weeks following induction chemotherapy. He refused to receive FLI and was maintained on monthly cyclical chemotherapy. He relapsed 13 months after diagnosis and achieved second remission. He is currently alive at 18 months, and receiving monthly cyclical chemotherapy.

DISCUSSION

The success of intensive chemotherapy in AML is influenced by several factors (Lister 1984) which include (a) the duration (3 to 10 days) and the number of effective drugs (2 to 4 drugs) used in the chemotherapy combination; (b) the availability of extensive and prolonged supportive therapy for the interim survival of those patients whose bone marrow is temporarily completely suppressed by these drugs; and (c) the "inherent characteristics of the patient populations". Further, the life span of the patients in remission will also be influenced by the usage of subsequent therapy in the form of consolidation and/or maintenance. Therefore, for comparative evaluation of different therapeutic schedules it is advisable to use the data from the same hospital.

As shown in Table 3, regimens employing Ara-C and 6 MP used by us earlier (Raina 1983) produced a response rate (complete and partial remission) of 68%; more intensive regimens but in lower dosage produced response rates of 44%. In the present study with Ara-C for 7 days and DNR for 3 days in full dosage, response rates were 27% without FLI and 50% with FLI. Although because of the small number of patients in each group, our data cannot yield statistically significant conclusions; it can, however, give some indications for further work which we are pursuing.

TABLE 3: Results of Different Therapeutic Schedules in AML at A.I.I.M.S.

Drugs, Dose Route, Duration	Total No. of Patients	Complete Remission	Median Survival (MS) Months	Partial Remission	(MS) Months	No. Remission MS	Remission Months	References
(1)								
Ara-C 100 mgm/m^2 12 hrly I.V. x 5 days	19	11 (58%)	8(1 alive)	2	4.5	6	1	Raina 1983
6 MP 100 mgm/m^2 12 hrly orally x 5 days								
(2)								
Ara-C 75 mgm/m^2 IV cont. infusion x 7 days	25	10(40%)	10(2 alive)	1	2.5	14	1.5	Raina 1983
DNR 35 mgm/m^2 IV push day 1,2,3								
(3)								
Ara-C 100 mgm/m^2 IV cont. infusion x 7 days	15	2(13%)	15(1 alive)	2	3.5	11	1	present work
DNR 45 mgm/m^2 IV push day 1,2,3								
(4)								
Chemotherapy as in No. (3) followed by FLI	10	4(40%)	21.5+ (3 alive)	1	3	5	1.5	present work

Case no. 1 in the present work demonstrates that female fetal liver cells are capable of complete engraftment in an adult male environment as indicated by the presence of XX chromosomes in all his bone marrow cells. Donor cells were engrafted in this case because apparently chemotherapy temporarily suppressed the patient's own stem cells. Occurence of Rh antigen in case no. 3 which was Rh negative prior to reinduction therapy and FLI, also suggests a similar phenomenon. Peripheral blood counts in both these cases were entirely normal at the time of donor engraftment. In these 2 cases engraftment, though complete, was only temporary. This was because total eradication of the host's cells was not aimed at due to inadequate support facilities. On recovery of patient's own cells, engrafted cells were rejected.

Engraftment of FL cells during induction therapy is important because it may improve the peripheral blood recovery and also the patient's chance of survival. Case no. 1, for instance, had normal peripheral blood counts within 19 days of start of chemotherapy; his own bone marrow cells took longer to regenerate.

During maintenance therapy, engraftment did not occur detectably in any patient even when there was a difference in sex of donor and recipeint. Chromosome studies on 7 occasions and HLA A and B and red cell antigens on 20 occasions in case numbers 1,3,4 and 11 failed to demonstrate any significant change following FLI. In a series of 30 severe aplastic anemia ceases not receiving immunosuppression, FLI could induce transient, partial mixed chimerism in 3 cases only associated with slow and not always complete recovery (Kansal 1979; Kansal 1981; Kochupillai 1984). Altogether it appears that FLI can induce complete engraftment if most stem cells are completely suppressed. If they recover or are partially suppressed the beneficial effect of FLI may not involve engraftment mechanisms.

The present study further suggests that the number of fetal liver cells infused is not important in determining the graft outcome (Kochupillai 1985). Cell dose of 3.0×10^8 (8.2×10^6/kg body weight), in case no. 1 was capable of producing complete engraftment.

Time interval between the last dose of chemotherapy

and fetal liver infusion, however, appears important. Six patients could be given FLI within 48 hours of the last dose of chemotherapy, 4 of whom responded (3 CR, 1 PR). Of the 3 who received FLI after 48 hours, but in less than one week, of the last dose of chemotherapy, 1 achieved CR, while of those 3 patients who received FLI on the 8th day, none achieved remission.

Fetal liver cell viability appears to be another important factor as indicated by cases 2 and 5 who received fetal liver cells with cell viability of less than 75% during induction therapy. Both died without achieving bone marrow remission. Importance of fetal liver cell viability was observed in aplastic anemia patients also (Kochupillai 1985).

It is unlikely that FLI by itself can maintain AML patients in remission. Thus in a study by Lucarelli, et al (Lucarelli 1980), all patients of acute leukemia treated with chemotherapy and FLI relapsed and died within 10 months. In the present study, when chemotherapy was given at 3 monthly intervals, both cases 1 and 3 relapsed; subsequently they received chemotherapy at monthly intervals. Cases 4 and 11 who received chemotherapy at more regular intervals have remained in remission.

Occurence of hepatitis in 3 complete remission patients following FLI on 8 occasions appears unrelated to FLI, as none of the 30 patients of severe aplastic anemia who recived FLI on 43 occasions had developed this complicaiton (Kansal 1979; Kansal 1981; Kochupillai 1984). It is more likely due to the following factors: (a) immunosuppression induced by chemotherapy; (b) repeated blood transfusions which were not always tested for the presence of Australia antigen; and (c) longer life span of these patients which permitted hepatitis to unfold.

The present work, though not conclusive, allows indication that fetal liver infusion may improve and extend the remission status in AML. This could be on account of a bettter tolerance to chemotherapy by the bone marrow or by the regulation of some immune mechanisms. The possibility exists that fetal liver cells may possess antitumor activity. The theoretical fear that fetal antigens may "enhance tumor" (Medawar 1983) does not seem applicable, at least to the present work which involves acute myeloid leukemia.

ACKNOWLEDGMENT

We extend our sincere gratitidue to Prof. N.K. Bhide, Professor and Head of the Department of Pharmacology, All-India Institute of Medical Sciences, for his valuable suggestions in the preparation of this manuscript.

REFERENCES

Coltman CA Jr., Bodey GP, Hewlett JS, et al (1978). Chemotherapy of acute leukemia. Arch Int Med 138:1342-1348.
Gale RP, Cline MJ (1977). High remission induction rate in acute myeloid leukemia. Lancet i:497-499.
Hamilton WJ, Boyd JI, Mohnan HW (1957). Human embryology. Cambridge, Heften and Sons, p 104.
Hughes A, Addison IB, Al-Hadithy H, Brozoric B (1981). Buffy coat and cell separator granulocyte concentrate. Vox Sang 41:1-5.
Kansal V, Sood SK, Batra AK, Adhar G, Malaviya AK, Kucheria K, Balakrishnan K (1979). Foetal liver transplantation in aplastic anemia. Acta Haematol 62:128-136.
Kansal V (1981). Fetal liver transplantation in aplastic anemia. J Soc Young Sci 2:8-9.
Kochupillai V (1984). Management of aplastic anemia. Ind J Haematol 3:149-154.
Kochupillai V, Sharma S, Francis S, Mehra NK, Nanu A, et al (1985, in press). Bone marrow reconstitution following human fetal liver infusion (FLI) in sixteen severe aplastic anemia patients. In: Fetal Liver Transplantation. Gale RP (ed). Alan R. Liss, New York.
Lister TA, Rohatiner AZS (1984). The management of acute myeloid leukemia. In: Hematology 1, Leukemias. Goldman IM, Preisler (eds). Butterworths International Medical Reviews, ; 136.
Lucarelli G, Izzi T, Porcallini A, et al (1980). Fetal liver transplantation in aplastic anemia and acute leukemia. In: Fetal Liver Transplantation: Current Concepts and Future Directions. Lucarelli G, Fliedner TM, Gale RP (eds). Amsterdam, Excerpta Medica, p 284-299.
Medawar PB, Hunt R (1983). Can fetal antigens be used for prophylactic immunization. In: Fetal Antigens and Cancer. Cuba Foundation, Pitman, London, p. 160-170.
Nanu A, Teneja N, Sood SK (1980). Preparation and standardization of platelet rich plasma and platelet concentrates in a developing blood bank. Ind J Med Res 71:661-667.

Raina V, Kochupillai V (1983). Acute myeloid leukemia in adults: experience at A.I.I.M.S. J Assoc Phys Ind 31(8):511-514.
Tijo JH, Whang J (1985). Direct chromosome preparations of bone marrow cells. In: Human Chromosome Methodology. Yunis JJ (ed). Academic Press, New York, p. 51.
Yates JW, Wallace HJ, Jr., Ellison RR, Holland JF (1973). Cytosine arabinoside (NSC-63878) and daunorubicin (NSC-83142) therapy in acute non-lymphocytic leukemia. Cancer Chemoth Rep 57:485-488.

ALLOGENEIC FETAL LIVER TRANSPLANTATION IN ACUTE LEUKEMIA

Pei-lin Meng, Rui-gao Fei, Ding-wei Gu, Wen-zheng Yie, Ben-tie Liu, Fang Yan, You-yu Yu, Zhi-guang Mai, Bao-zhen Chen, Ling-xian Zhu, Feng Guo, Xiao-hui Wang.

Department of Hematology, Changhai Hospital, Shanghai, China.

In recent years, chemotherapy has advanced quickly. Although complete remission (CR) of acute leukemia (AL) patients is more often seen, yet long-term survival of these patients is not. For the purpose of achieving long-term CR, a number of new protocols have been investgated.

Bone marrow transplantation (BMT) is more inspiring in the field, But the BMT donor is limited to HLA identical siblings or a partially HLA matched relative. Unfortunately, to obtain the bone marrow (BM) from HLA-matched related or unrelated donors is very difficult. Therefore, an other alternative source of hemopoietic stem cells (HSC) has been investigated . Many literatures (Lucarelli, et al 1980; Fei, et al 1982; Wu, et al 1982) have indicated that the properties and functions of the HSC from fetal liver (FL) are in the main similar to those of BM, capable of erythropoiesis and granulopoiesis, and that fetal liver transplantation (FLT) from animal to human has obtained some success (Yunis, et al 1976; Fliedner, et al 1980; Gale 1980). Recently successful FLT in acute leukemia has been reported (Lucarelli, et al 1982; Izzi, et al 1983). Therefore, FL may become another main origin of HSC in transplantation.

Here were reported 3 patients with acute leukemia in first CR who were transplanted with FL cells after conditioning regimen with cyclophosphamide and total body irradiation (TBI) from May 1983 to June 1984. Complete BM and peripheral blood (PB) hematological reconstitution was observed in each patient. There was definite proof of chimerism in 2 patients.

MATERIALS AND METHODS

ALLOGENEIC MARKERS

Cytogeneic studies of PB and BM from fetus and patient were performed by direct method (BM) and phytohemagglutinin (PHA) culture method (BM & PB) and Y chromosomes were confirmed by C-band staining technique. HLA typing for antigens of the A,B and C loci was determined using the thymocyte in fetus and PB in patient. Red cell isoenzyme phenotypes were performed by electrophoresis using agarose and starch substrate.

PREPARATION OF FL CELL SUSPENSION (FEI & WU 1983)

All fetuses were obtained from abortion induced by water bag. FL was taken out aseptically after laprotomy and cut in small cubes into a glass containing RPMI 1640 medium. Then it was stirred with a syringe core in double stainless steel wire net (pore size: 80 & 180 pore/inch) until a single cell suspension was obtained.

CASE REPORT

Case 1. The patient (H 194268), a 13-year-old boy, was admitted to our hospital on Feb. 24 1983 with complaints of fatigue, pallor and fever for one month. Laboratory examination: PB. HB 5.4g/dl, WBC 2.75×10^9/L, neutrophils 19%, lymphocytes 21%, lymphoblasts 14%, prolymphocytes 46%, platelets 49×10^9/L; BM. The nucleated cells exhibited hyperplasia with lymphoblasts 81%, prolymphocytes 12%; mixed rosetting method using erythrocytes and C3b sensitized yeast (Ey): T 65.5%, B 11%, D 2%, N 21.5%; E-Rosette forming cells (Et): 42%; E-Active Rosette forming cells (Ea): 22%; Lymphocyte transformation stimulation index (LT) was 29 (normal 700±300). the diagnosis of acute lymphocytic leukemia (ALL) was confirmed.

A CR was achieved with Vincristine (V) and Prednisone (P) protocol chemotherapy for 3 weeks. Spinal puncture was

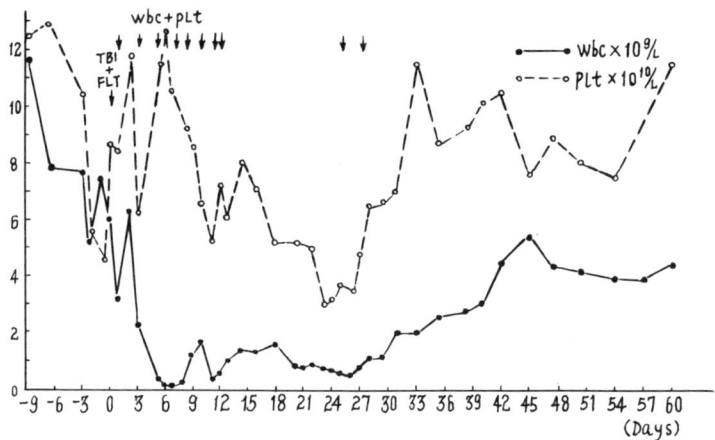

Figure 1: FLT in case 1

carried out as routine. The intracranial pressure was 235 H2O. Pandy's qualitative test of cerebral spinal fluid (CSF)+, protein 209mg/dl, leukocytes 6/ml. Central nervous system leukemia was considered. Thus the VP program was continued with additional intrathecal injection of methotrexate (MTX) and dexamethasone (Dex) for 4 times at interval of 5-7 days, CSF examination became normal. On April 14, BM examination revealed normal also. A CR was accomplished. The consolidation chemotherapy with VMTP (VCR, MTX, 6-thioguanine, pred) followed.

On May 3, 1983. The patient was transfered to sterilized ward. CTX 30mg/kg/day were given intravenously (day -3, -2). On day 0, the patient received TBI (600 rad) at a dose rate of 5.27r per minute from 60Co sourse, then, suspension of FL cells was transfused at P.M.. The recipient's blood group phenotype was A, CcDE, NP1, HLA type was A2, B15, CW3. The donor was a 21-week-old female fetus whose blood group phenotype was A, CcDE, MP2. The total number of nucleated cells of FL was 10.7×10^9 (2.6×10^8/kg) and the total CFU-C count, 6.45×10^6 (1.57×10^5/kg). The transformation rate of mixed lymphocyte culture (MLC) between patient and FL was 5% (morphological method).

After FLT, intravenous alimentation and suspension of WBC and platelets were transfused. WBC and platelet count decreased on day 1 and returned to normal gradually

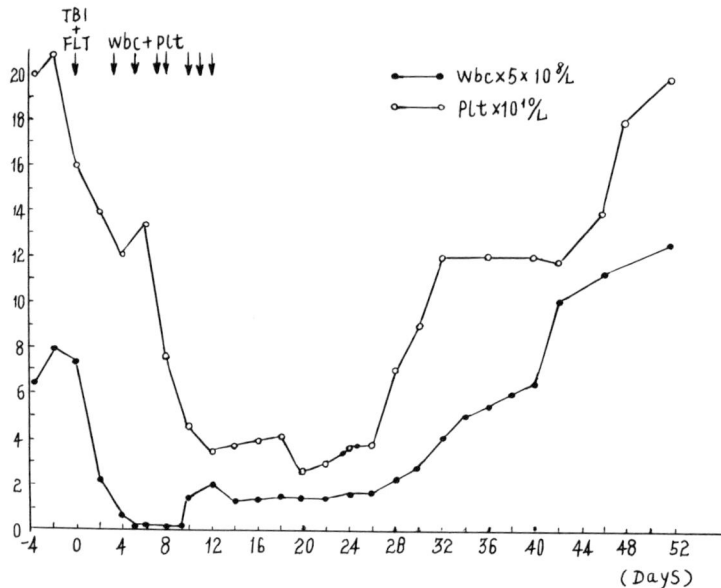

Figure 2: FLT in case 2

on day 42 (Fig. 1). On day 6 his temperature rose up to 39.2°C and dropped to normal on the second day without management. On day 5 Ey: T 62%, on day 11 Et: 51.5%, Ea: 49.5%, LT: 417, on day 18 Ey: T 86.5%, B 2%, D 1.5%, N 10%, Et: 52%, Ea: 46.5%, LT:151. these phenomena suggested cellular immune functions were more active than before FLT and returned to normal on day 31. BM examination on day 14, nucleated cells displayed severe hypoplasis. On day 14, chromosome analysis in BM by direct method: Karyotype, XX 6/8, XY 2/8. Cultural method with PHA: XX 11/16, XY 5/16. In PB on the same day, XX karyotype was 5/20, XY 10/20. Blood group phenotype on day 26 was A, CcDE, MN P1, HLA typing with the appearance of locus A9 was demonstrated.

BM examination on day 30 showed hypoplasia slightly. Karyotype of BM cells examined from PHA culture expressed XY in 18 and XX in 2 of 20 BM cells. Karyotype XY in PB was present in all of the 33 cells examined. The phenotype of RBC on day 52 was A, CcDE, MN P2, HLA: A2, B15, CW3. BM picture on day 90 revealed a normal cellularity. Chromosome analysis of BM using direct method 50 mitotic cells

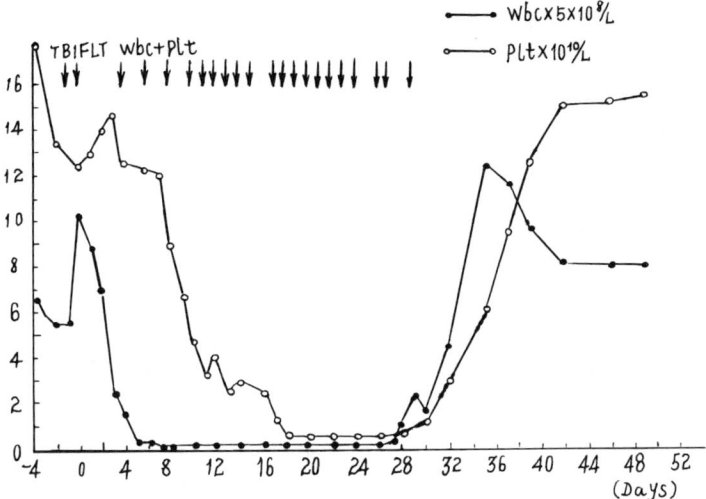

Figure 3: FLT in case 3

expressed karyotype of XY in 49, XX in 1 (2%).

Follow up: the patient was discharged on day 90. He had not received anti-leukemic therapy within 5 months after FLT and remained in CR. Clinical GVHD was not observed. On day 151 a relapse occured. A second CR was achieved following three courses of combination chemotherapy with VCR, Pred and 6-TG until day 360. The patient died of sepsis because of relapse on day 385.

Case 2. The patient (H 199983), a 6-year-old girl, was diagnosed as ALL (L1) in Augest 1982. A CR was achieved with VP protocol for 5 weeks. Then 2400 rad of cranial irradiation was given. A chemotherapy program with VCR, 6-MP, MTX and Pred was maintained.

On Sept 28, 1983, the patient in CR was admitted to our department and received 2 courses of reinduction program with VMP protocol. Ey: T 35%, B 39%, D 1%, N 34%; Et: 49%; Ea: 25%; LT: 229; Alpha-fetoprotein (AFP): hemagglutination (HA) (-); Rocket immunoelectrophoreses(RIE): 31µg/L; Blood group phenotype: O, CCDee, MN P1; HLA: A11, B13, B22, Bw4,6; Chromosome: 46, XX.

On October 28,1983, the patient entered laminar airflow room (LAFR). The conditioning regimen was CTX 40 mg/kg/day (day -3, -2) and TBI (600 rad, day 0) at a dose rate of 7.69r per minute. In the afternoon the patient received FLT (Nov 11, 1983) from a 24-week-old male fetus. The donor's phenotype of RBC was O, CcDee, MN P2, HLA: A9, A11, B40. Karyotype: 45, XYt (13;14). The total number of nucleated cells was 9.59×10^9 (5.64×10^8/kg). The transformation rate of MLC: 7%.

On day 6 after FLT, the patient had a fever from 38.5°C to 39°C for 4 days. On day 3: Et 2.5%, Ea 0.5%, Ey on day 6: T 15%, B 85%, Et and Ea on day 9 were 36% and 17% respectively. On day 17 they were 49% and 25% and LT was 416. On day 26 Ey: T 56%, B 3.5%, N 40.5%, Et 60%, Ea 36%. On day 39 their values returned to normal. AFP on day 3, HA 1:10 ++++, 1:100 ++++, 1:1000 +, RIE 125 µg/L; on day 10, HA 1:10 ++++, 1:100 ++++, 1:1000 (-), RIE 76 µg/L; on day 12, HA 1:10 ++++, 1:100 ++, 1:1000 (-), RIE 31 ug/L; on day 18, HA 1:10 +, RIE 31 µg/L; on day 40, HA 1:10 +, RIE 31 µg/L. The patient had an aplastic BM on day 14, but became normal on day 30. The nadir value of WBC was 0.04×10^9/L on day 9 and that of platelet, 26×10^9/L on day 19 (Fig. 2), chromosome on day 14, 30 and 60 was 46, XX.

Follow up: The patient was discharged on day 98 and has remained in CR up-to-date. The survival is 10 months.

Case 3. The patient (H 205980), a 9-year-old boy was diagnosed as acute myeloid leukemia (AGL, M2) on Nov 5, 1983. The patient was admitted on May 25, 1984 and a CR was accomplished with COAP (CTX, VCR, Ara-C, Pred) on June 12. Ey: T 38.5%, B 7.5%, D 1.5%, N 52.5%, Et:60%, Ea:24%, LT: 139, Blood type: O, CCDee, M, RBC isoenzyme: ESD 2-1, EAP A, PGM 1-1, AFP: (-), HLA: A33? B5, B12, chromosome: 46, XY.

The patient was prepared with CTX 40mg/kg/day x 2 and TBI (700 rad) at a dose rate of 6.83 rad per minute. On June 27, 1984 (day 0) he received 8.12×10^9 (3.12×10^8/kg) FL cells from a 21-week-old male fetus. the total CFU-C content was 1.97×10^6, average 7.58×10^4 CFU-C/kg. RBC phenotype: A, CCDee, MN. HLA: A11, A28? B13? B22. RBC isoenzyme: ESD 1-1, EAP B, PGM 2-1.

After FLT the value of AFP on day 2 was HA 1:10 ++++,

1:100 ++++, 1:1000 ++, RIE 450μg/L; On day 6 was HA 1:10 ++++, 1:100 ++++, RIE 125 μg/L; on day 13 HA 1:10 ++, 1:100 +, RIE 31 μg/L down; on day 20 (-). Ey on day 8 was T 38%, B 3%, N 59%; on day 15, T 75%, B 2%, N 23%; on day 29, T 20%, N 80%. Et on day 6,13, 20, 27 was 43%, 63%, 42%, 28%. While Ea was 9%, 21%, 30%, 5%. LT on day 6, 20, 27 was 28, 89, 5. The changes of BM picture were similar to those of the two above mentioned patient. The nadir count of WBC was 0.02×10^9/L on day 10 and that of platelet, 4.6×10^9/L on day 21 (Fig. 3). RBC phenotype was O, CCDee, MN on day 23 and 37. HLA on day 36 was A11, B22. RBC isoenzyme on day 37 was EAP: B-A, ESD: 2-1, PGM: 1-1.

Follow up: The patient was discharged on day 90 and has CR up-to-date. The survival is 90 days.

DISCUSSION

Recently on the basis of studying the properties of HSC from human FL, clinical trials of human FLT replacing BM in the treatment of hematological diseases have been extensively investgated (Lucarelli, et al 1980; Fei, et al 1982; Wu, et al 1982; Gale 1980; Kansal, et al 1979; Lucarelli, et al 1980). Although several reports have expressed some effective value of treatment, definite evidence of engraftment has not yet been achieved.

Successful engraftment of FLT for treatment of acute leukemia after TBI has been reported by Lucarelli and Izzi (Lucarelli, et al 1982; Izzi, et al 1983; Izzi, et al 1984). They reported that complete BM and PB hematological reconstitutions were observed in five cases and partial in another four and allogeneic markers were proven in six cases out of thirteen AL patients after FLT. The clinical outcome is promising.

In this paper it was indicated that the hemopoietic and immunological recovery was rapid and complete in each patient as expressed by the above data concerning BM, PB and immunology. There were evidence of chimerism in case 1 as demonstrated by the existence of the XX karyotype, new HLA-antigens and RBC antigens of donor origen and by the appearance of donor's HLA-antigens and RBC isoenzyme on day 36 in case 3. Obviously the engraftment was definite. however, on day 30 and 90 BM examination in case 1 discovered that the donor's XX karyotype reduced gradually, so the engraftment was unsustained. Although the serum AFP level increased and maintained for 40 days in case 2, which reflected the viability of FL cells following FLT (Touraine 1980), there had not definite proof of engraftment in case 2.

The factors of interfering sustained engraftment may be mainly that the doses in the conditioning regimen were too small to inhibit allogeneic resistance. FL derived stem cells are probably more sensitive to allogeneic inhibition (Gale 1980), thus the engraft cells in these patients were rejected gradually as showed by the non-infectious fever and the presence of active T-lymphocyte functions. While the rejection in case 2 may be also related to chromosome aberration of fetus. Another factor of rejection was that we did not give sufficient immunosuppressant promptly when immuno-fuctions were active and AFP levels were decreased indicated by laboratory data.

Beutler (1982) reviewed the literature of BMT and referred that whatever the type AL is, it should be transplanted in the first CR. In this stage the general condition of the patients is rather good, the leukemic cells are scanty in number and do not resist to antileukemic medicine. therefore we selected the patients of AL in the first CR. The transplantation went on smoothly and hemopoietic recovery was rapid. Possibly it was related to the opportunity of transplantation. We analyzed the relations between the clinical outcome and the opportunity of transplantation from Izzi's report (Izzi, et al 1983, 1984) as well as ours, 8 patients were transplanted in CR, complete BM reconstitution appeared in six of them and partial BM reconstitution in one and chimerism developed in six of them; while another 8 patients were transplanted in relapse, complete BM recostitution appeared in two of them and partial, in three of them and to two out of eight occured chimerism, thus it could be concluded that the selection of the opportunity of CR might be resonable.

4-5 month-old fetuses are suitable for FLT. Not only the CFU-C is abundant in this stage, but also keeps T-lymphocytes in 1-2 per cent (Lucarelli, et al 1980; Fei, et al 1982; Wu, et al 1982). Surely the data given here will be valuable to FLT, as to the number of FL transplanted needs further studies. An analysis of the outcome of 14 FLTs was made, 7 patients were transplanted with one FL, Among them complete and partial BM reconstitutions were evident in 5/7 and 1/7 respectively and chimerism was present in 4/7. Another 7 patients were transplanted with 2-4 FLs, among them 2/7 and 3/7 had complete and partial BM reconstitutions respectively, and 2/7 had chimerism. Therefore, there may be no particular advantage to transplant more than one FLs. On the contrary, it may increase the possibility of rejection.

Current problems of FLT are similar to those of BMT: relapse, interstitial pneumonia, allogeneic resistance and GVHD etc. Although GVHD was not observed in the above mentioned 16 patients, yet more data must be accumulated and further studies must be made. Among the 16 patients there were six patients died of relapse. Therefore relapse after FLT must be an important problem. If FL produces less GVHD, the action of graft versus leukemia will be small, which may not be of benefit. High doses of TBI may produce interstitial pneumonia, so the resonable preconditioning regimen still needs further investigation. Thus great efforts must be exerted to overcome the immunological barrier in allogeneic unrelated FLT and get sustained engraftment.

SUMMARY

Three patients with acute leukemia in first complete remission were transplanted with fetal liver cells from May 1983 to June 1984. A conditioning regimen of cyclophosphamide (60-80 mg/kg) and TBI 600-700 rads (a dose rate of 5-7r per minute) was taken. The hemopoietic and immunological recovery was rapid and complete in every patient. There was proof of chimerism in case 1 as demonstrated by the existance of the XX karyotype of donor fetus in 68.7% and 75% of marrow netaphases, in 25% of peripheral blood metaphases, by the appearance of new HLA-antigens and RBC blood type antigens of donor origin. The serum alpha-fetoprotein level increased and maintained for 40 days in case 2, but definite evidence of engraftment was not observed. The allogeneic marker, the donor's HLA-antigens and RBC isoenzyme, were detected in case 3.

A summary is reported in the following table.

Patient No.	1	2	3
Age/Sex	13/M	6/F	9/M
Diagnosis	ALL	ALL	AGL
Fetus Age (weeks)	21	24	21
Cell Dose $\times 10^8$/kg	2.6	5.6	3.1
BM reconstitution	Yes	Yes	Yes
Allogeneic Markers	Yes	No	Yes
Survival (days)	+385	300	90
Outcome	Relapse	CR.	CR.

REFERENCES

Beutler E, Mcmillan R & Spruce W (1982). The role of bone marrow transplantation in the treatment of acute leukemia in remission. Blood 59(6):1115.

Fei Rui-gao, Zhou Shu-zhen & Wu Chu-tze (1982). The proliferation and differentiation of hemopoietic cells from human bone marrow and fetal liver in vivo culture. Chinese J Hemat 3(1):5.

Fei Rui-gao & Wu Chu-tze (1983). Properties, storage and clinical application of hemopoietic stem cells from human fetal liver. In "The Progress of Hematology" (Chinese), Mudanjiang, p 29.

Fliedner TM, Grilli G, Calvo W, Nothdurft W, Haen M, Carbonell F (1980). Fetal liver as an alternative source of stem cells for hemopoietic reconstitution. A canine model. Exp Hemat 8 (Supple 7):23.

Gale RP (1980). Fetal liver transplantation in man. In Lucarelli G, Fliedner TM & Gale RP (eds): "Fetal Liver Transplantation, Current Concepts and Future Directions". Excerpta Medica, Amsterdam, p 268.

Gale RP (1980). Concepts of fetal liver transplantation in man. Ibid, p 247.

Izzi T, Porcellini A, Delfini C, Galimberti M, Polchi P, Moretti L, Manna A, Lucarelli G (1983). Fetal liver transplantation in acute leukemia. Exp Hemat 11 (supple 14):133.

Izzi T, Polchi P, Galimberti M, Delfini C, Moretti L, Porcellini A, Manna A, Sparaventi G, Giardini C, Angelucci E, Politi P, Lucarelli G. Fetal liver transplantation in aplastic anemia and acute leukemia. This volume.

Kansal V, Sood SK, Batra AK, Adhar G, Malviya AK, Kucheris K & Kalakrishnan K (1979). Fetal liver transplantation in aplastic anemia. Acta Hemat 62(3):128.

Lucarelli G, Fliedner TM & Gale RP (1980). "Fetal Liver Transplantation, Current Concepts and Future Directions". Excerpta Medica, Amsterdam, p 5-52.

Lucarelli G, Izzi T, Porcellini A, Delfini C, Galimberti M, Moretti L, Polchi P (1982). Fetal liver transplantation in 2 patients with acute leukemia after total body irradiation. Scand J Hemat 28:65.

Lucarelli G, Izzi T, Porcellini A, Delfini C, Polchi P, Moretti L, Manna A & Grilli G (1980). Fetal liver transplantation in aplastic anemia and acute leukemia. In Lucarelli G, Fliedner TM & Gale RP (eds): "Fetal Liver Transplantation, Current Concepts and Future Directions". Excerpta Medica, Amsterdam, p 284.

Touraine JL (1980). Value of alpha-fetoprotein determinations in the monitoring of patients with a fetal liver transplant for Fabry's disease or immunodificiency. Ibid, p 300.

Wu Chu-tze, Fei Rui-gao, Zhou Shu-zhen, Shi Fei-man, Li Chun-hai, Wang Bao-zhen (1982). Kinitic studies of hemopoietic progenitor cells (CFU-C) and T-lymphocytes in the liver of human fetus. Scientia Sinica (series B) 25(2):168.

Yunis EJ, Fernandes G, Smith J & Good RA (1976). Long survival and immunologic reconstitutions following transplantation with syngeneic or allogeneic fetal liver and neonatal spleen cells. Transp Proc 8:521.

FETAL LIVER TRANSPLANTATION IN HEMATOLOGIC DISORDERS

Robert Peter Gale, M.D., Ph.D.

Department of Medicine, Division of Hematology and Oncology
UCLA School of Medicine, Center for the Health Sciences,
Los Angeles, California 90024, U.S.A.

Concepts and animal models of fetal liver transplantation are reviewed in this volume. Studies in man have confirmed animal data indicating that fetal liver cells are a source of hematopoietic stem cells with decreased immune reactivity. These observations have led to limited trials of fetal liver transplantation in patients with severe combined immunodeficiency disease (SCID) and hematologic disorders. In this chapter I will briefly review the current status of fetal liver transplantation in hematologic diseases.

A literature review was performed using data bases from CANCERLIT, MEDLARS, and MEDLINE of the National Library of Medicine. Data were analyzed with regard to total patients, fetal age, number of cells transplanted, pretransplant conditioning, engraftment, evidence of engraftment, graft-versus-host disease (GvHD), response and survival.

Some reports were inadequate for critical analysis for several reasons. Individual patients were frequently not identified and many patients received more than one fetal liver transplant. Approximately one-third of transplants consisted either of multiple fetal livers. One major obstacle to critical analysis of these data was the lack of convincing evidence of fetal liver cell engraftment in most cases. For example, immune reconstitution does not necessarily indicate engraftment. Other studies reported engraftment based on the demonstration of new HLA antigens on recipient lymphocytes; of donor type red blood cell antigens or of hemoglobin F expression. These data are problematic since recipinets are frequently extensively transfused and since fetal hemoglobin synthesis occurs in the setting of bone marrow recovery in the absence of fetal liver. This evidence is questionable.

Results of fetal liver transplantation in aplastic anemia are reviewed in Table 1. Forty-four patients received these transplants between 1960-1985; approximately one-half had severe aplastic anemia. Age of fetal donors was 6-32 weeks; most were < 20 weeks. Total dose of nucleated fetal liver cells of hematopoietic origin was 0.2 - 13 x 10^8. Two patients received cyclophosphamide pretransplant.

Four of 44 patients (11%) were reported to have grafts; in all instances this was transitory. Engraftment was documented by cytogenetic analysis in 3 cases. In one case no convincing data were presented. None of the 4 patients developed GVHD. Complete or partial responses occurred in 15 patients (34%); survival ranged from < 1 - > 10 years.

Results of fetal liver transplantation in acute leukemia are reviewed in Table 2. Twenty-six patients received transplants for acute leukemia between 1978-1985. Fourteen had acute myelogenous leukemia (AML) and 12, acute lymphoblastic leukemia (ALL). Eight patients were in remission and 8 in relapse. Ten other patients were receiving induction chemotherapy with daunorubicin and cytarabine for AML. In 16 patients, pretransplant immune suppression was cyclophosphamide (60-120 mg/kg) and total body radiation (6-10 Gy).

Eight of 26 patients (31%) were reported to have transient grafts. Engraftment was documented by chromosome 5, RBC isoenzymes or antigens in 4, HLA-antigens in 2 and HbF synthesis in 3. No patient developed GVHD. Survival ranged from < 1 - > 2 years. Since in this setting antileukemic effect is generally attributed to chemotherapy and/or radiation it is not possible to determine if outcome or response is related to the transplantation of fetal liver cells.

Several important conclusions emerge from these data. First, it seems possible to achieve at least transient

Table 1. Fetal Liver Transplantation in Aplastic Anemia

Ref	Author	No.	Fetal Age(w)	No. Cell (x10⁸)	Conditioning	Graft	Evidence	GVHD	Response	Survival(m)
1	Scott	14	NI	20-200	-	1	NI	No	2	4-146+
2	Keleman	1	6	0.4	-	No	-	-	1	52+
3	O'Reilly	1	10-14	15	+	No	-	-	1	52+
4	Kansal	7	11-16	0.2-0.4	-	3	Chr (3)	No	3	1-52+
5	Izzi	5	10-25	0.8-13	+	No	-	-	1	<1- >36+
6.	Kochupillai	16	10-32	0.3-11	+(1)	No	-	-	7	<1- 95+
		44	6-32	0.2-13	2	4(11%)	-	-	15(34%)	<1-146+

Table 2. Fetal Liver Transplantation in Acute Leukemia

Ref	Author	No.	Fetal Age(w)	No. Cell (x10⁸)	Conditioning	Graft	Evidence	GVHD	Survival(m)
5	Izzi	13	12-22	0.3-7	+	4	Chr(3), RBC(1), HbF(3)	No	<1-27+
7	Kochupillai	10	10-24	0.7-34	+	2	Chr(1), RBC(1)	No	<1-28+
8	Meng	3	21-24	5.6-81	+	2	Chr(1), HLA(2), RBC(2)	No	3-12+
		26	10-24	0.3-81	26	8(31%)			<1-28+

hematopoietic engraftment following transplantation of fetal liver cells. This has been reasonably convincingly demonstrated by cytogenetic analysis in 5 cases of acute leukemia. The incidence of successful engraftment was higher in patients with leukemia than those with aplastic anemia (31% vs. 11%). In the 16 leukemia patients who received intensive pretransplant immune suppression, incidence of engraftment was 6 of 16 (38%). These data are consistent with data in rodents, dogs and man which indicate that fetal liver cells are immunogentic and likely to be rejected following transplantation to immune competent recipients. Patients with aplastic anemia generally have an intact immune system and would be expected to be at high-risk of rejecting fetal liver cells. Leukemia patients, both because of their disease and because of the use of high-dose, pretransplant chemotherapy and radiation are less likely to reject their grafts.

Graft-rejection or failure of engraftment remains the major obstacle to fetal liver transplantation in man. There are several reasons why fetal liver cells are likely to be rejected. First, relatively few hematopoietic stem cells are transplanted. Second, fetal liver transplants contain few, if any, T-lymphocytes. T-cells appear to be important in obtaining sustained engraftment. Several mechanisms may be operative including a direct interaction with hematopoietic stem cells, a graft-anti-host immune response, and possibly by serving a source of excess donor antigen in the host anti-donor response. Bone marrow transplants depleted of T-cells are at increased risk of graft-rejection. Because of these considerations it is not surprising that failure of engraftment and rejection are common following fetal liver transplantation. In dogs and preliminary clinical trials more intensive pre- and post-transplant immune suppression, primarily with higher doses of radiation, and a combination of methotrexate and cyclosporine.

GVHD has not been a problem following fetal liver transplantation in man. It is not possible to know if this relates to the immune incompetance of the fetal liver cells or to the high incidence of graft-failure. This issue will need to be addressed when a higher rate of successful, sustained engraftment is achieved. A second consideration is the possibility of an increased risk of leukemia relapse following transplants of T-cell depleted bone marrow transplants.

In summary, there has been progress in the application of fetal liver transplantation to hematologic diseases. The major problem is achieving sustained engraftment. Recent data in dog models suggests that this may be achievable with more intensive pre- and post-transplant immune suppression. When results in these animal models are optimized, it may be reasonable to apply these approaches in man.

Acknowledgment: Supported in part by grant CA 23175 NCI, NIH, USPHA, DHHS.

Kansal V, Sood SK, Batra AK, Adhar G, Malviya AK, Kucheria K, Balakrishnan K (1979). Fetal liver transplantation in aplastic anemia. Acta Haemat 62:128.

Kelemen E (1973). Recovery from chronic idiopathic bone marrow aplasia of a young mother after intravenous injection of unprocessed cells from the liver (and yolk sac) of her 22mm CR-length embryo. Scand J Haemat 10:305.

O'Reilly RJ, Pahwa R, Kagan W, Kapoor N, Sorell M, Meyers P, Good RA (1977). Reconstitution of hematopoietic function in post-hepatic aplasia following high-dose cyclophosphamide and allogenic fetal liver transplantation. Exp Hematol 5(suppl. 2):46.

Scott RB, Matthias JQ, Constandoulakis M, Kay HEM, Lucas PF, Whiteside JD (1961). Hypoplastic anemia treated by transfusion of fetal hemopoietic cells. Brit Med J 2:1385.

FETAL LIVER TRANSPLANTATION IN IMMUNODEFICIENCIES AND INBORN ERRORS OF METABOLISM

J.L. Touraine, M.G. Roncarolo, G.L. Marseglia, G. Souillet, B. Bétend, H. Bétuel, F. Touraine, C. Royo, N. Philippe and R. François
Transplantation and Immunobiology Unit, INSERM U80, Pav.P, Hôpital Edouard Herriot, 69374 LYON Cedex 08, FRANCE.

In our institution, forty transplants of fetal liver have been carried out in twenty patients (8 patients with severe combined immunodeficiency disease-SCID- and 12 patients with inborn errors of metabolism-IEM) over the last ten years. An associated transplant of fetal thymus from the same donor was performed in all patients with SCID.

Altogether, 15 of the 20 patients are alive and well. They have been either completely cured from their disease (children with SCID) or significantly improved (patients with IEM) by the treatment. The risks of fetal liver transplantation (FLT) are extremely low, as compared to bone marrow transplantation (BMT) from a mismatched donor. Despite the usual lack of any HLA antigen shared by cells of donor origin and cells of the host, stable chimerism was obtained, graft-versus-host disease (GvHD) was rare and functions of T lymphocytes were not restricted *in vivo* nor *in vitro*. SCID, Gaucher disease and Niemann-Pick disease are among the best indications for FLT. No significant ethical problem is encountered in FLT, as in any transplant from cadaver donor, provided that teams responsible for the therapeutic abortion and the transplant are separate.

FLT IN SCID

When no HLA-identical donor was available for BMT, we always resorted to fetal liver and thymus transplantation (FLTT) for the treatment of SCID patients. We have treated 8 patients thus (Table 1). Stem cells from the fetal liver can proliferate and differentiate after transplantation in the host, resulting in lymphocyte repopulation and immunological reconstitution.

TABLE 1
Fetal liver and thymus transplantation in 8 patients with SCID (Lyon, 1976-1985)

Patients	Treatment	Take	GvHD	Reconstitution	Outcome
S (male)	FLTT	+++	−	Full	Complete recovery
*B (male)	FLTT	?	−	No	Death (previous BCG infection)
C (female)	FLTT	+++	−	Full	Complete recovery
F (female)	FLTT	++	++	Partial	Death (meningitis)
M (male)	FLTT	+	+++	Initial	Death (GvHD and septicemia)
M (male)	FLTT	++	−	Subtotal and still progressing	Healthy, at home
M (male)	FLTT	+	++	Initial	Death (infection with Salmonella and catheter complications)
T (female)	FLTT	too early for evaluation			Healthy, in isolation

* Patient with ADA deficiency
FLTT = 1 to 5 fetal liver and thymus transplants per patient.

Because of their immaturity, stem cells confronted by allogeneic antigens acquire immunological tolerance to the latter. When the stem cell suspension is devoid of lymphocytes already involved in T-cell differentiation, no GvHD can occur initially. Following differentiation of some stem cells into T-lymphocytes, no or only minimal GvHD occurs, provided that the allogeneic antigens are present during this development.

It is suggested that the immune reconstitution provided by FLT is enhanced by simultaneous transplantation of thymus from the same donor (Bortin & Saltzstein 1969, Pahwa et al. 1977), which provides a syngeneic environment for T-lymphocyte differentiation of transplanted stem cells. Such an FLTT does not appear to result in an increased risk of GvHD (Bortin & Saltzstein 1969), at least when the thymus is at an early stage of fetal development.

For the above-mentioned reasons, we have used FLTT from 8 to 13 week-old (gestational age) fetuses, in all 8 patients. Thymuses which contained numerous thymocytes, i.e 13 week-old thymuses, were irradiated with 4000 rads prior to transplantation. The transplant consisted of the intraperitoneal injection of a suspension of fetal liver and thymus cells. A part of the cell suspension was also injected intramuscularly in the first 3 patients. Only fresh fetal tissues were used and the viability of all cell suspensions was found in every case to exceed 70%, as evaluated by the trypan blue method. The mean number of cells transplanted from an individual fetus was 8.2×10^8 nucleated cells, i.e. 1.2×10^8-per-kg of body weight. No attempt at HLA matching of the donor and recipient was made.

The patients received 1 to 5 sequential FLTT. Our initial approach was to repeat FLTT 5 months after the first FLTT only if results were felt to be insufficient. At present we carry out a systematic series of 3 FLTT a few months apart on each patient, a method which does not seem to have major drawbacks, but which increases the probability of graft "take" from at least one of the transplants.

All patients were isolated in a sterile "bubble" and decontaminated as much as possible prior to FLTT; isolation was prolonged until virtually full reconstitution was obtained, no matter how long this process took. One boy was left for 1.5 years in the isolator and one girl for 3.5 years. Adaptation of these young children to their limited environment has been remarkable and no significant psychological problem has been encountered either during isolation or after their removal from the "bubble".

Four patients, died due to previous BCG infection, to

GvHD associated with septicemia, to untractable Salmonella infection, and to neurologic sequellae of meningitis, respectively. Four patients are alive and very healthy. Three of them have immunological reconstitution, have left hospital and lead completely normal lives over a follow-up of 3 to 10 years after the transplant. The fourth patient has been transplanted recently and it is too early to evaluate immunological reconstitution.

Graft "take" could easily be documented by identification of cells with an HLA phenotype different from that of the host. HLA-typing also allowed determination of which of the sequential transplants had taken: the first FLTT in 2 patients, one of the further FLTTs in the others. Moderate GvHD occurred in 3 patients, transplanted with fetal tissues less than 13 weeks old. Two infants had infection prior to transplantation, the other had not. They were treated with prednisone. Two GvHDs improved under treatment but the infection lead to death. The other GvHD was virtually cured by prednisone, but neurologic sequellae following meningitis led to death more than 3 years after FLTT (Table 1).

Immunological reconstitution has developed progressively, but was much slower than that after HLA-identical BMT. In the patients attaining full reconstitution, it developed over approximately 2 years (Touraine et al. 1980, Touraine et al. 1982), stressing the need for decontamination and perfectly sterile isolation. If not isolated, patients with SCID treated by FLTT would not survive long enough for the development of immune defenses against micro-organisms. After 2 years, in the above-mentioned patients, numbers of T-lymphocytes and T-lymphocyte subsets, proliferative responses to various stimuli, and T-cell cytotoxic responses were virtually normal. Immunoglobulin levels, allohemaglutinins and antibody production following vaccination approached normal after only 3 years. IgG were first of restricted heterogeneity, then normal.

The first child had the following HLA phenotype: HLA A3 A33 B14 B47 DR4 DR5. The fetal donor from whom reconstituting cells derived (second donor) was HLA A1 A2 B18 B27 DR1 DR7. No HLA A, B, or DR specificity was therefore shared by donor and recipient. By separation of T- and B-lymphocyte populations, followed by HLA-typing, it was demonstrated that all T-lymphocytes were of donor origin, while B-lymphocytes were of host origin. The monocyte population included two varieties of cells: some monocytes derived from donor cells, others from host cells. Despite complete HLA mismatch at the A, B, and DR loci, T-lymphocytes did co-operate with B-lymphocytes and monocytes, resulting in antibody production toward thymus-dependent antigens. T-lymphocytes of donor origin could, in particular, recognize tetanus toxoid antigen presented by host monocytes and help host B-lymphocytes for anti-tetanus toxoid antibody synthesis *in vitro* (Roncarolo et al.1984). They also exerted effector functions on various other host cells. Defense against virus infections *in vivo* was normal and T-cell cytotoxic functions were present *in vitro* toward a large variety of target cells.

The second child was HLA A2 A11 B15 B35 DR5 DR6. The fetal donor was HLA A1 A33 B5 B16. No HLA A or B specificity was shared by donor and recipient. The DR phenotype of fetal cells has not yet been determined. By separation of T- and B-lymphocyte populations, followed by HLA-typing, it was demonstrated that (a) most T-lymphocytes were of donor origin, the others, being of host origin, remained immature; (b) approximately 50% of B-lymphocytes were of donor origin and 50% were of host origin. In this child, cell co-operation was also shown to be present but it is difficult to determine which type of B-cells co-operate with donor-type T-cells. From the study of SCID patients in this series, development of cell populations following FLTT can be envisioned as schematically represented in Figure 1.

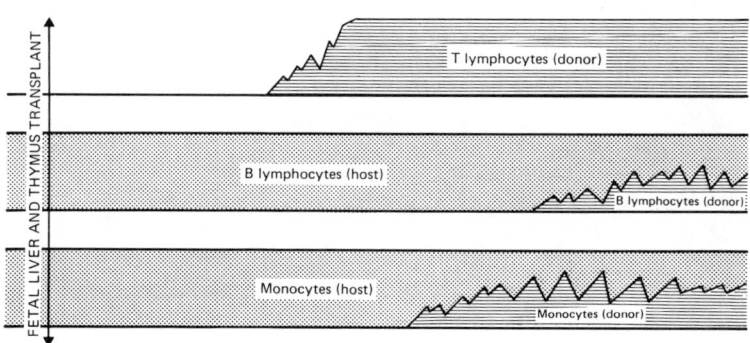

Figure 1. Schematic representation of the development of T-lymphocytes from transplanted fetal liver cells. Establishment of chimerism with both donor and host cells.

A survey of European results of FLT in SCID has gathered information in 23 cases (Touraine 1982). Five patients had been treated by FLT and 18 by FLTT. Ages of fetal donors ranged between 7 and 20 weeks. Six patients were alive with follows-up of 8-69 months at the time of the analysis, five of whom had total or sub-total reconstitution of the T-cell compartment. Except for one girl who recently developed acute lymphoblastic leukemia on the transplanted cells from a male fetus (Hugh-Jones and Hobbs, pers. comm.), all live patients were in very good clinical condition. Eleven of the 23 patients had T-cell reconstitution, 7 B-cell reconstitution and 14 documented chimerism. GvHD developed in 7 patients. The two main factors contributing to death of 17 patients were infection (vaccinia, BCG, pneumocystis, candida, measles virus, etc.) and GvHD. From this analysis, some factors could be considered as favorable for the outcome and are summarized in Table 2. Prevention of infection in the patient and use of fetal cells of good quality and in sufficient quantities were obviously favorable conditions. Male donors led to fewer GvHDs than females but the difference was not significant. Comparison between FLT and FLTT will also require the study of a larger series for several years before a definitive statement can be made. No difference in the outcome was seen whether few or no HLA antigens were shared by donor and recipient.

In the European survey, data on fetal thymus transplants was also collected and the analysis confirmed the poor results in patients with genuine SCID of fetal thymus transplantation alone.

TABLE 2

Favorable factors in fetal liver transplantation

Patient
- Early diagnosis, isolation & treatment
- Lack of infection
- *Prolonged* isolation in sterile environment

Transplant
- Fresh fetal tissue
- Fetal donor 7-12 weeks of age
- Repeated **trans**plants (2-6)
- No. of nucleated cells> 10^8/kg of b.w; of recipient
- IP or IV route
- Male donor?
- Syngenic thymus associated to liver?

Role of compatibility?

LACK OF IMPORTANT HLA RESTRICTION OF T-CELL FUNCTION IN CHIMERIC PATIENTS

Restriction of mouse T-cell function, dependent on major histocompatibility complex (MHC) determinants of T-cells and target cells, has led to the concept that T-cells have a dual specificity requirement for recognition: one for the foreign-X-antigen and one for self-MHC-determinants (Doherty & Zinkernagel 1975, Doherty et al. 1978, Zinkernagel 1978). Other studies also showed the lack of co-operation between allogeneic T- and B-cells (Katz et al. 1973). The necessary recognition of self-MHC-determinants by T-cells for interaction with other cells has been reported in several species, including man (Thorsby 1979, Goulmy et al. 1977).

In SCID patients treated by allogeneic FLTT, T-lymphocytes derive from transplanted stem cells and, in most cases, do not share any HLA determinant with the other host cells. Experimental data predicted a low or absent interaction of T-lymphocytes with various cells of the HLA-mismatched host, in such cases. It was stated that for such treatments "transplant and host must share the HLA-D region and at least one HLA-A or -B region. This match must occur whether one is considering either transplanted thymus epithelium of the host vs transplanted stem cells from fetal liver, T-cell depleted bone-marrow cells, or both thymus and stem cells when transplanted simultaneously" (Zinkernagel 1978).

In contrast with predictions, we observed that, following the slow reconstitution induced by FLTT, no important restriction of T-cell function was imposed by either donor or host MHC. *In vivo* defense mechanisms against virus infections were normal. *In vitro* T-cell cytotoxic responses toward target cells with a variety of MHC-determinants were present. In addition T-B-cell co-operation could develop, although at a later date. Antibody production in response to vaccination with thymus-dependent antigens became optimal more than one year after demonstration of normal T-cell function *in vitro*. This T-B-cell co-operation across a major histocompatibility barrier was demonstrated *in vitro* and *in vivo*, and it even occurred in a patient in whom all T-cells were of donor origin and all B-cells of host origin. In this interaction, monocytes also derived from host cells.

Although we could not determine whether donor stem cells differentiated into host or donor thymus, these results suggest that the restriction of T-cell response by the MHC may not be absolute in human transplantation. Several explanations for this lack of significant restriction in long-term human chimeras can be postulated (Touraine 1980): a) partial *in vivo* restriction when more absolute restriction appears to exist *in vitro* by lack of very discriminative assay; b) absolute restriction in short experiments as in the mouse, but a partial one in long-term T-cell reconstitution; c) restriction partially imposed by the thymus MHC, partially by the lymphoid-cell MHC; d) absolute restriction in inbred animals, but a partial one in outbred individuals, in which many cross-reactions between MHC determinants have been demonstrated; e) possibility to circumvent the restriction, e.g. by progressive development of allo + X recognition ("allo + X" hypothesis).

The apparent discrepancy between experimental data and results in patients following allogeneic FLTT does not appear to result from a species difference nor from a major difference between inbred and outbred individuals. Even in classic, inbred mice, evidence is now accumulating to suggest that restriction is not a systematic, absolute phenomenon, but rather reflects a relative "preference" of T-cells for syngeneic cells in several types of interactions (Zinkernagel 1982, E. Klein, pers. comm.). When recognition of self + X is not proposed to T-cells, alternative mechanisms of recognition (possibly of the "allo + X" type) may develop. These hypotheses can be further analyzed experimentally.

THE "ALLO + X" HYPOTHESIS

This hypothesis (Touraine & Bétuel 1981) has been based on the following facts: a) in most models where MHC restriction has been unequivocally demonstrated, the control experiments with allogeneic target cells show a low, but present, response; b) in our chimeric patients, T-cells become progressively capable of all types of interaction with allogeneic host cells; c) in circumstances where MHC restriction is not observed, MHC products are still necessary, suggesting that the presence of these molecules at the surface of target cells is important even when they are of a different specifity (Lipinski et al. 1979).

In the thymus there may be development of T-cell subsets, each of which has a primary recognition structure for a given type of histocompatibility antigen. In normal circumstances, only those T-cells with recognition for self-histocompatibility antigens are solicited (because the alloantigens are not encountered), induced to proliferate and develop a full repertoire of recognition of the large variety of antigens in association with self-recognition. In chimeric patients, a given set of other histocompatibility antigens is also continuously presented to T-cells. Those T-cells with recognition for the given alloantigens are then solicited, expand by proliferation and develop the repertoire of antigen recognition in association with alloantigen recognition. The molecule for recognition of either self or alloantigens may be the MHC products themselves at the surface of T-lymphocytes, as suggested by the severe immune incompetence of T-lymphocytes devoid of HLA molecules in the Bare Lymphocyte Syndrome (Touraine 1981).

Schematic representation of these two types of T-cells is given in Figure 2. Each individual would develop the repertoire of antigen recognition mainly in association with the MHC products available in areas of T-cell differentiation.

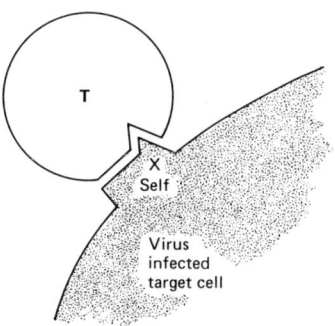
Recognition for «Self + X»

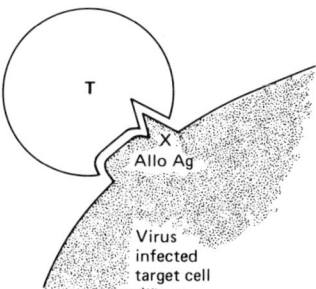
Recognition for «Allo + X»

Figure 2. Hypothesis of two types of T-lymphocytes differentiating in the thymus, one with "Self+X" recognition structures the other with "Allo+X" recognition structures.

However each one would have the capacity to considerably expand any of the other T-cell subsets with recognition for any other MHC product and then develop an additional spectrum of antigen recognition. (figure 3). Possibilities of development of the repertoire of recognition may thus be in the order of one hundred times that spontaneously solicited in natural conditions.

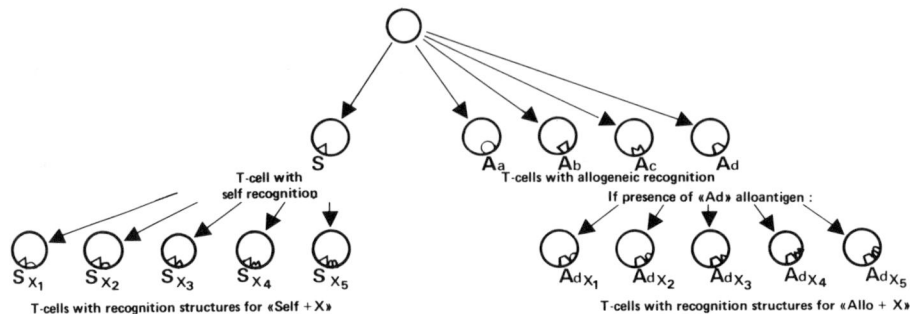

Figure 3. Intra-thymic development of T-lymphocytes. From the stem cells, a first degree of diversity may be represented by the acquisition of the capacity to recognize histocompatibility antigens. In normal conditions, pre-T-cells with recognition structures for self(S) histocompatibility antigens are likely to be stimulated to expand and to acquire additional recognition structures for all antigens of the repertoire (X1, X2, X3, X4, X5). In chimeric patients, pre-T-cells are confronted in the thymus with distinct alloantigens, e.g. Ad. It is postulated that such cells are then stimulated to expand and to acquire further diversity, thus becoming responsible for the recognition of all antigens of the repertoire in the context of, and in association with the given alloantigen.

Alternatively, rather than postulating different types of pre-determined and then co-existing T-cells, the hypothesis of one type of T-cell developing into different T-cells in the thymus due to contact with alloantigens can be put forward. T-cells would acquire simultaneously tolerance and recognition for the given alloantigens. This latter theory would not, however, account for the low, but present, cytotoxic response of normal T-cells toward infected allogeneic cells.

FLT IN IEM

BMT has been shown to be effective at correcting, at least in part, a number of enzyme deficiencies (Hobbs et al

1981, Hugh-Jones et al 1982). Out of 19 patients treated, 10 are alive and well, while the other 9 patients died of graft-versus-host reaction, hemorrhages or infection during the post-transplant period. To avoid the high risk of complications associated with the pre-transplant conditioning and bone marrow aplasia, and to develop treatments also applicable to patients lacking of HLA -identical sibling, we have initiated the study of FLT as an alternative form of therapy for IEM.

Fetal livers were obtained from therapeutic abortions performed at gestational ages ranging from 7 to 18 weeks. The suspension of fetal liver cells in culture medium was injected intraperitoneally. Twelve patients with a variety of enzyme deficiency have been treated : 3 Fabry, 4 Gaucher, 2 Fucosidosis, 1 Niemann-Pick, 1 Hurler, 1 San Filippo B.

Clinical evaluation
Three adult patients with Fabry disease received 5 FLTs in association with azathioprine and prednisone treatments. Clinical results have been encouraging and remain satisfactory after follow-ups of 5-9 years. Sweating appeared for the first time, becoming and remaining normal ; pains completely disappeared ; no neurological manifestation occured since FLT ; renal involvement appeared to be stabilized except in one patient who already had a partial renal failure on the time of FLT ; the blood creatinine of this patient was transiently stabilized for a period of 4 years, then it rose again with a slow progression. Cutaneous lesions seemed slightly decreased. The first patient apparently developed two rejection crises ; the first one was successfully treated with an increased dosage of steroids; after the second rejection, pains reappeared but vanished again following a second FLT. The α-galactosidase A activity has not been significantly increased in either leucocytes or sera. Trihexosylceramides were decreased in urines and in sera. The long-term effect of FLT on Fabry disease itself is still uncertain and no complete correction can be expected since a kidney with glycosphingolipid deposits is not cleaned out even after transplantation into a non-Fabry recipient. The best results that can be hoped from this form of therapy should not even attained the condition of heterozygote females who have a few clinical symptoms.

Two patients received a total of 5 FLTs (+ azathioprine+ prednisone) over the last two years for a fucosidosis with neurological involvment. Their clinical condition is presently good. Levels of α-fucosidase were not significantly increased in serum. Despite the very optimistic impression of the parents and neurologists on their clinical status, we feel that is is too early to evaluate the long-term benefit of the treatment. In addition, uncertainly exists on the passage of enzymes across the blood-brain barrier.

Four patients with Gaucher disease (one adult type and three severe forms in children) recently received one FLT each. A noticeable clinical improvement and a mild diminution of spleen and liver enlargement have been recorded. Only partial correction of thrombocytopenia was observed.

The condition of one patient with Niemann-Pick disease has been significantly improved during the years following FLT. A noticeable decrease of hepatomegaly and of the digestive manifestations enabled the child to go back to school and to live a virtually normal life, at the present time.

The patient with S. Filippo B disease also appeared to be partially ameliorated, although the neurological involvement is probably irreversible.

The patient with Hurler disease was treated at a very late stage and the brain deterioration could not be reversed.

Biological evaluation

The viability of the transplanted fetal liver cells was monitored by measuring serum levels of α-fetoprotein (AFP) which rose sharply, then decreased progressively while cells matured (figure 4) . In all patients, the serum level of enzyme was not dramatically increased. However, the level of the various substrates was decreased and tissue deposits were stabilized.

In parallel, *in vitro* studies have demonstrated a partial incorporation of lysosomal enzymes in deficient cells, when co-cultured with normal cells (Veyron et al. 1982).

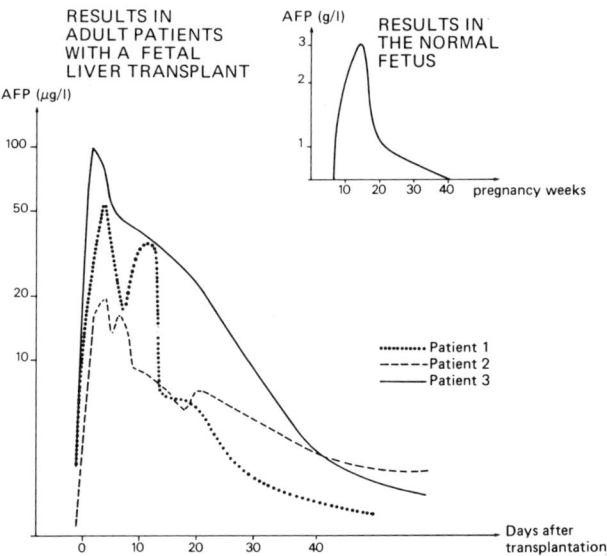

Figure 4. Variations of α-fetoprotein (AFP) levels in the serum of three patients with Fabry disease following fetal liver transplantation. Comparison with levels in the normal fetus, according to Gitlin's results.

In conclusion, FLT appears to be a very valid form of therapy in patients with SCID when no compatible donor is available for a bone marrow transplant. HLA matching is not necessary and a full immunological reconstitution can develop despite HLA mismatch. FLT is also able to improve the condition of patients with congenital enzyme deficiencies. No particular risk is associated with the transplant. This mode of therapy should also become applicable to a large number of hemopathies when methods leading to a more rapid hematological reconstitution will be developed.

These studies were conducted in accordance with recommendations of the Ethical Committee of Claude Bernard University and, more recently, of the French National Ethical Committee. Organ procurement from fetal cadavers, in the hours following extraction and death of the fetus, is very comparable to organ procurement from adult cadavers and therefore does not raise any specific ethical problem. It is, however, the opinion of the authors that some precautions should warrant the lack of interference between the decision of pregnancy interruption and the method of abortion on the one hand, and the use of fetal tissue on the other hand. The teams must therefore remain separate and under the control of Ethical Committees.

REFERENCES

Bortin, M.M. & Saltzstein, E.C. (1969) Graft-versus-host inhibition : Fetal liver and thymus cells to minimize secondary disease. Science 164, 316.

Doherty, P.C., Biddison, W.E., Bennink, J.R. & Knowles, B.B. (1978) Cytotoxic T cell responses in mice infected with influenza and vaccinia viruses vary in magnitude with H-2 genotype. J. Exp. Med. 148, 534.

Doherty, P.C. & Zinkernagel, R.M. (1975) A biological role for the major histocompatibility antigens. Lancet 1, 1406.

Goulmy, E., Termijtelen, A., Bradley, B.A. & Van Rood, J.J. (1977) Y-antigen killing by T-cells of women is restricted by HLA. Nature (Lond.) 266, 544.

Hobbs, J.R., Hugh-Jones, K., Barrett, A.J., Byrom, N. Chambers, D., Henry, K., James, D.C.O., Lucas, C.F., Rogers, T.R., Benson, P.F., Tansley, L.R., Patrick, A.D., Mossman, J. & Young, E.P. (1981). Reversal of clinical features of Hurler's disease and biochemical improvement after treatment by bone marrow transplantation. Lancet, 2, 709.

Hugh-Jones, K., Kendra, J. James, D.C.Q., Rogers, T.R., Williamson, S., Desai, S., Patrick, A.D. & Hobbs, J.R. (1982) Treatment of Sanfilippo B disease (MPS 111 B) by bone marrow transplant. Exp. Hematol. 10, suppl. 10, 50.

Katz, D.H., Hamaoka, T., & Benacerraf, B. (1973) Cell interactions between histoincompatible T- and B-lymphocytes. II. Failure of physiologic co-operative interactions between T- and B- lymphocytes from allogeneic donor strains in humoral response to hapten-protein conjugates. J. Exp. Med. 137, 1405.

Lipinski, M., Fridman, W. H., Tursz, T., Vincent, C., Pions, D. & Fellous, M. (1979) Absence of allogeneic restriction in human T-cell-mediated cytotoxicity to Epstein-Barr virus-infected target cells. Demonstration of an HLA-linked control at the effector level. J. Exp. Med. 150, 1310.

Pahwa, R., Pahwa, S., Good, R. A., Incefy, G. S. & O'Reilly, R. J. (1977) Rationale for combined use of fetal liver and thymus for immunological reconstitution in patients with variants of severe combined immunodeficiency. Proc. Natl. Acad. Sci. USA 74, 3002.

Roncarolo, M. G., Touraine, J. L. & Banchereau, J. (1984) In vivo and in vitro anti-tetanus toxoid antibody production in patients with HLA-mismatched T-cells following fetal liver and thymus transplantation. In: Progress in Immunodeficiency Research and Therapy I, eds. C. Griscelli & J. Vossen, p. 179. Elsevier Science Publ., Amsterdam.

Thorsby, E. (1979) The human major histocompatibility complex HLA : some recent developments. Transpl. Proc. 11,616.

Touraine, J.L. (1980) Co-operation between thymus and transplanted precursor cells during reconstitution of immunodeficiencies with bone marrow or fetal liver cells. In Immunobiology of Bone Marrow Transplantation, eds. S. Thierfelder, H. Rodt & H.J. Kolb, p.141, Springer-Verlag, Berlin.

Touraine, J.L. (1981) The Bare Lymphocyte Syndrome : Report on the Registry . Lancet 1, 319.

Touraine, J.L (1983) European experience with fetal tissue transplantation in severe combined immunodeficiency (SCID) In : Primary Immunodeficiency Diseases, Birth Defects, The National Foundation-March of Dimes, eds. R.G. Wedgwood F.S. Rosen, N.W. Paul, 19, p. 139.

Touraine, J.L., & Bétuel H.(1981) Immunodeficiency diseases and expression of HLA antigens. Human Immunology, 2, 147.

Veyron, P., Maire, I., Zabot, M. T., Mathieu, M., Bonneau, M. & Touraine, J. L. (1982) Fabry's disease: Attempted correction of alpha galactosidase A deficiency in cell cultures. In: Advances in the Treatment of Inborn Errors of Metabolism, eds. M. d'A. Crawfurd, D. A. Gibbs & R. W. E. Watts, p. 333. John Wiley & Sons, Chichester.

Zinkernagel, R. M. (1978) The Thymus: Its influence on recognition of "Self-Major-Histocompatibility Antigens" by T-cells and consequences for reconstitution of immunodeficiency. Springer Semin. Immunopathol. 1, 405.

Zinkernagel, R. M. (1983) HLA and cell interactions. Transplant. Proc. 15,48.

TRANSPLANTATION OF T LYMPHOCYTE DEPLETED BONE MARROW TO PREVENT GRAFT-VERSUS-HOST DISEASE: ITS IMPLICATIONS FOR FETAL LIVER TRANSPLANTATION

Richard E. Champlin, M.D.
Ronald T. Mitsuyasu, M.D.
Robert Peter Gale, M.D., Ph.D.
For the UCLA Transplantation Biology Program
Division of Hematology/Oncology
UCLA Center for the Health Sciences
Los Angeles, California 90024

Bone marrow transplantation is an effective treatment for a number of hematologic and immunologic diseases (Champlin 1984; Gale 1982; Thomas 1975; O'Reilly 1983). Unfortunately, allogeneic marrow transplantation is frequently complicated by acute and chronic graft-versus-host disease (GVHD) a life threatening complication that occurs in more than 50% of patients even if the donor and recipient are HLA-identical. The pathophysiology of GVHD is incompletely defined but current data suggests it is mediated by donor T lymphocytes which react against HLA and non-HLA antigens on host tissues (Van Bekkum 1980). The problem of GVHD has largely restricted the clinical use of bone marrow transplantation to patients who have an HLA-identical sibling donor.

Because of the problem of GVHD following transplantation of bone marrow, other sources of stem cells with a lesser capacity to produce GVHD have been considered for transplantation studies. The fetal liver contains abundant numbers of hematopoietic stem cells but few, if any, mature T lymphocytes (Champlin 1980). Transplantation of fetal liver cells can reconstitute hematopoiesis and immunity in lethally irradiated rodents. The ensuing graft-versus-host disease is mild and delayed compared to that seen with bone marrow even if transplantation occurs between major histocompatibility complex (MHC) incompatible donor-recipient pairs (Uphoff 1958; Lowenberg 1975).

The success of fetal liver cell transplantation in rodents has led to human trials with this approach.

Preliminary studies of human fetal liver cell transplantation for severe combined immune deficiency (SCID) or hematologic disease have revealed several major problems (O'Reilly 1978; Lowenberg 1977; Lucarelli 1980). Failure of engraftment is common and immunologic recovery has been incomplete despite sustained lymphoid engraftment in many patients transplanted for treatment of SCID. Graft failure and leukemic relapse have frequently occurred in patients receiving fetal liver transplantation for acute leukemia.

Human fetal liver transplantation has several practical limitations. Fetal liver tissue can only be obtained following spontaneous or prostaglandin induced abortion and is not routinely available. The viability of fetal liver cells obtained from post-mortem abortuses is inconsistent and the cells may be unsuitable for transplantation. Even under optimal circumstances human fetal liver at 14-16 weeks gestation contains only 10^8-10^9 nucleated cells, approximately 10% of that routinely obtained from an adult donor for bone marrow transplantation. The cloning efficiency of committed hematopoietic progenitors BFU-E and CFU-GM in fetal liver is similar to that of bone marrow although it is unclear whether the number of pluripotent stem cells relavent to transplantation are increased or decreased (Champlin 1980). If fresh fetal liver is to be utilized, transplantation must generally occur into an HLA-mismatched recipient. Since it is difficult to accurately predict when fetal liver cells will become available, it is often necessary to cryopreserve the cells. This requires an additional manipulation which results in cell loss and compromises cell viability. Transplantation of cryopreserved fetal liver has only rarely been successful.

Recently a number of techniques have been developed to selectively eliminate T lymphocytes from donor bone marrow prior to transplantation. These include physical separation by density gradients, agglutination with lectins, treatment of the marrow with drugs, or treatment with monoclonal anti T cell antibodies either alone, with complement or linked to toxins such as ricin (immunotoxins) (Mitsuyasu 1984; Prentice 1984; Filipovich 1984; Reisner 1980). In uncontrolled studies, transplantation of T-lymphocyte depleted bone marrow has been associated with a relatively low incidence of acute GVHD (Mitsuyasu 1984; Prentice 1984; Filipovich 1984; Reisner 1980). The use of T-lymphocyte depleted bone marrow has logistical advantages over fetal liver cells. A larger number of cells can be routinely procured; 2-3 x 10^{10} bone marrow cells can typically be obtained from an adult donor. The marrow procurement can be scheduled and the cells are consistently viable. Lastly, an HLA-identical or -haploidentical bone marrow donor (parent or sibling) can be identified for most patients.

We performed a prospective controlled clinical trial to critically evaluate whether ex vivo depletion of T lymphocytes from donor bone marrow with monoclonal anti T-lymphocyte antibody and complement would decrease the incidence and severity of graft-versus-host disease. We also sought to determine if this technique would affect other important outcomes of transplantation, including engraftment, immunologic recovery, infections and leukemic relapse and to determine its overall impact on survival. Furthermore, since antibody and complement treated bone marrow is devoid of T lymphocytes, similar to fetal liver cells, we hoped to gain insight into the possible problems that might follow fetal liver cell transplantation in man.

MATERIAL AND METHODS

Patients with acute leukemia in remission or chronic myelogenous leukemia (CML) in chronic phase were eligible for study entry. Bone marrow donors and recipients were identical for HLA-A, B, C and DR antigens. Patients were stratified by diagnosis and age, (greater or less than 20 years), and randomized to receive or not to receive ex vivo treatment of donor bone marrow with monoclonal anti T-lymphocyte antibody (CT-2) and complement. CT-2 is a murine monoclonal IgM antibody developed by Drs. R. Billing and P. Terasaki which is reactive with the E rosette receptor of mature T-lymphocytes. The study design was approved by the UCLA Human Subject Protection Committee and informed consent was obtained from all patients.

The pretransplant conditioning regimen for patients with CML consisted of cyclophosphamide, 60 mg/kg/day intravenously on day -4 and -3 followed by total body irradiation 11.25 Gy in 5 fractions over 2 1/2 days.

Patients with acute leukemia received high-dose cytosine arabinoside, 3 gram/m^2 intravenously every 12 hours for 8 doses followed by total body irradiation the same dose and schedule.

Mononuclear cells (MNC) of the donor marrow were separated on a Ficoll/hypaque density gradient in all patients. For patients randomized to receive T-lymphocyte depleted bone marrow, donor bone marrow (2 x 10^7 MNC/ml) was treated with 1 mg CT-2 for 30 minutes at 24°C followed by incubation with normal rabbit serum (1:6 dilution) as a source of complement for 60 min. at 37°C. Patients randomized to the control group received untreated bone marrow cells that were maintained in the laboratory for an identical period of time as the treated specimens.

The efficacy of T-lymphocyte depletion was determined by E-rosette formation, indirect immunoflourescence with non-cross reactive monoclonal anti-T cell antibodies leu 1 and leu 4, proliferative response to phytohemagglutinin (PHA) and formation of T lymphocyte colonies (CFU-TL) in semisolid agar (Rozenszajn 1975). CT-2 antibody and complement treatment was nontoxic to myeloid and erythroid colony forming cells as assayed by myeloid (CFU-GM) and erythroid (BFU-E) stem cell assays respectively (Pike 1970; Ogawa 1977).

Patients in both arms of the study received identical post-transplant GVHD prophylaxis. Patients treated before April 5, 1984 received methotrexate, 15 mg/m^2 on day +1 and 10 mg/m^2 on days +3, +6, +11 and then weekly to day +102. Patients transplanted after this date received cyclosporine, 6 mg/kg as a loading dose followed by 3 mg/kg/day by constant intravenous infusion for 21 days. Oral cyclosporine, 3 mg/kg every 12 hours, was administered from day +21 to day +90. Cyclosporine doses were reduced in patients with hepatic or renal dysfunction. Patients with grade $\geq$ 2 GVHD received high-dose corticosteroids slowly tapered as tolerated to control symptoms. Patients, medical staff and investigators responsible for evaluation of outcome were not informed of the treatment assignment. Engraftment was documented by increasing peripheral blood counts, bone marrow morphology, and chromosome and red blood cell isoenzyme analysis (Sparkes 1977). GVHD and interstitial pneumonia were evaluated by previously reported criteria (Thomas 1975; Hershko 1980; Bortin

1982). Patients with evidence of engraftment were
evaluable for analysis of GVHD. Patients surviving > 30
days were evaluable for analysis of interstitial
pneumonitis.

Statistical comparisons of clinical factors were
performed by the Fisher exact test. Survival and freedom
from relapse were determined by the Kaplan-Meier method;
comparisons of the two groups were performed by the
generalized Wilcoxan and Mantel-Savage tests.

RESULTS

Forty patients were entered in the study and have been
followed for greater than 60 days, including 20 recipients
of CT-2/complement treated bone marrow and 20 controls
receiving untreated bone marrow. Pretreatment
characteristics are summarized in Table 1. The two groups
were comparable for age and diagnosis. The median number
of mononuclear cells infused was 4.9 x 10^7/kg in the CT-2
treated group and 6.8 x 10^7/kg in controls. Treatment of
bone marrow with CT-2 and complement consistently reduced
the number of T cells to < 1%, below the level of detection
of the E-rosette assay and immunoflourescence with
non-cross reactive anti-T cell antibodies. The median
(range) proportion of T-lymphocytes transplanted in the
controls was 28% (18-42%). PHA reactivity was reduced from
a median stimulation index of 2.4 to 0.3 and CFU-TL colony
formation was reduced by more than 99% in all cases. CFU-C
and BFU-E were unaffected by treatment with CT-2 and
complement.

Table 1   PATIENT CHARACTERISTICS

	CT-2 Treated	Control
Number	20	20
Age	31(7-46)	33(6-45)
M:F	13:7	14:6
Diagnosis		
AML	7	6
ALL	6	8
CML	7	6

The clinical outcome of the marrow treatment and

control groups is summarized in Table 2. All 20 control patients engrafted promptly. In contrast, 2 of 20 patients in the CT-2 treatment group failed to reestablish hematopoiesis following transplantation. These additional patients in the CT-2 treatment group had initial engraftment but developed delayed graft failure after 2-4 months. These patients had an acellular or hypocellular marrow without morphologic evidence of recurrent leukemia. Cytogenetic studies in all 5 patients with graft failure detected small numbers of cells with the identical chromosome abnormality present in the patient's leukemic cells prior to initial treatment. The mechanism of graft failure in these patients is unclear. The tempo of engraftment was somewhat delayed in the CT-2 treated group with median time to granulocytes $> 0.5 \times 10^9/l$ of 23 days and platelets $> 50 \times 10^9/l$ of 29 days compared to 19 days and 22 days respectively in the untreated patients ($P = 0.04$). Two patients in the treatment group and one in the control group died of early infection before engraftment could be fully established.

Table 2   OUTCOME OF BONE MARROW TRANSPLANTATION

	CT-2 Treatment	Control	P
N	20	20	
Graft Failure	5	0	P < 0.05
Acute GVHD $\geq$ 2	3	12	P < 0.01
Fatal GVHD	0	5	P = 0.05
Relapse	10*	2	P = 0.05
Fatal Infection	2	1	NS
Interstial Pneumonia	3	3	NS
Alive	9	11	NS
Actuarial Survival (1 yr)	37%	54%	NS

*Includes 5 overt relapses and 5 patients with hypocellular marrows and cytogenetic evidence of persistant or recurrent leukemia, if only the 5 patients with overt relapses are considered P = 0.40.

Three of 18 evaluable patients in the treatment group at risk for graft-versus-host disease developed grade 2 GVHD confined to skin which responded promptly to corticosteroid treatment; no patients had fatal GVHD. In contrast, 13 of the 19 evaluable controls developed grade $\geq$ 2 GVHD which was fatal in five. The difference both in the incidence and mortality of acute GVHD is significant ($P \leq$

0.01). It is premature to draw any conclusions regarding chronic graft-versus-host disease. The incidence and mortality from infections and intersitial pneumonia is similar in each group.

There have been 5 overt leukemic relapses in the CT-2 treatment group. As noted above cytogenetic evidence of persistant or recurrent leukemia was noted in an additional 5 other patients in the CT-2 treatment group who had graft failure without morphologic evidence of relapse. Only two control patients have relapsed. This difference in recurrent leukemia between the CT-2 treatment and control groups is significant ($P < 0.05$). If only overt leukemic relapses are considered the difference between the two groups is not significat ($P = 0.40$). The median time to relapse was 4 months post transplant. Nine patients in the treatment group and 11 control patients are alive. Actuarial survival at ≥ 1 year is 37% and 54% respectively ($P = 0.53$).

DISCUSSION

These data indicate that ex vivo treatment of bone marrow with the monoclonal anti-T-lymphocyte antibody CT-2 and complement is effective in removing > 99% of T-lymphocytes from the donor bone marrow as assayed by phenotypic and functional assays. Patients undergoing allogeneic bone marrow transplantation from HLA-identical siblings who were randomized to receive T lymphocyte depleted bone marrow had a significantly lower incidence and severity of acute graft-versus-host disease compared to controls receiving untreated marrow. Unfortunately the risk of graft failure was increased in patients receiving T cell depleted marrow. This is consistant with animal data in which depletion of T lymphocytes enhanced graft rejection (Vallera 1982). T cells may facilitate engraftment either by a graft versus host effect abrogating residual host lymphocytes that survive the immunosuppressive conditioning treatment or by providing cellular or humoral factors which stimulate hematopoiesis. Graft failure in these patients may have been caused by immunologic rejection, lack of T cell mediated stimulation of hematopoiesis or injury to pluripotent hematopoietic stem cells of the donor marrow by the T-lymphocyte depletion procedure. Alternatively, the graft may have been suppressed by persistant or recurrent leukemia. In all, 5 patients had graft failure with an extremely hypocellular marrow and no morphologic evidence of recurrent leukemia; all 5 of these patients did have small numbers of cells with cytogenetic abnormalities characteristic of their original leukemia. A similar syndrome of pancytopenia with a hypocellular marrow does not typically occur, however, with leukemia relapse after transplantation of untreated marrow.

In this preliminary analysis the incidence of leukemia relapse was higher in the patients receiving CT-2 and complement treated bone marrow than in controls. Relapse was not related to bone marrow cell dose, age, or diagnosis. It is possible that in addition to its effect on GVHD, depletion of T lymphocytes from the donor marrow may have abrogated any graft-versus-leukemia effect associated with allogeneic marrow transplantation (Gale 1984). Other factors such as inability of treated bone marrow to effectively repopulate marrow, impaired recovery of immunity, or de novo reinduction of leukemia, could also be responsible for the higher rate of leukemia relapse in the treatment group.

These data highlight the problems encountered with the use of T-lymphocyte depleted hematopoietic transplants for treatment of leukemia. Even when the donor cells are HLA-identical to the recipient and large numbers of cells are transplanted, graft failure is a major problem. Preliminary data from several centers indicate that the use of T-lymphocyte depleted marrow transplants for HLA-nonidentical recipients is associated with an even higher risk of graft failure. More effective immunosuppressive conditioning regimens are presumably required to prevent graft rejection in this setting. In addition, T-lymphocyte depleted grafts may be unable to confer a graft-versus-leukemia effect and may be associated with a high risk of leukemia relapse.

The results of this study have major implications for fetal liver cell transplantation where relatively small numbers of HLA-mismatched cells that are inherently devoid of T lymphocytes are transplanted. From the data presented, it is not surprising that fetal liver cell transplants for treatment of aplastic anemia or leukemia have frequently been complicated by graft failure. These studies have typically utilized either cyclophosphamide alone or in combination with 10 Gy total body irradiation. More intensive immunosuppressive conditioning therapy is probably required to prevent rejection of fetal liver transplants for patients with hematologic diseases (Lucarelli 1980). Preliminary data in dogs support this hypothesis (Champlin, this volume).

The use of fetal liver or T-lymphocyte depleted bone marrow grafts is a promising approach to allow hematopoietic transplantation without severe graft-versus-host disease. Because of the logistical considerations favoring the use of T-lymphocyte depleted bone marrow, substantial qualitative advantages must be demonstrated for fetal liver over bone marrow derived stem cells to justify the clinical use of fetal liver transplantation to treat hematologic diseases. Major problems must still be overcome with transplantation of T-lymphocyte depleted bone marrow or fetal liver cells, notably graft failure and recurrent leukemia, before either modality of treatment can be routinely recommended. Hopefully more effective conditioning regimens can be developed such that this approach will ultimately allow hematopoietic transplants in patients who are not currently eligible for bone marrow transplantation.

Supported by grants CA-23175 and AM 30296 from the National Institutes of Health

USPHS grant RR-00865, and CICR grant G830332

R.C. is a recipient of a New Investigator Research Award from the National Institutes of Arthritis, Diabetes, Digestive and Kidney Diseases

R.M. is a recipient of a Clinical Investigator Award from the National Cancer Institute and Junior Faculty Clinical Fellowship from the American Cancer Society

Champlin RE, Gale RP (1984). The role of bone marrow transplantation in the treatment of hematologic malignancies and solid tumors: a critical review of syngeneic, autologous and allogeneic transplants. Cancer Treat Rep 68:145-161.

Gale RP (1982). Progress in bone marrow transplantation in man. Surv Immunol Res 1:40-66.
Thomas ED, Storb R, Clift RA, et al (1975). Bone marrow transplantation. New Engl J Med 292:832-843, 895-902.
O'Reilly RJ (1983). Allogeneic bone marrow transplantation: Current status and future directions. Blood 62:941.
Van Bekkum DW (1980). Immunologic basis of graft-versus-host disease. IN Gale, Fox (eds). The Biology of Bone Marrow Transplantation, Academic Press, New York, p 175-194.
Champlin RE, Gale RP (1980). Hematopoiesis and immune reactivity of human fetal liver cells. IN Lucarelli G, Fleidner TM, Gale RP, (eds). Fetal Liver Transplantation. Excepta Medica, Amsterdam p 117-125.
Uphoff DE (1958). The precusion of secondary phase of irradiation syndrome by innoculation of fetal hematopoietic tissue following lethal total body irradiation. J Natl Cancer Inst 20:625-632.
Lowenberg B (1975). Fetal liver cell transplantation - role and nature of the fetal haemopoietic stem cell. Publication of the Radiobiological Institute of the Organization for Health Research TNO, Rijswijk (Z.H.), The Netherlands.
O'Reilly RJ, Pahwa R, Dupont B, Good RA (1978). Severe combined immunodeficiency: Transplantation approaches for patients lacking an HLA genotypically identical sibling. Transplant Proc 10:187-199.
Lowenberg B, Vossen JMJJ, Dooren LJ (1977). Transplantation of fetal liver cells in the treatment of severe combined immunodeficiency disease. Blut 34:181-195.
Lucarelli G, Izzi T, Porcellini A, et al (1980). Fetal liver transplantation in aplastic anemia and acute leukemia. IN Lucarelli G, Fleidner T, Gale RP (eds). Fetal Liver Transplantation: Current Concepts and Future Directions. Excepta Medica, Amsterdam p 284-299.
Mitsuyasu R, Champlin R, Ho WG, et al (1984). Prospective randomized controlled trial of ex vivo treatment of donor marrow with monoclonal anti T cell antibody and complement for the prevention of graft-versus-host disease: a preliminary report. Transplant Proc (in press).
Prentice HG, Blacklock HA, Janossy G, et al (1984). Depletion of T lymphocytes in donor marrow prevents significant graft-versus-host disease in matched

allogeneic leukemic marrow transplant recipients. Lancet 1:472-475.
Filipovich AH, Vallera DA, Youle RJ, Quinones PR, Neville DM, Kersey JH (1984). Ex vivo treatment of donor bone marrow with anti T cell immunotoxins for prevention of graft-versus-host disease. Lancet 1:469-471.
Reisner Y, O'Reilly RJ, Kapoor N, Good RA (9180). Allogeneic bone marrow transplantation using stem cells fractioned by lectins: in vitro analysis of soy bean agglutinin. Lancet ii:1320-1324.
Rozenszajn LA, Shoham D, Kalechman I (1975). Clonal proliferation of PHA stimulated lymphocytes on soft agar. Immunol 1975; 29:1041-1055.
Pike B, Robinson WA (1970). Human bone marrow growth in agar gel. J Cell Physiol 76:77-84.
Ogawa M, Grush OC, O'Dell RF, Hara H, MacEachern MD (1977). Circulating erythroid progenitors assessed in culture: characterization in normal men and patients with hemoglobinapathies. Blood 1977; 50:1081-1092.
Sparkes MC, Crist MG, Sparkes RS, Gale RP, Feig SA and the UCLA Bone Marrow Transplant Team (1977). Gene markers in human bone marrow transplantation. Vox Sang 33:202.
Hershko C, Gale RP (1980). GVHD scoring system for predicting survival of specific mortality in bone marrow transplant recipients. IN Gale RP, Fox CF (eds). The Biology of Bone Marrow Transplantation, Academic Press, New York 1980; 59-68.
Bortin MM, Kay HEM, Gale RP, Rimm A (1982). Factors associated with interstitial pneumonitis after bone marrow transplantation for acute leukemia. Lancet 1982; 1:437-439.
Vallera DA, Soderling CCB, Carlson GJ, Kersey JH 1982). Bone marrow transplantation across major histocompatibility barriers in mice: T cell requirement in total lymphoid irradiation-conditioned recipients. Transplantation 1982; 33:243-248.
Gale RP, Champlin RE (1984). How does bone marrow transplantation cure leukemia? Lancet 1984; 2:28-30.
Champlin RE, Cain G, Stitzel K, Gale RP. Fetal liver transplantation in dogs (this volume).

A COMPARATIVE REVIEW OF THE RESULTS OF TRANSPLANTS OF FULLY ALLOGENEIC FETAL LIVER AND HLA-HAPLOTYPE MISMATCHED, T-CELL DEPLETED MARROW IN THE TREATMENT OF SEVERE COMBINED IMMUNODEFICIENCY

Richard J. O'Reilly, Dahlia Kirkpatrick, Neena Kapoor, Nancy Collins, Joel Brochstein, Nancy Kernan, Neal Flomenberg, Marilyn Pollack, Bo Dupont, Carlos Lopez and Yair Reisner

Memorial Sloan-Kettering Cancer Center, New York, NY 10021

INTRODUCTION

Between 1975 and 1983, the Marrow Transplant Program at Memorial Sloan-Kettering Cancer Center has treated 31 patients with severe combined immunodeficiency. Of these patients, 8 received transplants of fully allogeneic fetal liver with irradiated allogeneic fetal thymus. Twelve patients, including 2 of the 8 fetal tissue graft recipients who failed to achieve functional reconstitution, were transplanted with HLA haplotype-mismatched parental marrow depleted of T cells by differential agglutination with the lectin soybean agglutinin and E-rosette depletion according to the technique of Reisner et al (1,2). In this brief review, we compare the results achieved with each type of transplant. These results indicate that either type of transplant abrogates severe graft vs. host disease. However, the incidence of durable engraftment and functional reconstitution appears to be increased in those patients treated with SBA^-E^-, parental, T cell depleted marrow grafts.

METHODS

Eighteen patients with SCID who were transplanted with either allogeneic fetal liver and thymus (6), lectin-separated, E-rosette depleted parental marrow (10) or both (2) constitute the subjects of this study. The diagnosis of SCID was based on the absence of tonsils and nodal tissue, severe T-lymphocytopenia, the absence of in vitro transformation responses to mitogens, antigens or allogeneic cells and the failure of the patient to generate antibody or a delayed type hypersensitivity response following in vivo immunization.

In vitro transformation responses to mitogens, bacterial antigens and allogeneic cells were measured as previously described (3), and compared with the responses of a battery of normal controls, at least 3 of whom were tested concurrently at each test point. Serum immunoglobulin levels and antibody titers to tetanus, blood group substances, and polio vaccine were performed according to standard techniques (4-7). Serological typing for HLA A,B,C and Dr were performed on separated peripheral blood E^+ and E^- populations. Assignment of fetal HLA phenotypes was performed on cultured fetal lung or brain fibroblasts (8,9), with assignments of materal haplotypes based on typing of PBL derived from the consenting mother of the transplanted fetal tissue.

Fetal livers were derived from dead fetuses of < 12 weeks gestation which were the product of elective abortion. The informed consent of the mother of the aborted fetus was obtained prior to use of these tissues. Fetal liver cells were made into single cell suspensions by aspirations of the minced liver fragments through 18 gauge needles. The fetal liver grafts were administered intravenously. Recipients of fetal liver received fetal thymus from either the same or a separate donor. Thymuses derived from 16-20 week gestational aged elective abortions, were irradiated (800-1000r) prior to transplantation. All thymus grafts were surgically implanted into the rectus abdominal sheath.

Parental, HLA-haplotype disparate marrow grafts, were depleted of T lymphocytes by differential agglutination with SBA, followed by E-rosette depletion, according to the technique of Reisner et al (1,2). Irradiated thymus grafts were not administered to recipients of T-cell depleted marrow.

None of the patients received any immunosuppressive therapy prior to their initial transplant. Ultimately, 2 fetal liver recipients and 3 recipients of SBA^-E^- marrow required treatment with Cyclophosphamide (100-200 mg/Kg) and either Busulfan (2 mg/Kg X 4) (2 patients) or antithymocytic globulin (30 mg/Kg X 4 i.v.) (3 patients) prior to a secondary or tertiary graft before they achieved durable engraftment.

RESULTS

The results of transplants of allogeneic fetal liver and thymus and of heminoallogeneic SBA^-E^- parental marrow grafts are compared in Table 1.

Table 1
Comparison of the Results of Fully Allogeneic Fetal
Liver and Thymus Transplants and HLA Haplotype
Mismatched Parental SBA⁻E⁻ Marrow Transplants
in the Treatment of Severe Combined Immunodeficiency

	Fully Allogeneic Fetal Liver & Thymus		Haplotype Mismatched SBA⁻E⁻ Marrow	
Patients	8		12	
Number of Transplants	23		16	
Avg. number of Transplants/Patient	2.8		1.8	
Cell Dose X 10^8/Transplant	4.6	(0.27-40)	5.7	(2.5-13.4)
Patients Engrafted After 1° Transplant	4		8	
Patients Durably Engrafted	6		12	
Time to Engraftment	7-32	weeks	4-6	weeks
Reconstitution of T cell Function:				
Full	2 $^\Delta$		9	
Partial	2		3	(1 early)
None	2		0	
Reconstitution of B cell Function	1	(full) (1±)	7	(4 full) (3 partial)
Longterm Survival with Reconstitution	2*	(1 partial reconstit.)	10	(1 partial reconstit.)
Acute GvHD	1	(1+)	1	(1+)

$^\Delta$ In 1 of the 2 patients, T cell function deteriorated after 16 months: the child died of a presumed viral encephalitis.

*   2 additional patients survive, but achieved reconstitution only after transplants of SBA⁻E⁻ parental marrow.

Between 1975 and 1981, 23 separate transplants of liver with or without thymus were consecutively administered to 8 patients with SCID. Engraftment of lymphoid precursors was documented by HLA phenotype or karyotype following 9 of the 23 transplants. However, sustained engraftment of lymphoid precursors was documented in only 6 cases, each of which was engrafted from a single fetal source. In comparing those fetal transplants which did or did not engraft, we were unable to discern differences in the type of abortion (prostoglandin or hysterectomy-induced), gestational age, cell dose, viability or degree of HLA homology between donor and recipient to distinguish transplants which did or did not achieve sustained engraftment. However, concurrent administration of liver cell and thymus epithelium from the same <12 week gestational aged fetus appeared to be more effective than the administration of liver cells alone followed by a transplant of irradiated lymphoid thymus from a second, older fetus. In our series, 3 of 5 transplants of liver and thymus from the same fetus engrafted, but only 3/18 transplants of fetal liver alone achieved durable chimerism. In addition, our finding that 2 patients who had failed to engraft following multiple transplants without immunosuppression, did engraft after being prepared for a fetal transplant with cyclophosphamide and anti-thymocyte globulin, providing initial evidence that patients with SCID, although they lack allospecific T lymphocytes, do possess other cell systems capable of resisting engraftment of allogeneic hematopoietic cells.

Of the 6 patients durably engrafted with fully allogeneic fetal-liver derived T cells, 2 developed normal transformation responses to mitogens. These patients and an additional 2 patients developed near normal responses to allogeneic cells in mixed leukocyte culture and to antigens of Candida Albicans, an agent to which all had been heavily exposed. Of these 4 patients, 3 developed DTH responses to DNCB challenge. One of these patients also generated an effective granulomatous response and thereby eradicated a disseminated M. avium infection. Although these indicators of T cell function suggested that reconstitution of cell-mediated immunity had been achieved, they have been sustained over 2 years by only 1 patient. The other 5 patients remained engrafted, but their cell-mediated immune functions deteriorated.

Of the 6 patients durably engrafted with fetal cells, 2 developed transient rashes which were pathologically consistent with Grade I GvHD. One of these patients died of pneumonia within 2 months of engraftment, the other is clinically stable, but remains with a very limited reconstitution of cellular immune functions. The contribution of a subclinical form of GvHD to the patients' continued immune deficiency is difficult to estimate, but may be significant.

Only 2 of the 8 patients transplanted with fetal liver tissues survive with engraftment of fetal cells. One of these patients is fully reconstituted 9 years post transplant. The other remains engrafted 6 years post transplant but the fetal T cells exhibit in vitro responses to mitogens and allogeneic cells which are only 10% of normal. She is also severely hypogammaglobulinemic. She has been maintained on gamma globulin and antibiotic prophylaxis. In the interval since transplant, she has lived at home but has had recurrent pneumonias, oral monilisis, and poor growth and weight gain. Recently, she developed a Mycobacterium avium infection. She has been admitted for an SBA^-E^- marrow transplant from her mother. Four patients died of interstitial pneumonia (2), adenovirus-induced hepatitis (1) or encephalitis (1). Two other patients, including 1 patient who had been engrafted with fetal liver-derived lymphocytes for more than 9 months without functional reconstitution, survive with full immunologic reconstitution following successful transplants of SBA^-E^- parental marrow.

In September, 1980, we administered a transplant of HLA-haplotype mismatched, maternal marow, depleted of T cells by E-rosette depletion and subsequent agglutination with soybean agglutinin according to the original technique of Reisner et al (1), to a patient with SCID, complicated by adenovirus pneumonia and refractory stage IV neuroblastoma. This patient engrafted, developed partial reconstitution of T cell function, but ultimately died of the adenovirus infection 3 months post transplant. Subsequent to this initial case, the technique was modified to include an initial SBA lectin agglutination to concentrate hematopoietic precursors and achieve a partial T cell depletion, followed by two depletions of T-cells forming rosettes with unmodified and, thereafter, neuraminidase treated sheep red cells (2). This technique was then used to deplete T-cells from parental marrow for transplantation of 2 patients with SCID who had failed to achieve engraftment (1 case) or functional reconstitution (both cases) following multiple fetal liver and thymus transplants. These patients and their transplant courses have been previously described (10). Both patients are now more than 4 years post transplant. They are persistently chimeric with T cells of donor type and B cells of both donor and host origin. Both patients have full cell-mediated and humoral immune function.

We have now transplanted 12 patients with marrow depleted of T cells by the technique of Reisner et al (1,2). Results of these transplants are summarized in Table 1.

Each of the 12 patients transplanted for SCID ultimately achieved a durable engraftment of donor lymphoid precursors with development of T cells of donor origin. In all but 3 cases, engraftment and functional reconstitution was achieved following transplants for which no immunosuppressive therapy was administered. However, for 7 of the 12 patients, multiple grafts were administered before immunologic reconstitution was achieved. Of the 12 patients, 8 were engrafted following the primary transplant administered without immunosuppression; however, only 5 of these patients developed T cell function without further manipulation. Four patients underwent secondary transplants from the same donor without immunosuppression, 2 of whom had been primarily engrafted without functional reconstituion. Three of these 4 patients thereafter developed full T cell function. Three patients, including 1 patient who was subsequently shown to have been engrafted from his original donor, underwent secondary transplants from the other parent after immunosuppression with cyclophosphamide and anti-thymocyte globulin. Each of these patients achieved durable chimerism, 2 with a full reconstruction of the T cell system. These experiences again strongly suggested the possibility that selected patients with SCID were capable of restricting the engraftment or proliferation of T cell depleted histoincompatible marrow transplants, even though none of these patients exhibited any evidence of a capacity for allospecific immune reactions.

We prospectively examined natural killer functions in patients with SCID as a possible contributor to the graft resistance observed. In an analysis of patients who had been transplanted for SCID with either fetal liver and thymus, or SBA^-E^- parental marrow and were not already materno-fetal chimeras, we observed that those patients with normal or high natural killer activity, as defined by cytotoxic activity against K562, commonly failed to achieve initial engraftment or, if engrafted, exhibited extreme delay in immunologic reconstitution. In contrast, only 1 of 5 patients who exhibited deficient natural killer functions failed to achieve immediate engraftment and immunologic reconstition following a primary transplant.

SBA^-E^- marrow transplants, once engrafted, have, in 9 of the 12 cases, engendered a full and durable reconstitution of T cell function. These 9 patients maintain a normal number and distribution of T lymphocytes, in vitro responses to mitogens, antigens and allogeneic cells that are within the range of responses generated by concurrently tested normal controls, and delayed type hypersensitivity responses to the hapten DNCB and/or to antigens encountered through prior infection or in vivo sensitization, such as PPD and candida.

Despite this development of normal T cell functions, graft vs. host disease, limited to a transient Grade I skin rash, was observed in only 1 patient, a patient who had manifested evidence of materno-fetal graft vs. host disease (GvHD) in the pretransplant period and was successfully reconstituted following an SBA^-E^- marrow graft from the mother. Chronic GvHD was not observed in any case. The donor type T cells, which have developed within each patient differ strikingly from the donor's own lymphocytes in that they fail to respond in mixed lymphocyte culture or in allospecific cell mediated lympholysis assays against host cells. Engrafted donor cells exhibit appropriate normal responses in these assays, when challenged by third party cells.

Of the 12 patients, 3 who have been engrafted have achieved only a partial reconstitution of T-cell function. One of these patients is the first in our series, the patient who succumbed to adenovirus pneumonia in the early stages of development of T cell functions. The second patient, 1 of 2 patients with adenosine deaminase deficiency, never achieved a functional reconstitution, and ultimately lost the graft 2 years following his first transplant. Thereafter he succumbed to an EBV^+, B-cell lymphoma of host type. The third patient, a child with SCID associated with short-limbed dwarfism, remains engrafted with a partial reconstitution mediated by phenotypically normal, and mature paternal T lymphocytes. The basis of this child's persistent immune deficiency is under intensive study.

Ten of the 12 patients are evaluable for reconstitution of B cell function. As shown in Table 2, 7 patients have developed increments in the circulating concentrations of each of the major immunoglobulin classes; however, only 3 patients have achieved normal levels of these major classes of immuneoglobulins. Similarly, only 4 of the 10 evaluable patients have demonstrated a capacity to generate antibody in response to an antigenic stimulus. Determinations of the genetic origin of B cells in the post-transplant period have confirmed durable engraftment of donor B cells in only 4 of the 12 cases, 3 of whom have exhibited normal immunoglobulin

Table II
Factors Influencing Selection of
SBA⁻E⁻ Haplotype Mismatched Parental Marrow Grafts

	Parental Fetal Liver Grafts	SBA⁻E⁻BMT
Graft Accessibility	Low	High
Hematopoietic Cell Population	High	High
Potential for Lethal GvHD	<12 Week Gestation: Low >16 Week Gestation: High	Minimal
Donor/Recipient HLA Homologies	Few, Variable	Haploidentity

levels and appropriate antibody responses. Of the 6 patients who have been shown to have only host B cells in the circulation following transplantation, all but 1 has remained severely hypogammaglobulinemic, and none has produced antibody in response to immunization. Thus, those patients left with host B cells have failed to achieve a reconstitution of humoral immune function.

DISCUSSION

In the last 9 years we have accumulated a limited but significant experience with the use of HLA-mismatched fetal liver and thymus grafts and T-cell depleted HLA-haplotype disparate parental SBA$^-$E$^-$ marrow grafts in the treatment of children with SCID. A comparison of our results with these 2 techniques (Table 1) and a review of the attributes of each approach has underscored several limitations to the use of fetal tissue transplants and led us to abandon this approach for all but exceptional cases.

A major limitation to the use of fetal tissue grafts is their limited accessibility. In murine models the potential of fetal hematopoietic and lymphoid cells to induce severe GvHD has been correlated with the development of the thymus and its infiltration with lymphocytes, an event which, in man occurs between the 12th and 14th week of gestation. Indeed, lethal GvHD has been observed in recipients of fetal thymus of 16 weeks gestation. Thus, fetal tissues should be of less than 12 weeks gestation if serious GvHD is to be avoided. However, elective abortions at this stage rarely yield intact fetuses suitable for procuring fetal liver or thymus. While large banks have been developed to cryopreserve fetal liver and thymus for transplantation purposes, to our knowledge, no human has ever been demonstrated to have been engrafted with cryopreserved fetal liver or thymus, suggesting that these cells when cryopreserved may be considerably more fragile than their marrow counterparts. Because of limited accessibility, fetal tissue grafts may be delayed for months before a suitable graft is available. The prospect of such delays almost prohibits the pretransplant use of cytoreductive agents to overcome host resistance and thereby potentiate engraftment.

Fetal liver transplants of <12 weeks gestation and SBA$^-$E$^-$ marrow grafts are both enriched for hematopoietic progenitors and relatively depleted of T cells. Both types of transplant abrogate the risk of a severe GvHD. In our series, only Grade I skin GvHD was observed, and at low frequency (1/6 durably engrafted fetal liver and thymus grafts; 1/12 SBA$^-$E$^-$ marrow grafts) with either approach.

Furthermore, following either type of transplant, we have demonstrated that engrafted, donor type T cells may be fully responsive to third party alloantigens, yet are unable to respond to the alloantigens specific to the engrafted host. Thus, the donor type T cells developing within an allogeneic host are tolerant of the host. Whether this tolerance is based on selective clonal deletion or suppression of host-reactive T cell populations is as yet unknown.

Engraftment of fetal liver with or without thymus is less consistent and much slower when achieved, than that observed following SBA$^-$E$^-$ parental marrow transplants. This disadvantage of fetal liver/thymus grafts likely reflects, in part, the greater degree of genetic disparity existing between fetal donor and host and possibly other variables such as the smaller number of mature T cells in the fetal liver/thymus graft, or damage to fetal cells due to hypoxia and liver cell lysis between the time of death of the fetus and its subsequent abortion. However, repeated SBA$^-$E$^-$ marrow grafts have also been necessary in certain patients, sometimes with pretransplant cytoreduction of the host, before functional reconstitution has been achieved.

The biologic basis of the resistance exhibited by patients with SCID against the engraftment or functional differentiation of HLA disparate donor lymphoid elements derived from fetal liver and thymus or SBA$^-$E$^-$ marrow grafts is still poorly understood. Assuming the grafts themselves are an adequate source of lymphoid progenitors, a failure of engraftment could be based on at least two mechanisms: 1) an abnormality of the host microenvironment which precludes normal lymphoid development; or 2) an active resistance mechanism presumably mediated by host cells which limit engraftment and functional reconstitution. Our studies to date favor the latter basis for the initial graft failures observed. Prospective analyses suggest a strong correlation between the presence of natural killer cell functions in the host and the occurrence of graft failure or delayed functional reconstitution of engrafted donor T cells. Furthermore, the resistance observed can be overcome if the patient is prepared for transplantation with cytoreductive agents such as cyclophosphamide and anti-lymphocyte globulin. Characterization of the resistance mechanisms available to a given host should ultimately permit immediate identification of patients who should be considered for intensively immunosuppressive therapy prior to their primary transplant.

An analysis of the functional reconstitutions of cell-mediated immunity achieved by patients durably engrafted wth fetal liver/thymus or with SBA⁻E⁻ T-cell depleted parental marrow again strongly favors the use of the latter transplant approach. In our series, only 1 of 6 patients durably engrafted with fetal liver and thymus has achieved a full and sustained reconstitution of T cell function, as compared to 9 of 12 recipients of SBA⁻E⁻ parental marrow grafts. A similar disparity in the incidence and quality of T cell functional reconstitution has been observed in murine transplant models in which recipients of T-cell depleted fully allogeneic or haplotype disparate marrow grafts have been studied and compared. Early studies by Zinkernagel et al (11) documented reconstitution of T cell function in only a small proportion of lethally irradiated mice durably engrafted with fetal liver from fully allogeneic donors, but full function in F1 hybrid recipients of parental fetal liver. They suggested that the absence of genetic homologies between donor and recipient within the major histocompatibility region, precluded effective education of donor T cell precursors by host thymus and/or accessory cells within the thymus for the generation of antigen-specific T cell responses. However, in similar murine models, Singer et al (12), have been able to repeatedly generate long-term fully allogeneic chimeras possessing T cells capable of interacting with both host and donor cells by manipulating the recipient animal so that T lymphocyte progenitors migrating to the thymus are educated by thymic dendritic cells of both donor and host origin.

Our group (13) and Touraine et al (14) have demonstrated that fully allogeneic fetal liver cells can be educated to interact effectively with host cells both in the generation of host-restricted virus-specific cytotoxic cells and the development of T-cell dependent virus-specific antibodies of host type. Indeed, the one patient in our series who has achieved a full immunologic reconstitution, and remains chimeric and functional 10 years following a fetal liver and thymus graft, has fetal-type T cells which, upon stimulation with a virus such as influenza, will generate MHC-restricted virus-specific cytotoxic cells which will kill virus-infected cells bearing host, but not fetal HLA determinants. However, unlike this patient, most recipients of fetal liver and thymus grafts have achieved only a limited reconstitution of T cell functions. It is possible that these limited reconstitutions are due to an inadequate migration of fetal T-cell precursors to the fetal thymus or an ineffective or limited interaction between host dendritic cells within the thymus and donor T cell precursors. An active inhibition of donor T cell functions mediated by donor or host cells participating in a subclinical form of graft vs. host must also be considered. Indeed graft vs. host reactions characterized only by a slow attrition of T cell functions have been well described in murine transplant models by Hurtenbach et al (15), and have also been implicated as a major cause of mortality following allogeneic fetal liver transplants in mice by Lowenberg (16).

The residual deficiencies of humoral immune function obserbed at high frequency in recipients of either fetal liver/thymus grafts or haplotype disparate T cell depleted marrow transplants are more difficult to interpret. It is clear that patients developing donor B lymphocytes following transplantation have regularly achieved a reconstitution of humoral immunity, whereas those patients in whom donor B lymphocytes have not developed, have remained antibody deficient. Based on this observation, we have recently initiated therapeutic trials in which patients with SCID are prepared for transplantation with myeloablative doses of busulfan and cylcophosphamide to insure engraftment of both T and B cell lineages. Each of the first 2 patients has been durably engrafted and functionally reconstituted with the hematopoietic system of the donor, including lymphoid precursors of both the T and B cell lineages, suggesting the validity of this approach.

However, if indeed donor B lymphocyte precursors must develop if humoral immunity is to be restored to these patients, we must also address and explain an important distinction in the functional reconstitutions achieved by patients with SCID transplanted from HLA identical siblings and that observed in patients engrafted with fetal liver or HLA unfractionated or T cell depleted marrow. Indeed, persisting deficiencies of humoral immune function cannot be completely explained by a failure to engraft or differentiate donor B cell precursors. Analysis of the chimeric state of patients transplanted for SCID with unfractionated marrow from HLA identical siblings at our Institution has demonstrated that development of donor B cell progenitors is observed in no more than 50% of such cases. Nevertheless, humoral immunity has been regularly reconstituted. With rare exceptions (17), this has also been observed at other centers where the presence of donor B cells has been documented in fewer than 30% of cases (18). This suggests that in most patients with SCID, host B lymphocytes are intrinsically normal and can be induced to generate appropriate antibody responses in the presence of appropriate help from donor T lymphocytes. In our early experiences with fetal liver transplants (13), we suggested the possibility that residual humoral immune deficits might be based on the incapacity of fully allogeneic donor T cells to interact effectively with host B cells in the generation of antibody responses. However, based on current concepts of genetic restrictions, residual humoral immune deficits would not be expected in recipients of haploidentical T cell depleted marrow grafts, nor recipients of unfractionated marrow from HLA D compatible donors. Our observations thus suggest the possibility that the requirement for HLA homologies between T and B cells in the generation of an effective humoral immune response may be considerably more stringent than that required for effective interaction of T cells with macrophages and other host cells in the generation of functional cell mediated immunity and delayed type hypersensitivity. Alternatively, it may be found that donor-derived helper T cells necessary for antibody generation are not developed to the numbers or function necessary to insure an effective interaction with antigen primed host B lymphocytes. We have not been able to demonstrate suppressors of polyclonally-activated normal B cells. However, it is possible that T-B interactions in these cases are subject to more subtle allospecific suppressor mechanisms. Immune deficiencies have been ascribed to a subclinical form of GvHD in selected mouse models of fetal liver transplants, and transplants from selected parent strains into lethally irradiated F1 hybrid recipients (15,16). However, the mouse models differ significantly from the patients transplanted for SCID, in that all of the hematopoietic and lymphoid cells generated in the post-transplant period are of donor type, whereas in the patient with SCID, only donor T cells develop in the engrafted host. Furthermore, in the murine models, the immune deficiency observed is not selective for the B cell as it is in patients with SCID, suggesting that in patients with SCID, more selective abnormalities of immune regulation must be impugned.

In summary, we have briefly reviewed the clinical and immunologic findings in 18 patients with SCID who have been transplanted with fully allogeneic fetal liver and thymus of less than 12 weeks gestation (6), $SBA^- E^-$ T-cell depleted HLA haplotype disparate parental marrow (10) or both (2). Both transplantation approaches induce durable chimerism and reconstitution of immunologic functions without risk of severe or lethal GvHD. Both types of T-cell depleted transplants may be susceptible to non-immune systems of host resistance, particularly natural killer cell systems, which may restrict initial engraftment or subsequent development of donor lymphoid precursors. However, comparing the 2 approaches, transplants of T-cell depleted parental marrow, which are at least haploidentical with the recipient, appear to offer significant advantages over fully allogeneic fetal liver and thymus grafts in their accessibility, consistency and speed of engraftment, and the quality of the T cell reconstitution usually achieved. The superior accessibility of T-cell depleted parental marrow grafts also permits the use of cytoreductive agents to prepare the patient with SCID for transplantation, thereby enhancing the possibility of engrafting donor B lymphocyte precursors and achieving reconstitution of both T and B cell function in the post-transplant period.

REFERENCES

1. Reisner Y, Kapoor N, O'Reilly RJ, Good RA: Allogeneic bone marrow transplantation using stem cells fractionated by lectins: VI. In vitro analysis of human and monkey bone marrow cells fractionated by sheep red blood cells and soybean agglutinin. Lancet 2:1320-1324, 1980.

2. Reisner Y, Kapoor N, Kirkpatrick D, Pollack MS, Dupont B, Good RA, O'Reilly RJ: Transplantation for acute leukemia with HLA-A and B non-identical parental marrow cells fractionated with soybean agglutinin and sheep red blood cells. Lancet 2:327-331, 1981.

3. Cunningham-Rundles S, Hansen JA, Dupont B: Lymphocyte transformation in vitro in response to mitogens and antigens. Clin Immunobiol 3:151-194, 1976.

4. Mancini G, Carbonara AO, Heremans JF: Immunochemical quantitation of antigens by single radial immunodiffusion. Immunochemistry 2:235-259, 1965.

5. Applied Blood Group Serology. 1975, p. 255, In: P.D. Issitt, C.H. Issitt (eds). Division of Becton, Dickinson and Co., Oxnard, California, U.S.A.

6. Diagnostic Procedures for Viral and Rickettsial Infections. 1969, p. 583. In: H. Lennette, N.J. Schmidt (eds). Amer. Public Health Assn., New York.

7. Schubert JH, Cornell RG: Determination of diptheria and tetanus antitoxin by hemagglutination test in comparison with tests in vivo. J Lab Clin Med 52:737-743, 1958.

8. National Institute of Allergy and Infectious Diseases. Manual of Tissue Typing Techniques. Washington, D.C., NIH DHEW Publication 76-545, 1976, p. 22.

9. Pollack MS, Kapoor N, Sorell M, Kim SJ, Christansen FR, Silver DM, Dupont B, O'Reilly RJ: DR-positive maternal engrafted T cells in a severe combined immunodeficiency patient without graft-versus-host disease. Transplantation 30:331-334, 1980.

10. Reisner Y, Kapoor N, Kirkpatrick D, Pollack MS, Cunningham-Rundles S, Dupont B, Hodes MZ, Good RA, O'Reilly RJ: Transplantation for severe combined immunodeficiency with HLA-A,B,D,DR incompatible parental marrow cells fractionated by soybean agglutinin and sheep red blood cells. Blood 61:341, 1983.

11. Zinkernagel RM, Althage A, Callahan G, Welsh RM: On the immunocompetence of H-2 incompatible irradiation bone marrow chimeras. J Immunol 124:2356, 1980.

12. Singer A, Hathcock KS, Hodes RJ: Self recognition in allogeneic radiation bone marrow chimeras. A radiation-resistant hot element dictates the self specificity and immune response gene phenotype of T-helper cells. J Exp Med 153:1286-1301, 1981.

13. O'Reilly RJ, Pollack MS, Kapoor N, Kirkpatrick D, Dupont B: Fetal liver transplantation in man and animals. In: R.P. Gale (ed). Recent Advances in Bone Marrow Transplantation. Alan R. Liss, Inc., New York, pp 799-830, 1983.

14. Touraine JL: Transplantation of both fetal liver and thymus in severe combined immunodeficiencies: Interaction between donor's and recipient's cells. In: G. Lucarelli, T.M. Fliedner, R.P. Gale (eds): Fetal Liver Transplantation. Exerpta Medica, Amsterdam, pp 276-283, 1980.

15. Hurtenbach U, Shearer GM: Analysis of murine T lymphocyte markers during the early phases of GvH-associated suppression of cytotoxic T-lymphocyte responses. J Immunol 130:1561-1566, 1983.

16. Lowenberg B: Foetal liver transplantation. Ryswijk, Radiobiological Institute. pp 56-58, 1975.

17. Geha RS: Is the B-cell abnormality secondary to T-cell abnormality in severe combined immunodeficiency? Clin Immunol Immunopathol 6:102-106, 1976.

18. Vossen J, Buckely R. Personal communications.

Index

AB Rh-negative serum, 122, 125–126
Acid isoferritin, 37
ADA deficiency, 300, 333
Adenovirus, 331
Adherent cells
  depletion, erythroid and myeloid progenitor, isolation from human fetal liver, 136, 139–140
  hemopoietic ontogeny, baboon liver, 44, 48–50, 53
Adjuvant fetal liver transplants. *See* Leukemia *entries*
AFP monitoring, inborn errors of metabolism, FLT for, 310–311
Age, fetal, 258, 261, 262
Alanine aminotransferase, 179, 187, 190
Alkaline phosphatase, 179, 187, 190
Allogeneic FLT. *See* SCID, FLT with thymus vs. HLA mismatched T-cell depleted parental BMT
Alveolar pneumonia and hemorrhage, mini-pig, 210, 212, 213
Alveolitis, fibrosing, dogs, 199, 201
Antibiotics, AML, 270, 272
Antigen data confounded by transfusions, 294
Anti-HbA and -HbE, mouse, 22–23
Antithymocyte globulin, FLT, 102–103
  SCID, 328, 330, 332, 336, 338
Aplastic anemia, fetal liver transplants, 102–103, 238, 239, 242, 244, 245, 251–262
  age factor, 258, 262
  cf. BMT, 251, 260, 261
  case histories, successful immune reconstitution, 256–258
  current status reviewed, 294–296

cyclophosphamide, 257, 259, 260
fetal age, 261
fetal hemopoiesis, predominance of erythropoiesis, 260–261
fetal liver procurement, preparation, infusion, 252, 254
GVHD, 252, 261–262
Hb, 253, 256–258
HLA typing, 253, 258
infections, 262
no chimerism or engraftment, 259–260
patient characertistics, listed, 254
prednisone, 253, 256, 258
pure red cell aplasia, 252, 253, 257
survival, 258
thymoma, 258
Ara-C, 31, 34, 35, 276–277, 286, 318
L-Asparaginase before TBI, 239
Australia-antigen-positive hepatitis, 273, 277
Azathioprine, 309

Baboon. *See* Hemopoiesis, changes in growth requirements during ontogeny, baboon liver
BALB/c mice, THSC donor, 9–11
BA-1 mAb, 76–78, 138
B1 and B2 mAbs, 76–78
Bare lymphocyte syndrome, 307
B cell lymphoma, host, 333
B cells
  development, human fetal liver, 74–78
  fetal liver transplant, dogs, 180, 184–185, 189–190
  reconstitution, SCID, 330, 332–333, 335–339

343

BCG infection in SCID, 300, 301
beige genotype, mouse, 4, 6
BFU-E
  assay, 115, 117–118
    BMT for leukemia, 318
    inhibiting factors, 117, 118
    changes in rquirements during ontogeny, baboon liver, 44–52
    granulopoiesis in vitro, regulation by fetal liver stromal cells, 163
    human liver, sequential morphology, 63–66, 69
    isolation from human fetal liver, 138, 141–143
    mouse, 24
  eBFU-E, changes in requirements during ontogeny, baboon liver, 45, 46, 52
Birds, bursa of Fabricius, 75
Blastogenesis, in vitro, 185–186, 189
Blood-brain barrier, inborn errors of metabolism, FLT for, 310
Blood component transfusions, AML, 270
Bone marrow
  adult
    fetal liver culture on, granulopoiesis, 115–118
    granulopoiesis in vitro, cf. regulation by fetal liver stromal cells, 158–161, 163
    stem cells, cf. human fetal liver, 98
  culture, Dexter long-term, 113, 157, 164
  fetal, regulators of stem cells, cf. fetal liver, 31–32
  cf. liver, changes in requirements during ontogeny, baboon, 44–50, 52, 53
Bone marrow transplant cf. FLT
  acute leukemia, 281, 289
  aplastic anemia, 251, 260, 261
  inborn errors of metabolsim, 308–309
  in SCID, 302
  see also SCID, FLT with thymus vs. HLA mismatched T-cell depleted parental BMT

Bone marrow transplant, T-cell depleted cf. nondepleted, leukemia, 315–323
  abrogation of graft-vs.-leukemia effect, 322
  acute leukemia in remission, 317
  Ara-C, 318
  assays for CFU-TL, CFU-GM, BFU-E, 318
  CML, 317
  conditioning with cyclophosphamide and TBI, 317–318, 321, 323
  depletion with mAb CT-2 and complement, 318–321
  engraftment failure, 320, 321, 323
  cf. FLT limitations, 316, 322–323
  HLA matching, 317, 321
  interstitial pneumonia and infections, 318–321
  pancytopenia with hypocellular marrow, 322
  prevention of GVHD, 315, 317–323
    MTX and cyclosporine, 318
  relapses, 321, 322
  survival, 320
BPA, human liver, sequential morphology, 69
"Bubble," isolation, in SCID, 301, 302, 304
Bursa of Fabricius, birds, 75
Busulfan, SCID, 328, 330, 332, 336, 338

CALLA
  and B cell development, human, 76–78
  fetal progenitor purification, 138
CANCERLIT, 293
Candida albicans, 330
C57BL/6 mice, THSC donors, transplantation into *W*-mutant mouse fetuses, 9–11
CFU. *See also* Stem cell *entries*
CFU-E
  baboon liver, ontogeny, 44–50, 52

human liver, sequential morphology,
58, 66, 69
mouse, 23, 24
eCFU-E, baboon liver ontogeny, 43–46,
52
CFU-G, isolation from human fetal liver,
138, 141–143
CFU-GEMM
baboon liver ontogeny, 44–48, 52–53
isolation from human fetal liver,
139, 141–143
CFU-GM (GM-CFC)
assay
BMT for leukemia, 318
cryopreservation, human fetal liver,
123, 124, 130
fetal liver transplant, dogs, 179–180
human fetal liver, 99, 100, 109
fetal liver transplant, dogs, 177–179,
182, 183, 185, 187–188, 190
DLA-compatible and -incompatible,
199, 201
elevated blood levels, 183–184
granulopoiesis in vitro, regulation by
fetal liver stromal cells, 157,
159–163
human liver, sequential morphology,
58, 61–63, 66, 68, 69
eosinophils, neutrophils, 63
regulators, fetal liver, 29–30, 35, 36
inhibitor, 37
stimulator, 38
see also, Cryopreservation, human
fetal liver, CFU-GM survival
CFU-M, 30, 31
human liver, sequential morphology,
58, 60, 62
CFU-S, fetal liver, 29, 30, 38
development and differentiation, 74, 97
inhibitor, 31–36
stimulator, 36, 37
CFU-TL
assays, BMT for leukemia, 318
and immune development, human fetal
liver, 81, 82

Chimerism, 259–260
allogeneic adjuvant FLT in acute
leukemia, 281–282, 287–289
fetal liver transplants, mini-pig,
207, 210, 214
in SCID, 303, 304
Chromosome analysis
allogeneic adjuvant FLT in acute
leukemia, 284–285, 287–288
sex, AML, 271, 272, 276
Coated vesicles and pits, human liver,
morphology, 66
Collagenase treatment, 23, 24
Complement, BMT T-cell depletion,
318–321
Cryopreservation, 239, 240, 242
DMSO, 177–179, 187
Cryopreservation, human fetal liver, CFU-
GM survival, 121–131
CFU-GM assay, 123, 124, 130
cooling rate, 126–127, 130
DMSO, 122, 125–127, 130
freezing method, 122
AB Rh-negative serum,
122, 125–126
number of nucleated cells, 123, 124
osmotic variations in medium, 130
preparation of cell suspension, 122
storage, ampoules vs. bags, 128–129
thawing, 122–123
washing, effects of, 127–128, 130–131
CSA, fetal liver transplant, dogs, 179
CSF-GM, in vitro granulopoiesis, human,
158–163
CT-2 mAb, BMT T-cell depletion,
318–321
Cyclophosphamide,
107–109, 238, 239, 244, 245, 294
aplastic anemia, 257, 259, 260
dogs, DLA-compatible and -
incompatible, with TBI, 202
leukemia

BMT, 317–318, 321, 323
   FLT, 281, 286
   SCID, 328, 330, 332, 336, 338
Cyclosporine, 318
Cytosine arabinoside, 31, 34, 35,
   267–277, 286, 318

Daunorubicin, 267–277
Dexamethasone, 282
Dexter long-term bone marrow culture,
   113, 157 164
diffuse Hb locus, mouse, 13
DLA. *See* Fetal liver tansplants, dogs,
   DLA compatible and incompatible
DMSO and cryopreservation,
   122, 125–127, 130, 177–179, 187
DNA synthesis, 31, 33–35
Dogs. *See* Fetal liver tansplants, dogs
   entries
Dwarfism, short-limbed, with SCID, 333

Embryonic fluid in culture, 20
Engraftment
   allogeneic adjuvant FLT in acute
      leukemia, 281–282, 287–289
   AML, 271–273, 276
   failure, 259–260, 296
   BMT for leukemia, 320, 321, 323
   cf. immune reconstitution,
      293–294, 296
   markers, 238–244
      fetal Hb, 243
   SCID, 327, 330, 331, 336
Enzyme deficiencies. *See* Inborn errors of
   metabolism, FLT for
Environment. *See* Hemopoietic-inductive
   microenvironment
Eosinophils, human liver, sequential
   morphology, 63
Erythrocyte
   isozymes, 282, 286, 287, 289
   -specific antigen Ft, 12, 13

Erythroid maturation nest, human liver,
   sequential morphology, 63, 64, 68
Erythropoiesis
   and fetal liver transplants
      dogs, 182, 187, 189
      mini-pig, 208
   predominant in fetal hemopoiesis,
      167–170, 260–261
   shift to granulopoiesis in vitro, fetal
      liver, 113
   see also BFU-E; CFU-E
Erythropoietic system ontogeny, mouse,
   17–26
   anti-HbA and -HbE, 22–23
   BFU-E, 24
   CFU-E, 23, 24
   collagenase treatment, 23, 24
   embryonic fluid in culture, 20
   erythropoietin and spleen-cell
      conditioned medium, culture,
      18–23, 25
   fetal liver, 17–19
   HbA, 18–23
   HbE I-III, 18–23
   IEF, 22
   TPA induction of early progenitor
      cells, 19
   yolk sac, 17–18, 21–25
      and pluripotent progenitors, 20–21
      two separate developmental lines,
      25
Erythropoietin
   eCFU-E and eBFU-E, 43–46, 52
   changes in requirements during
      ontogeny, baboon liver,
      43–46, 48, 52, 53
   -conditioned medium, 18–23, 25
   human liver, sequential morphology, 69
   -like substance, clinical transfusion of
      fetal liver, cells, 103
   nonsensitivity phase, 29
Ethical issues, FLT, 311–312

Fabry disease, 309, 311

FC-conditioned medium, granulopoiesis in vitro, 162–163
Ferritin, 66
Fetal age and FLT, 261, 288
Fetal hemopoiesis, predominance of erythropoiesis, 167–170, 260–261
Fetal liver cells, procurement, storage, preparation, and transfer, 177–179, 197–198, 252, 254
Fetal liver transplants, dogs, 175–191
  alanine aminotransferase, 179, 187, 190
  alkaline phosphatase, 179, 187, 190
  CFU-GM,
    177–179, 182, 183, 185, 187, 188, 190
    assay, 179–180
    elevated blood levels, 183–184
  chimerism of circulating lymphocytes, 180, 186
  CSA, 179
  DLA-matched sibling donors, 177, 187
  erythropoiesis, 182, 187, 189
  fetal liver cells, procurement, storage, and transfer, 177–179
    DMSO cryopreservation, 177–179, 187
    intravenous transfusion, 179, 181, 187
  granulopoiesis and monocytopoiesis, 181–182, 188
  GVHD, 178, 187, 190
  Igs, serum, 180, 185, 190
  in vitro blastogenesis, 185–186, 189
  lymphocytes, B and T, 180, 184–185, 189–190
  malnutrition, pancreas-related, 181, 190
  megakaryopoiesis, 182, 189, 190
  MNC, 177–180, 183, 185–186, 190
  platelet transfusion, 182
  cf. rodents and humans, 176, 196
  TBI, 178–179, 181, 184, 186, 187
Fetal liver transplants, dogs, DLA compatible and incompatible, 195–202

CFU-GM, 199, 201
  fetal liver cell procurement and transfusion, 197–198
  fibrosing alveolitis, 199, 201
  GI toxicity, 200, 202
  graft rejection/failure, 200
  GVHD, 196, 200, 202
    possible T-cell mediation, 196
  myasthenia gravis, 199–201
  pancreas toxicity, 199
  schema of study design, 198
  TBI, 197, 199–202
    cyclophosphamide, 202
    plus MTX, 200, 202
Fetal liver transplants, humans, 102–109, 237–245
  acute leukemias. *See* Leukemia *entries*
  aplastic anemia. *See* Aplastic anemia, fetal liver transplants
  cf. dogs, 176, 196
  engraftment markers, 238–244
    fetal Hb, 243
  ethical issues, 311–312
  fetal liver suspension, 239–241
    cryopreservation and thawing, 239, 240, 242
  hematologic diseases, current status, 293–297
  in inborn errors of metabolism. *See* inborn errors of metabolism, FLT for
  pretreatment with cyclophosphamide, 107–109, 238, 239, 244, 245
  in SCID. *See* SCID *entries*
  TBI, 239, 244, 245
    vincristine and L-asparaginase before, 239
Fetal liver transplants, mini-pigs, 205–215
  alveolar pneumonia and hemorrhage, 210, 212, 213
  chimerism, 207, 210, 214,
  E rosettes, 207, 209, 210
  erythropoiesis, 208
  Igs, 207, 210, 213, 214

mitogen tests of PBL or fetal liver, spleen, or thymus, 206–207, 209, 210, 213
  by gestational age, 209
  no MSLA typing, 206
  platelets, 207, 208
  reconstitution, 213–215
  survival, 210–212
  TBI, 207, 210, 212
Fetal liver transplants, rodents cf. dogs, 176, 196
Fetal liver transplants, sheep. *See* Hemoglobin switching, fetal liver transplants, sheep
Fetal skin cells, granulopoiesis in vitro, regulation, 158–163
Fetus-specific antigen Ft, 12, 13
Febroblastic stromal cells. *See* Granulopoiesis in vitro, regulation by human fetal liver stromal cells
Fibrosing alveolitis, dogs, 199, 201
Fleece loss, sheep, 226
Ft, erythrocyte- and fetus-specific antigen, 12, 13
Fucosidosis, 309–310

Gastrointestinal toxicity, TBI and MTX
  dogs, 200, 202
  sheep, 225–226, 230
Gaucher disease, 299, 309, 310
Germ-free environment, fetal liver, 170
Globin synthesis, fetal liver transplants, sheep, 220–222, 227–231
  "time clock," 221, 229–230
  see also Hemoglobin *entries*
GM-CFC. *See* CFU-GM (GM-CFC)
Golgi zones, 141, 142, 144
Graft resistance, NK cells and, 332, 333
Graft-vs.-host disease, 82, 83, 170
  aplastic anemia, 252, 261–262
  BMT for leukemia, 315, 317–323
    MTX and cycolosporine, 318
  clinical transfusion of fetal liver cells, low incidence, 95–96, 107

current status, 293, 294, 296
dogs, 178, 187, 190
  DLA-compatible and -incompatible, 189, 200, 202
  T-cell mediation, 196
in SCID, 301, 302, 304, 329–331, 333–335, 337, 339
Granulopoiesis, dogs, FLT, 181–182, 188
Granulopoiesis in vitro, fetal liver, 113–118
  culture conditions, 114
  culture on adult marrow stroma, 115–118
  lack of erythropoiesis (BFU-E assay), 115, 117, 118
  inhibiting factors, 117, 118
  shift from erythropoiesis in vitro, 113
  see also CFU-GM
Granulopoiesis in vitro, regulation by human fetal liver stromal cells, 157–164
  cf. BFU-E, 163
  CFC-GM, 157, 159–163
  culture methods, 158
  cf. Dexter LTBMC, 113, 157, 164
  fetal skin cells, 158–161, 163
  fibroblastic stromal cells, 157, 159–163
  normal adult lBM cells, 158–161, 163
  stimulation of granulopoiesis by GM-CSF, 158–163
    FC-conditioned medium, 162–163
    in human placenta conditioned medium, 158–162
Growth requirements. *See* Hemopoiesis, changes in growth requirements during ontogeny, baboon liver

H-2 control, THSC transplantation into *W*-mutant mouse fetuses, 10–11, 13–14
Hemoglobin
  diffuse locus, THSC transplantation into *W*-mutant mouse fetuses, 13
  fetal, 243

fetal liver tansplant, aplastic anemia, 253, 256–258
mouse, HbA and HbE I-III, 18–23
synthesis, human liver, sequential morphology, 66–67
variants, monitoring THSC transplantation into W-mutant mouse fetuses, 5–6, 9–10
Hemoglobin switching, fetal liver tansplants, sheep, 219–231
donors and recipients, 222–223
effect of adult hemopoietic microenvironment, 221, 229
engraftment, 224–225, 230
experimental design, 220–222
globin synthesis, 220–222, 227–231
time clock, 221, 229–230
cf. human Hb switching, 219, 221
no histocompatibility matching, 223, 230
platelets, 224
TBI, 223–226, 231
with MTX, 224
with other agents, 231
toxicity and complications of preconditioning, 225–226, 228
Hemopoiesis, changes in growth requirements during ontogeny, baboon liver, 43–53
adherent cells, 44, 48–50, 53
cf. adult, 43, 46–48, 50, 52
BFU-E, 44–52
eBFU-E, 45, 46, 52
cf. BM, 44–50, 52, 53
CFU-E, 44–50, 52
eCFU-E, 43–46, 52
CFU-GEMM, 44–48, 52–53
Ep, changes in requirements, 43–46, 48, 52, 53
PBLs, 45, 48, 51
see also specific compartments
Hemopoiesis, embryonic, sequential morphology, human liver, 57–70
BFU-E, 63–66, 69

BPA, 69
CFU-E, 58, 66, 69
CFU-GM, 58, 61–63, 66, 68, 69
eosinophils and neutrophils, 63
CFU-M, 58, 60, 62
coated vesicles and pits, 66
cytochemistry, 58
Ep, 69
erythroid maturation nest, 63, 64, 68
Hb synthesis, 66–67
HIM, 69–70
light and electron microscopy, 58
megalobasts, YS-derived, 59–60, 66, 67
monoclonal cf. biclonal model, 67–68
sinusoids, 59–60
cf. yolk sac, 57–59, 66–69
Hemopoietic cell ratios, fetal liver, predominance of erythropoiesis, 167–170, 260–261
Hemopoietic-inductive microenvironment
adult, and fetal liver transplants, sheep, 221, 229
human liver, sequential morphology, 69–70
THSC, transplantation into W-mutant mouse fetuses, 12
Hemopoietic stem cells. *See* CFU *entries*; Stem cells *entries*
Hepatitis, Australia antigen positive, 273, 277
HLA
and B cell development, human 77, 78
-DC, 138, 143, 144
-DR, 141, 143, 144
HLA typing, 109–110
aplastic anemia, 253, 258
inborn errors of metabolism, mismatch, 311
leukemia, 271, 272, 276
allogeneic adjuvant FLT, 282–284, 286–287, 289
BMT, 317, 321
in SCID, 302, 303, 328

sheep, 223, 230
see also SCID, FLT with thymus cf.
  HLA-mismatched T-celldepleted
  parental BMT
HLA typing of fetal lymphocytes with α-interferon, 149–154
  class I HLA (-A and -B),
    149, 151, 153–154
  clinical applications, 149, 154
  α-IFN induction assay, 150
  immunofluorescence staining (FITC),
    150–153
  liver, spleen, thymus, 150–153
  β_2-microglobulin, 149–153
  mAbs, 150
Hurler disease, 309, 310
Hypogammaglobulinemia, SCID, 331
Hypokalemia and hyponatremia, AML,
  272, 274

Igs
  and B cell development, human,
    75, 77–79
  fetal liver transplants, mini-pig,
    207, 210, 213, 214
  reconstitution, SCID, 330, 332–333,
    335–339
  serum, fetal liver transplant, dogs,
    180, 185, 190
Immune development, human fetal liver,
  73–84
  B cells and pre-B cells, 74–78
    HLA, 77, 78
    Ig, 75, 77–79
    mAbs, 76–78
    β2-microglobulin, 77
  lymphoid cells, 73–74
  NK cells, 81–82, 84
    cf. K cells, 82
  regulation, 82–83
  T cells, 79–83
    CFU-TL, 81, 82
    cf. dogs, 80–81, 83
    thymocytes, 83

transplantation, 78
  thymocytes, 83
  transplantation, 78
  GVHD, 82, 83
  SCID, 73, 78, 81
  "veto" cells, 82
  cf. yolk sac, 73
Immune reconstitution
  allogeneic adjuvant FLT in acute
    leukemia, 281, 287
  case histories, 256–258
  cf. engraftment, 293–294, 296
  mini-pig, FLT, 213–215
  SCID, 330, 332–333, 335–339
Immunofluorescence staining
  erythroid and myeloid progenitor
    isolation from human fetal liver,
    139, 141–142
  HLA-typing of fetal lymphocytes, α-interferon, 150–153
  indirect, mAb, 91
Inborn errors of metabolism, FLT for,
  299, 308–312
  AFP monitoring, 310–311
  with azathioprine and prednisone, 309
  blood-brain barrier, 310
  cf. BMT, 308–309
  Fabry disease, 309, 311
  fucosidosis, 309–310
  Gaucher disease, 299, 309, 310
  HLA mismatch, 311
  Hurler disease, 309, 310
  Niemann-Pick disease, 299, 309, 310
  San Filippo B disease, 309, 310
Infection, 330, 331
  BMT for leukemia, 318–321
  FLT, 228, 262
  see also specific infections
α-Interferon. *See* HLA typing of fetal
  lymphocytes, α-interferon
Interstitial pneumonia, 318–321
Irradiation. *See* Total body irradiation
Isoelectric focusing, 22

K cells, 82

Kinetics studies, human fetal liver, 99–102

Leukemia
-associated inhibitor, 37
CALLA, 76–78, 138
see also Bone marrow transplant, T-cell depleted cf. nondepleted, leukemia
Leukemia, acute lymphocytic, adjuvant fetal liver transplantation, allogeneic, 103, 104, 107, 239–245, 281–290
cf. BMT, 281, 289
case reports, 282–287
chemotherapy regimens, 239, 282, 283, 285, 286
chimerism and engraftment, 239–244, 281–282, 287–289
chromosome analysis, 284–285, 287–288
complete remission, 239, 242, 243–245
current status reviewed, 294, 295, 296
cyclophosphamide, 239, 244, 281, 286
dosage, 288
fetal age, 288
fetal Hb, 243
HLA typing, 282–284, 286, 287, 289
immune reconstitution, 281, 287
red cell isozymes, 282, 286, 287, 289
relapsed, 239, 240, 242–244
TBI, 239, 244, 281, 283, 286, 287, 289
Leukemia, acute myelogenous, adjuvant fetal liver infusion, 239–241, 243–244, 267–277, 286
antibiotics, 270, 272
blood component transfusions, 270
case histories, 272–274
chemotherapy schedule and FLI, 269, 271
maintenance therapy, 270, 272, 273, 276
cf. other regimens, 274, 275
complete remission, 271, 272

engraftment, 271–273, 276
fetal liver viability, 277
hepatitis, Australia antigen positive, 273, 277
HLA typing and sex chromosomes, 271, 272, 276
partial remission, 271, 272, 274
patient data at diagnosis, 268–269
septicemia, hyponatremia, hypokalemia, 272, 274
survival, 272
tuberculosis, 273
Leu 1, Leu 5, Leu 10, and Leu M1 mAbs, fetal progenitor purification, 138
Liver
HLA-typing of fetal lymphocytes, α-interferon, 150–153
mAb characterization, 89, 90, 92–94
mitogen tests, fetal liver transplants, mini-pig, 206–207, 209, 210, 213
Lymphocytes
bare, 307
chimerism, fetal liver transplant, dogs, 180, 186
fetal liver, low levels, 167–170
and immune development, human fetal liver, 73–83
lineage, monoclonal derivation, THSC transplantation into W-mutant mouse fetuses, 7–8
see also B cells; HLA typing of fetal lymphocytes with α-interferon; T cells
Lymphoma, host B cell, 333
Lysosomal granules, large, 4, 6

Malnutrition, TBI-related, 181, 190, 226
Markers, engraftment, 238–244
fetal Hb, 243
MEDLARS asnd MEDLINE, 293
Megakaryocytes, fetal liver, none in, 167–170; see also CFU-M

Megakaryopoiesis, fetal liver transplant, dogs, 182, 189, 190
Megaloblasts, YS-derived, human liver, sequential morphology, 59–60, 66, 67
Meningitis in SCID, 300, 302
Metabolism. *See* Inborn errors of metabolism, FLT for
Methotrexate, 200, 201, 224, 282, 283, 285, 318
β_2-Microglobulin
 and B cell development, human, 77
 HLA typing of fetal lymphocytes, α-interferon, 149–153
 mAbs, 150
Microinjection technique, THSC transplantation into *W*-mutant mouse fetuses, 4
Mini-pig. *See* Fetal liver transplants, mini-pig
Mitogen tests, fetal liver transplants, mini-pig, 206–207, 209, 210, 213
Monoclonal antibodies
 and B cell development, human, 76–78
 erythroid and myeloid progenitor isolation from human fetal liver, 136, 138, 139, 141
 fetal progenitor purification, 136, 138, 139, 141
 listed, 138
 see also specific antibodies
Monoclonal antibodies, characterization of human fetal tissues, 89–94, 150
 B cells, 92–93
  mAbs B1, HLA-DR, CALLA, 90–93
 indirect immunofluorescence, 91
 liver, 89, 90, 92–94
 multilineage, mAb OKT10, 90–91, 93–94
 spleen, 89, 90, 92–94
 T cells, 91–92
  mAbs OKT3, OKT4, OKT8, 90–92
 thymus, 89–94

Monoclonal cf. biclonal model, human liver, sequential morphology, 67–68
Monoclonal derivation, myeloid and lymphoid lineages, dog, 7–8
Monocytopoiesis, fetal liver transplant, dogs, 181–182, 188
Mononuclear hemopoietic cells, fetal liver transplant, dogs, 177–180, 183, 185–186, 190
Morphology. *See* Hemopoiesis, embryonic, sequential morphology, human liver
6-MP, 285
MSLA typing, fetal liver transplants, mini-pig, 206
Myasthenia gravis, 199–201
Mycobacterium avium, 330, 331
Myeloid precursor cells
 fetal liver, low, 167–170
 monoclonal derivation, mouse, 7–8
 see also Stem cells, erythroid and myeloid, isolation from human fetal liver

Neutrophils, human liver, sequential morphology, 63
Niemann-Pick disease, 299, 309, 310
NK cells
 and graft resistance, 332, 333
 and immune development, human fetal liver, 81–82, 84
 cf. K cells, 82

OKT3, OKT4, and OKT8 mAbs, 90–92
OKT10 mAb, 90–91, 93–94
Ontogenetic barrier, human fetal liver, 109–110
Ontogeny. *See* Hemopoiesis, changes in growth requirements during ontogeny, baboon liver
Oxymethalone, 256, 257

Pancreas, 181, 190, 199, 226, 230
Pancytopenia with hypocellular marrow, 322

Panning, erythroid and myeloid
progenitors, isolation from human
fetal liver, 135, 141–144
PBLs
changes in requirements during
ontogeny, baboon liver, 45, 48,
51
mitogen tests, fetal liver transplants,
mini-pig, 206–207, 209, 210,
213
Peripheral reticulocyte count, 103–106
Pig. See Fetal liver transplants, mini-pig
Placenta-conditioned medium,
granulopoiesis in vitro, 158–162
Platelets
dog, 182
mini-pig, 207, 208
sheep, 224
Pluripotent progenitors. See Stem cells,
totipotent hemopoietic entries
Pneumonia
alveolar, 210, 212, 213
interstitial, 318–321
Prednisone, 282, 285, 286
aplastic anemia, 253, 256, 258
inborn errors of metabolism, 309
Progenitors. See CFU entries; Stem cells
entries
Prostaglandin E, 37

Radiation. See Total body irradiation
RBF-1 mAb and B cell development,
human, 76–78
Reconstitution, immune. See Immune
reconstitution
Red cell isozymes, allogeneic adjuvant
FLT in acute leukemia, 282, 286,
287, 289
Rejection, 296; see also Engraftment
Reticulocytes, peripheral, FLT, 103–106
R.18 mAb, fetal progenitor purification,
138

San Filippo B disease, 309, 310

SCA, 219
SCID, 73, 78, 81, 293
SCID, FLT with thymus, 299–307, 311,
316
BCG infection, 300, 301
cf. BMT, 302
bubbles, isolation, 301, 302, 304
chimerism, 303, 304
graft take, 300–302
GVHD, 301, 302, 304
meningitis, 300, 302
T cells, 302–304
"allo + X" hypothesis, 306–308
intrathymic development, 308
lack of HLA-restriction in chimeric
patients, 305–306
SCID, FLT with thymus vs. HLA-
mismatched T-cell depleted parental
BMT, 327–340
ADA deficiency, 333
cyclophosphamide, Busulfan,
antithymocyte globulin, post-
transplant, 328, 330, 332, 336,
338
diagnosis of SCID, 327
engraftment, 327, 330, 331, 336
GVHD, 329–331, 333–335, 337, 339
HLA typing, 328
host B-cell lymphoma, 333
hypogammaglobulinemia, 331
infections, 330, 331
cf. liver cells alone, 330
NK cells and graft resistance, 332, 333
no immunosuppressive
preconditioning, 328, 332, 336
prenatal marrow, 327, 328
reconstitution, immune
B cells and Igs, 333, 335, 338–339
T-cell mediated, 330, 332, 333,
336–339
results summarized, 329
SCID with short-limbed dwarfism, 333
source of fetal tissues, 335

T cell depletion with soybean
agglutinin and E-rosette, 327,
328, 331, 332, 334
Self-renewal, THSC transplantation into
W-mutant mouse fetuses, 3, 4
Septicemia, AML, 272, 274
Sheep. *See* Hemoglobulin switching, fetal
liver transplants, sheep
Sickle cell anemia, 219
Sinusoids, human liver, sequential
morphology, 59–60
Skin cells, fetal, and granulopoiesis in
vitro, 158–163
SPF mice, 33–34
Spleen
-cell-conditioned medium, 18–23, 25
HLA-typing of fetal lymphocytes, α-interferon, 150–153
mAb characterization, 89, 90, 92–94
mitogen tests, fetal liver transplants,
mini-pig,
206–207, 209, 210, 213
steel mutant, 12–13
Stem cells. *See also* CFU *entries*
Stem cells, erythroid and myeloid,
isolation from human fetal liver,
135–145
BFU-E and CFU-G, 138, 141–143
CFU-GEMM, 139, 141–143
immunofluorescence staining, 139,
141–142
initial characterization of progenitors,
141–142
Golgi zones, 141, 142, 144
HLA-DC, 138, 143, 144
HLA-DR, 141, 143, 144
in vitro short term cultures,
138–139, 141
negative selection by panning, 135,
141–143
cf. other techniques, 143–144
purification, 136–138, 140–141
adherent cell depletion, 136,
139–140

mAbs, 136, 138, 139, 141
schema, 137
Stem cells, hemopoietic, fetal liver,
human, 95–110
background, 95–96
biological studies, 96–99
cf. adult BM, 98
schema of CFU-S development and
differentiation, 74, 97
clinical transfusion. *See* Fetal liver
transplants, humans
histocompatibility, 109–110
kinetics studies during development,
99–102
CFU-GM assay, 99–100, 109
ontogenetic barrier, 109–110
T cells, 99, 101, 102
Stem cells, hemopoietic, regulators, fetal
liver, 29–38
cf. adult stem cells, 30–31
Ara-C effect, 31, 34, 35
CFC-GM, 29–30, 35, 36
inhibitor, 37
stimulator, 38
See also Granulopoiesis in vitro,
regulation by human fetal
liver stromal cells
CFU-M, 30, 31
CFU-S, 29, 30, 38
inhibitor, 31–36
stimulator, 36–37
DNA synthesis, 31, 33–35
effect of SPF mice, 33–34
cf. fetal BM, 31–32
Stem cells, totipotent hemopoietic, mouse
yolk sac, 20–21
Stem cells, totipotent hemopoietic
(THSC), transplantation into *W*-mutant mouse fetuses, 3–14
adult bone marrow THSC, 10–11
autonomous vs. environmental control
of development, 12–13
HIM, 12
steel mutant, 12–13

beige genotype (large lysosomal granules), 4, 6
C57BL/6 cf. BALB/c donor, 8-9, 11
fetal liver THSC, 5-10
    clonal succession leads to THSC heterogeneity, 8-10
    monoclonal derivation of myeloid and lymphoid lineages, 7-8
    reserve compartment, 9-10
    H-2 control, 10-11, 13-14
    microinjection in utero, in vivo technique, 4
    progressive developmental heterogeneity, 11-12
    RBC, hemoglobin variant monitoring, 5-6, 9-10
    diffuse Hb locus, 13
    self-renewal capacity, 3, 4
    $w^f w^f$, 5, 7
Storage, human fetal liver, 128-129; *see also* Cryopreservation *entries*
Stromal cells. *See* Granulopoiesis in vitro, regulation by human fetal liver stromal cells
Suspension, fetal liver, 239-241

T cells
    engraftment failure, 296
    fetal liver transplant, dogs, 180, 184-185, 189-190
    human fetal liver, 99, 101, 102
    and immune development, human fetal liver, 79-83
    mAb characterization, 90-92; *see also* specific mAbs
    mediation of GVHD, 196
    in SCID, 302-304
        "allo + X" hypothesis, 306-308
        intrathymic development, 308
        lack of HLA-restriction in chimeric patients, 305-306
    see also Bone marrow transplant, T-cell depleted cf. nondepleted, leukemia

TdT mAb and B cell development, human, 76-78
TG-1 mAb, fetal progenitor purification, 138
β-Thalassemia, 219
6-Thioguanine, 286
Thymocytes and immune development, human fetal liver, 83
Thymoma, 258
Thymus
    HLA-typing of fetal lymphocytes, α-interferon, 150-153
    mAb characterization, 89-94
    mitogen tests, fetal liver transplants, mini-pig, 206-207, 209, 210, 213
    see also SCID, FLT with thymus cf. HLA-mismatched T-cell depleted parental BMT
Total body irradiation, 107-109, 239, 244, 245, 294
    dogs, 178, 179, 181, 184, 186, 187
        cyclophosphamide, 202
        DLA-compatible and -incompatible, 197, 199-202
        with MTX, 200, 202
    in leukemia
        allogeneic adjuvant FLT, 281, 283, 286, 287, 289
        BMT, 317-318, 321, 323
        mini-pig, 207, 210, 212
        sheep, 223-226, 231
            with MTX, 224
            other agents, 231
        vincristine and L-asparaginase before, 239
Totipotent hemopoietic stem cells. *See* Stem cells, totipotent hemopoietic *entries*
TPA, 19
Transfusions
    blood component, AML, 270
    confounding effect on antigen data, 294
Tuberculosis, 273

Vesicles, coated, human liver, sequential morphology, 66
Veto cells, 82
Vincristine, 239, 282, 283, 285, 286

Washing and cyropreservation, human fetal liver cells, 127–128, 130–131
W mutant mouse. *See* Stem cells, totipotent hemopoietic (THSC), transplantation into W-mutant mouse fetuses

Yolk sac
-derived megaloblasts, human liver, 59–60, 66, 67
cf. liver, humans
and immune development, 73
sequential morphology, hemopoiesis, 57–59, 66–69
mouse, 17–18, 21–25
pluripotent progenitors, 20–21
two separate developmental lines, 25

PETERS HEALTH
SCIENCES LIBRARY
Rhode Island Hospital